AF294859

Membership Book

Springer

Berlin
Heidelberg
New York
Barcelona
Budapest
Hong Kong
London
Milan
Paris
Santa Clara
Singapore
Tokyo

International Skeletal Society

Membership Book

2nd Edition

Compiled on Behalf of the Society by
Morrie E. Kricun M.D.

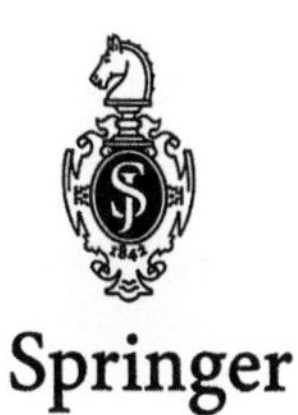

Springer

Professor Morrie E. Kricun M.D.
Hospital of the University of Pennsylvania
Department of Radiology
3400 Spruce Street
Philadelphia, PA 19104
U.S.A

ISBN-13: 978-3-642-72122-9   e-ISBN-13: 978-3-642-72120-5
DOI: 10.1007/978-3-642-72120-5

Library of Congress Cataloging-in-Publication Data

International Skeletal Society. ISS membership book / International Skeletal Society ; compiled and edited on behalf of the Society by Morrie E. Kricun ; Preface 1997 by Morrie E. Kricun. Preface 1987 by Heinz Götze and Friedrich H.W.Heuck.–2nd ed. p. cm. Rev. ed. of:Book of members. c1989,ISBN-13: 978-3-642-72122-9(alk. paper). 1. Orthopedics – Directories. I. Kricun, Morrie E., 1938–   . II. Internation Skeletal Society. Book of members. III. Title. [DNLM: 1. International Skeletal Society. 2. Orthopedics directories. WE 22.1 I61b 1998]. RC930. I545 1998. 616.7' 1'00601 – dc21. DNLM/DLC. for Library of Congress. 98-9192 CIP

Cover design: Anna Deus, Heidelberg
Typesetting: Fotosatz-Service Köhler OHG, Würzburg

SPIN: 10573623   21/3135 – 5 4 3 2 1 0 – Printed of acid-free paper

Preface 1987

The International Skeletal Society is now fifteen years old and as measured in human terms has outgrown its childhood. During this time the ISS has earned worldwide respect and praise for succesful work. The International Skeletal Society is an interdisciplinary working group concerned with skeletal disease, their pathogenesis, diagosis, and treatment at all ages.

At the Annual Closed Meetings of the ISS prominent scientists representing many countries from all over the world gather to exchange ideas in the fields of radiology, pathology, orthopedic surgery, nephrology, and endocrinology. Following these meetings Refresher Courses are offered for students, physicians in training, and interested collegues from the various medical specialities. The purpose of these courses is to present the latest developments in clinical practice and research with regard to skeletal diseases. The Society's internationally well-known journal "Skeletal Radiology", which is published by Springer-Verlag, Heidelberg adds in exchanging updated developments in the field of skeletal disorders.

The hereby presented first *Book of Members* contains a record summarizing the most important milestones and events of the history of the International Skeletal Society up to 1987 in the form of short biographies regarding the members of the Society. The task of gathering all important informations for this book was accomplished by one of the members during his term as President of the ISS. The other one – honorary member – took upon himself the tasks related to publication.

We would like to acknowledge the determination and untiring support given to us by the Society's Cofounder and first President Harold G. Jacobson, M.D. of New York and by the experienced Secretary-Treasurer and current President-Elect Akbar Bonakdarpour, M.D. of Philadelphia. Brigitte Bast provided valuable and dedicated support in compiling the questionaires. Heino Matthies and the staff of Springer-Verlag prepared the book for publication. We are endebted to all of them.

We hope that this first edition of the *Book of Members* will be followed by many others, further documenting the Society's history and keeping information about the membership up to date. The more we know about one another, the better we will be able to understand each other. We extend to the *International Skeletal Society* our sincere wishes for continued success.

Heinz Götze
Heidelberg

Friedrich Heuck
Stuttgart

Contents

The International Skeletal Society: How it Began

Introduction

Three radiologists with a special interest in skeletal radiology (one from Great Britain and two from the United States) laid the groundwork for the inception and development of The International Skeletal Society and its official Journal – *Skeletal Radiology*. The concept of such a Society was introduced first in an idle moment of conversation in 1970 between the British radiologist and one of the two American radiologists – a conversation in which the British radiologist queried "would it not be a great idea to have a society of international scope dedicated to the concept of studies in depth of disorders of the skeleton?" The American radiologist attended a meeting of the Fleischner Society (dedicted to the study of diseases of the chest) sometime later in Montreal. He came away imbued with the idea that a similar Society in bone could be established. The American radiologist, upon his return to New York after the Fleischner meeting in Montreal, decided that in order for such a venture to be succesful it required the skill, talents and sagacity of the radiologist in Great Britain who had introduced the concept and another radiologist in the United States whose reputation and organization skills were such that no skeletal society could really be founded without his being an intimate part of the beginnings. And so, Ronald Murray from Great Britain, Jack Edeiken from Philadelphia and Harold Jacobson from New York, working with Mrs. Rosalyn Levine as the secretary of the group, agreed by phone to move ahead.

Formation of the ISS

A letter was sent by Mrs. Rosalyn Levine early in 1972 to Dr. Leo G. Rigler which stated "As you undoubtedly know, Drs. Jacobson, Edeiken and Murray and several other radiologists with a major interest in skeletal radiology are interested in forming an International Skeletal Society which would function somewhat like the Fleischner Society which is dedicated to the dissemination of information related to the chest. The meeting which Dr. Jacobson attended in Montreal in May of 1972 impressed him so much that the idea of forming a Skeletal Society became intriguing. In order to establish the groundwork for such a society, I wonder if it would be possible for you to send me a copy of the by-laws of the Fleischner Society, its charter (if any) and any other pertinent information which might serve as guides for us."

A letter was written simultaneously by Dr. Sidney W. Nelson who was the Professor and Chairman, Department of Radiology, Ohio State University Medical Center in Columbus, Ohio on June 22, 1972 to Mr. William C. Stronach, the Executive Director of the American College of Radiology, which stated, "We are in the process of forming a society devoted to the study of skeletal diseases and would like to hold the organizational meeting at the time of the ARRS meeting in Washington, D.C. this fall... We would like to ask your help in obtaining the use of a room that will hold about 40 people. We would like to have it from 4:30 p.m. – 6 p.m. on Wednesday, October 4th".

The first meeting conerning the proposed International Skeletal Society was held at the Washington Hilton Hotel during the American Roentgen Society Meeting on 4 October, 1972 from 4:30 – 6:00 p.m. Present were Drs. Jack Bowerman of Baltimore, Maryland, Murray Dalinka of Philadelphia, Pa., Jack Edeiken of Philadelphia, Pa., Frieda Feldman of New York, Richard Gold of San Francisco, George B. Greenfield of Chicago, Ill., Philip Hodes of Miami, Fla., Harold G. Jacobson of the Bronx, New York, Herbert J. Kaufmann of Philadelphia, Pennsylvania, John Kirkpatrick, then of Philadelphia, Pennsylvania, Gwilym Lodwick of Columbia, Missouri, Ronald O. Murray of London, England, Sidney W. Nelson of Columbus, Ohio, Maurice Reeder of Washington, D.C., Stanley Siegelman of the Bronx, New York, Thomas W. Staple of St. Louis, Missouri and Elias G. Theros of Bethesda, Maryland – a total of 17 in all. The meeting was held to discuss the possible formation of an organization devoted to the discipline of skeletal radiology. Preliminary inquiries had been made in letters from Drs. Harold G. Jacobson and Jack Edeiken that were addressed to a number of physicians in the United States known to have made significant contributions to the field of skeletal disorders. At the same time similar inquiries were undertaken in Europe by Dr. Ronald O. Murray of London.

Following a short preliminary discussion, the desirability of forming such a society was unanimously agreed upon by those present. Dr. Jacobson was then invited to take the chair.

The following tentative decisions were made:

1) *Name.* The provisional name of the "International Skeletal Society" was agreed upon.
2) *Object.* It was decided that the objective of the Society was the advancement of the science and art of radiology of the skeleton with cooperation from and participation by associated disciplines.
3) *Membership.* Whereas the initial intention had been to confine the membership to between 50 and 100, it was pointed out that many more might want to join. It was decided by unanimous vote that two classes of membership should be established.
   a) *Fellows* – to be individuals of considerable seniority, who contributed significantly to the advancement of knowledge in this speciality.
   b) *Members* – to be similar individuals of junior status, but already with established staff or consultant positions and reasonable bibliography. The possibility of creating another junior group of Associate Members was considered and left open until it was established whether or not such a demand existed.
4) *Types of Member.* The organization is to be basically radiological, but other disciplines of similar interest were to include orthopaedic surgeons, skeletal pathologists, pediatric physicians with special interest in bone disease, metabolic physicians and rheumatologists. An epidemiologist would be an asset.
5) *Meetings*
   a) An Annual Meeting for one or two days should take place for intimate discussion between members only on problems of diagnosis (unusual and difficult cases).

b) The Annual Meeting could be followed by a 3-day Instructional Course which would be open for registrants. The belief was expressed that such a course would attract a large number of registrants in the U.S.A., (and abroad) paying a fee to be established. (The Fleischner Society attracted almost 600 registrants at its previous meeting). Should similar success be achieved by this new society, it could be possible to finance meetings in other parts of the world with travel expenses for participating members.

A Steering Committee was then elected to draw up Bylaws and consider the details of administration of such a Society. The Steering Committee consisted of: Dr. Harold G. Jacobson as Acting Chairman, Dr. Jack Edeiken, Dr. Ronald O. Murray as the European representative, Dr. Elias G. Theros of the Armed Forces Institute of Pathology in Washington, Dr. Herbert Kaufmann of the Children's Hospital, Philadelphia, Pa. and Dr. Gwilym Lodwick of the Columbia University Medical Center in Missouri.

This Steering Committee was to meet in Chicago in November and to present to this meeting at the RSNA a proposed constitution and rules of the new Society. Authority was given to the Steering Committee for the selection of founding Fellows and Members.

Incidentally, the original signatures of the individuals attending this first meeting on 4 October, 1972 are on file.

The Minutes of this Inaugural Meeting held on October 4th, 1972 were taken by Dr. Murray and submitted to Mrs. Levine who then in turn submitted the Minutes to Dr. Jacobson. (see "Exhibit A").

Also on file is a letter from Dr. Murray to Dr. Jacobson dated 13 October, 1972 in which he states "I have written to many people about the International Skeletal Society and I will be in touch with you as soon as I get replies from them. Meanwhile, I enclose a copy of the Constitution of the British Orthopaedic Association which I think might be of considerable value to you in drawing up a similar Constitution for a new Society".

On hand as well is a copy of a letter sent by Drs. Edeiken and Jacobson to invited Founding American members of the new Society. This letter in the first paragraph deals with the issue of the importance of forming a Society that will concern itself with disorders of the skeleton and would be "international in scope, would have a strong radiological thrust in its dedication to the dissemination and exchange of information and to a consideration of the advances in this field and would abviously include in its membership authorities in skeletal pathology, physiology, clinical orthopaedics, etc.". The letter goes on to say "a good case in point, which might well serve as a model is the Fleischner Society, which was started only about two years ago and is already a huge success. The Fleischner Society, with an International membership limited to a total of sixty, meets in a different city each year, holding its business and scientific meetings on a weekend, followed by a three day postgraduate course in Diseases of the Chest.

In line with the concept of a limited and select membership we have drawn up a tentative list of individuals who are either outstanding leaders in the field of skeletal disorders and/or majorally interested in the field. You, of course, are one of these individuals and we ardently hope that you will join us in this new endeavor.

The Steering Committee of this Society has decided to hold the first (formal) meeting of this International Skeletal Society at the Washington Hilton Hotel from

March 23rd to the 27th, 1974 at which time a regular Society meeting would be held to be followed by a three day postgraduate course in skeletal diseases.

The Society dues for the first year have been set at $ 75.00.

We believe that you will lend much toward the growth and future development of this Society and we hope that you will indicate your interest and acceptance of a role in this new Society by returning the enclosed form to either Dr. Edeiken or me as soon as possible."

The letter was signed by Jack Edeiken who had been elected Secretary-Elect by the Steering Committee and Harold G. Jacobson who had been elected as President-Elect by the Steering Committee.

Below are the names of the physicians contacted and offered Founding Membership in the new Society:

UNITED STATES

Ernest Aegerter, M.D.
James B. Arey, M.D.
John W. Beabout, M.D.
John Caffey, M.D.
David Dahlin, M.D.
Murray Dalinka, M.D.
Anthony F. DePalma, M.D.
Howard Dorfman, M.D.
Jack Edeiken, M.D.
Frieda Feldman, M.D.
Barnett Finkelstein, M.D.
Robert Freiberger, M.D.
Richard H. Gold, M.D.
Irving M. Greenberg, M.D.
George B. Greenfield, M.D.
Philip Hodes, M.D.
John C. Ivins, M.D.
Harold G. Jacobson, M.D.
Henry L. Jaffe, M.D.
Lent C. Johnson, M.D.
Herbert Kaufmann, M.D.

Theodore E. Keats, M.D.
John Kirkpatrick, M.D.
Walter M. Levy, M.D.
Louis Lichtenstein, M.D.
Gwilym Lodwick, M.D.
William Martel, M.D.
Wallace T. Miller, M.D.
Victor A. McKusick, M.D.
Sidney W. Nelson, M.D.
Alex Norman, M.D.
David Pugh, M.D.
Stanley Siegelman, M.D.
Robert Siffert, M.D.
Harlan J. Spjut, M.D.
Thomas W. Staple, M.D.
Howard L. Steinbach, M.D.
Elias G. Theros, M.D.
Joseph P. Whalen, M.D.
Philip Wilson, M.D.
George T. Wohl, M.D.

GREAT BRITAIN

Edward H. Allen, M.D.
Philip Jacobs, M.D.

Ronald O. Murray, M.D.
Hubert Sissons, M.D.

Of this entire group initially invited (numbering 45), only four did not reply (Dr. Pugh, because of illness, was unable to join).

Dr. Murray, representing the European contingent of the new Society, then suggested a list of European members (in addition to the 4 listed) whom he considered suitable and eligible for membership in the International Skeletal Society. The radiologists he listed were: J.T. Patton, D.J. Stoker, W.M. Park, J.K. Davidson, F.H. Doyle, E.J. Roebuck and C.K. Warrick. Dr. Murray wrote to these individuals numbering 7 and all accepted. He also suggested for membership the following in pathology – Dr. J. Ball; in Medicine – Professor C.E. Dent; in Rheumatology – Dr. D.A. Brewerton; and the following orthopaedic clinicians – Professor Burrows, Drs. Newman, Yeoman and Professor Fairbanks. A letter written by Dr. Murray to Dr. Jacobson on 17 August, 1972 states "Jocelyn McDonald has prepared the enclosed list of possible members of the International Skeletal Society made from our mutual discussion. I rather doubt whether all these radiologists would in fact qualify if a condition of membership is to be that of at least fifty percent of their time is to be spent in orthopaedic radiology. I think this condition is in fact essential.

Representation from other disciplines should, in my opinion, only be made by special invitation. In regards to European (non British) radiologists, the only ones I can think of personally to recommend are Norgaard from Denmark, Professor Van Ronnen from Leiden, Holland, Olaf Norman from Lund, Sweden and possibly Victor Segelstadt from Oslo, Norway. All of these people to my knowledge are fluent in English. You will recall that I suggested the names to you of Richard Schreiber at the Orthopaedic Hospital in Los Angeles and John Moseley at the Mount Sinai Hospital in New York".

On file are letters of acceptance from Herbert Kaufmann, John Kirkpatrick, Dennis Stoker, C.K. Warrick, John Sutcliffe, C.H.G. Price, E.J. Roebuck, Reginald Nassim, William M. Park, Philip Yeoman, Richard H. Gold, George B. Greenfield, Howard Steinbach, Elais G. Theros, George Wohl, Robert Siffert, Alex Norman, Sidney Nelson, Joseph Whalen, Tom W. Staple, Gwilym Lodwick, Louis Lichtenstein, Walter M. Levy, Theodore E. Keats, John C. Ivins, Philip Hodes, Professor J.R. von Ronnen, Frederic N. Silverman, E.B.D. Neuhauser, Professor J.H. Middlemiss, Henry L. Jaffe (from his wife), Philip Jacobs, Murray Dalinka, Lent Johnson, Mr. T.J. Fairbank, John K. Davidson, Olaf Norman, Hubert Sissons, Wallace T. Miller, William Martel, Stanley Bohrer, Terry Patton, Akbar Bonakdarpour, Corinne Farrell, T.J. Fairbanks, J. Leland Sosman, John P. Dorst, Richard R. Schreiber, C.J. Karibo, Morris Kricun, Peter G. Bullough, Daniel Wilner, David Dahlin, Bryan Preston, Malcolm Chapman, W.J. Weston, Professor Kosinskaya (of the Leningrad Institute), John L. Gwinn, Professors F.H.W. Heuck and C.E. Dent.

In their letters of acceptance, a number of individuals proposed ideas and concepts for the new organization.

Of interest is a note from Dr. Ivins in accepting membership in which he wrote to Dr. Jacobson:

"Your friend and my colleague, Dave Dahlin, said you certainly would not be offended by a comment or two.

My practice is very largely limited to orthopedic oncology, including lesions of soft tissues, in bone and of the skin. It is very hard to justify the formation of yet another medical organization, but I can see where this would be a very valuable group if it was indeed limited and select in its membership and, perhaps, international in scope."

The eminent Dr. E.B.D. Neuhauser in his note of acceptance also stated "Is it too late to alter the name? I doubt it is correct English usage".

Also of great interest is that Dr. Henry L. Jaffe inserted 2 check marks opposite the question of whether he was interested in the formation of a Society and wanted to be included in the charter group (two checks instead of one for greater emphasis). Also included is a letter from Mrs. Clarisse Jaffee who stated:

"Your letter of July 19th arrived and greatly pleased Dr. Jaffe. He warmly agrees with you that a Society such as the contemplated one dealing with skeletal disorders has long been overdue in formation. It constitutes an essential area of study with its ramifications of pathology, radiology, physiology and clinical orthopaedics.

Dr. Jaffe is willing to enter into such a Society and give whatever good may accrue from the use of his name towards the goals you have envisaged. However, it must be understood that he cannot do any work or assume responsibility for the work that must necessarily accompany the effort for organization and projection of ideas until he is completely recovered from his illness. Then he may use his energies toward the achievement of the Society's objectives."

Dr. Dahlin wrote, "I am honored to be asked and shall plan to join".

The Steering Committee met again on November 8th, 1972 at the office of Dr. Harold Jacobson in the Bronx. Present were Drs. Jack Edeiken, Herbert Kaufmann, Maurice Reeder, Elias Theros and Harold G. Jacobson. Gwilym Lodwick could not attend and he was contacted by telephone for consultation during the meeting.

A decision was made to have a set of Bylaws and Constitution for the proposed International Skeletal Society prepared for presentation at the next meeting of the Steering Committee to be held in Chicago on November 28, 1972 at the time of the RSNA meeting. Dr. Edeiken agreed to undertake this task.

The matter of categorization of members was raised and was decided that those of considerable prestige who either because of age or limited activity would not be able to participate actively but who would like to be part of the Society would be named as follows:

1) *Distinguished Fellows*
2) *Fellows*
   Those who have written at least 5 significant publications, a significant monograph, or those who have made outstanding conribution to trainees in Radiology (or allied fields) on a national and/or international level.
3) *Honorary Fellows*
   Those who satisfy the above criteria, but who have reached the age of 68.
4) *Members*
   Those of junior status who are already of established staff or consultant position and who show great promise in the field of skeletal radiology.

It was decided that each member must spend a significant part of his/her professional day devoted to skeletal radiology, pathology, physiology, etc.

Dr. Luther Brady of Philadelphia was added to the original list, having been inadvertently omitted. He accepted membership.

The designation of status of membership was evaluated by the Steering Committee. It was the opinion of the Steering Committee in that meeting that membership in the Society should be kept to a limit of 80 members or Fellows during the first year, with the possibility of membership being increased to 100 the second year.

It was agreed unanimously that the Steering Committee should act as the Nominating Committee for the first slate of officers to be presented to the next regular membership committee.

The matter of the type of the first Refresher Course was considered. The date, April, 1974, was tentatively agreed upon as the time for the first course. Drs. Edeiken, Theros and Reeder agreed to investigate an appropriate site for this first course and it was agreed that there would be a one and a half or two day weekend Closed Meeting to be followed by a three day postgraduate course on Skeletal Radiology.

The next meeting of the Steering Committee was held on Tuesday, November 28, 1972 at 5:30 p.m. at the Palmer House in Chicago during the time of the RSNA Meeting in the ACR College Suite. Present were Drs. Edeiken, Kaufmann, Lodwick, Reeder, Theros and Jacobson. Dr. Murray could not attend. The time and place for the first formal meeting and refresher course still were being considered. It was unanimously agreed that is should be sometime in 1974. No definite decision was reached as to the exact date and place.

The issue of category of memberships again was discussed.

A proposal was made to limit initially membership to no more than 80 to 100 active members or Fellows. Drs. Edeiken and Lodwick were selected as a Committee to review the current membership roster as to status. It was decided that the initial dues for all members be set at $ 50.00 for the first year, with the proviso that the amount would be changed thereafter, if it was found necessary to do so.

It was decided that there be no age limit for regular members and it was also decided that only one class of membership would exist.

The next meeting of the Steering Committee took place on February 15, 1973, in Dr. Edeiken's office in Philadelphia. Present were Drs. Edeiken, Kirkpatrick, Dalinka, Reeder, Kaufmann, Jacobson and an attorney selected by Dr. Edeiken for help in incorporating the Society – Mr. Herbert R. Weiman. Absent were Drs. Theros, Murray and Lodwick.

The current membership roster was reviewed. It was noted that the membership to date included 55 Active Members and 5 Honorary Fellows. It was decided that the latter category was not to be included in the final count of members and would not affect the number of people who could be added to the current membership listing.

Dr. Edeiken had prepared the ByLaws of the Society and Mr. Weiman reported that these were essentially accurate and in good form, but that minor additions and/or corrections would have to be included. It was indicated that a "main office" would have to be established in the State of Pennsylvania, but subsidiary offices could be set up in any other State. When review of the By-Laws was completed by Mr. Weiman, they would be submitted for ratification to the membership.

The issue of the number of members to be permitted then was discussed. Dr. Kaufmann believed that membership should be limited to no more than 100. Dr. Edeiken suggested that the idea of limited membership be deleted and that an "Authors' Club" composed of select individuals within the Society, be formed and that this "Author's Club" would meet at the time of the ISS meeting. The basic requirements for membership in this intra-society group would be that these individuals *must* have authored or co-authored a minimum of 12 articles or a text dealing with skeletal diseases. It was suggested that Mr. Weiman include this provision in the By-Laws.

It was also the consensus of the group that anyone not attending a meeting of the Society at least once every two years would be dropped, but this prerequisite would be waived for those individuals who reside in the country other than the one in which the meeting was being held.

Dr. Edeiken had been named to head the Program Committee of the first meeting; he recommended that the *First Postgraduate Program be held from March 23rd to March 27th, 1974 at the Washington Hilton Hotel in Washington, D.C.*

The general format of the meeting and the Refresher Course was submitted by Dr. Edeiken.

The issue of dues again was discussed and it was decided unanimously that the annual dues for all members for the first year be $ 75.00, subject to change and that all members would be allowed to attend the Postgraduate Course free of charge. The fee of $ 160.00 for physicians and $ 80.00 for resident physicians was set as the fee for attendance at the first Refresher Course; it was decided that this sum would include three lunches and one cocktail party.

The Steering Committee agreed to assume the transportation fare for Dr. Ronald Murray for his attendance at the forthcoming meeting.

Additional recommendations for membership were approved. These included W. Paul Britt of Montreal, Rolf Noer of Arlington, Va., Professor E.A. Uehlinger of Switzerland, Mary Fisher of Philadelphia, Robert Wilkinson of Boston, Robert Rosen of Los Angeles, Richard Rosen of New York, Stanley Craig of New York, Henry Pendergrass of Boston, Professor Hanno Poppe of Germany, Theodore Van Rijssel of the Netherlands (pathologist), Professor R.G. van der Heul, Netherlands (pathologist), Philip Wood of Great Britain, Jacob Jerushalmay of Berkeley, California, Sven-Olaf Ahlbock of Sweden, Akbar Bonakdarpour of Philadelphia, Michael Pitt of Tucson, Arizona, Martin Gelman of Salt Lake City, Utah, Leland Sosman of Boston, Wan Kulik of Los Angeles, Jack W. Snarr of Manitoba, Canada, John Weston of New Zealand, Leonard Langer of Minnesota, Professor Jurgen Spranger of Germany, Andrew Poznanski of Ann Arbor, Michigan, John Holt of Ann Arbor, Michigan, Hooshang Taybi of Oakland, California, John Dorst of Baltimore, Maryland, Peter Cockshott of Ontario, Stanley Bohrer of Nigeria, W.P. Pattinson of London, England, Robert Gorlin of Minneapolis, Jack Reynolds of Dallas, Robert Sherman of New York, Philip Palmer of Davis, California, Robert Ormond of Michigan, Harold Frost of Michigan, Robert Allman of Washington, D.C., Richard Cavanagh of Washington, D.C., Colonel LeRoy Thompson of Washington, D.C., and George Simon of London, England.

Most of the individuals named accepted membership in the Society.

The next meeting of the Steering Committee was held in the office of Dr. Edeiken at the Thomas Jefferson University Hospital in Philadelphia on May 25, 1973. Present were Dr. Reeder, Edeiken, Kaufmann and Jacobson.

Dr. Reeder gave his report on the arrangements for the first meeting and the Refresher Course to be held on March 23rd to 27th, 1974 at the Washington Hilton Hotel in Washington, D.C.

Dr. Edeiken informed the Steering Committee that the Refresher Course had received approval under Category I of the American Medical Association. Detailed recommendations for the Closed Meeting, the Refresher Course and the social activities were presented and accepted. The format for the Scientific Program was considered. The cost also was stated.

A phone call arrived from Mr. Weiman, the attorney for the ISS, informing the Committee that the International Skeletal Society now was incorporated officially under the laws of the State of Pennsylvania.

The registration fee to be charged for the first course was set at $ 200.00 and $ 100.00 for residents, with the charge including lunches.

Dr. Jacobson recommended that all proceedings be recorded and sent to the membership. Dr. Edeiken believed that a "Proceeding Journal" should be published recording the scientific sessions of the Closed Meetings and put on the open market for sale. Williams & Wilkins and perhaps W.B. Saunders were to be approached regarding price, etc., according to Dr. Edeiken.

At this meeting plans for the second meeting of the ISS to be held in London in 1975 with a tentative date of June 17th to the 21st were discussed.

Another Steering Committee meeting was held in Montreal during the American Roentgen Ray Society meeting in September, 1973. The major topic of discussion was the annual meeting to be held in March, 1974 in Washington, D.C. Present at this meeting were Drs. Theros, Kaufmann, Reeder, Edeiken and Jacobson.

It was decided by the Steering Committee that most of the Scientific (Closed) Meeting would consist of showing interesting cases. It was suggested that each member should bring a minimum of three cases but it was urged strongly that at least seven cases be prepared by each member. The cases should be well prepared with good original films and good photographs as well as microscopic slides when possible. It was decided that the cases would be worked up into some sort of an annual "Proceedings Journal", since they would make a fince collection. The editors would be Drs. Edeiken, Murray and Jacobson, together with a large Editorial Board.

Considerable discussion took place about the meeting to be held in London in April, 1975. Dr. Ronald Murray would be in charge of the proceedings at that meeting.

The By-Laws of the Society were received. They had been reviewed by the lawyer and they were now part of the incorporated organization. A vote for approval of these By-Laws was to be taken at the annual meeting.

It was reiterated that the officers recommended by the Steering Committee for the first meeting would be: President – Dr. Jacobson; President-Elect – Dr. Murray: Secretary-Treasurer – Dr. Edeiken. Nominations would be accepted from the floor.

It was decided that members of the faculty of the Refresher Course did not have to pay the $ 50.00 tuition.

The next meeting of the Steering Committee was held on November 29th, 1973 in Chicago. Attending were Drs. Edeiken, Theros, Reeder, Lodwick, Kaufmann and Jacobson.

The Steering Committee approved in principle that a Journal be published six times a year and that this Journal would include the cases presented at the Annual Meetings of the ISS, in addition to articles on skeletal radiology and allied disciplines.

Dr. Edeiken recommended the admission of additional physicians who were out-standing in the field of skeletal disorders and maintained that the limitation of 100 members placed too great a restraint on the Society. In response the Steering Committee agreed that 125 members should be the new figure.

The Steering Committee agreed that the President-elect should serve for two years, so that in the future, the terms of the President and President-elect would be 2 years. Because in the first year of the founding of the Society, Dr. Jacobson had been the Founding President, it was decided that there would be Co-Presidents – an American and European President – Dr. Jacobson from the United States and Dr. Murray from London for the second year.

It was decided to request $ 2000 from each of about six important x-ray companies in the United States, including General Electric, Dupont, Phillips, etc.

It was decided that Dr. Jacobson act as a Scribe for the Scientific Sessions (Closed Meetings) of the ISS at their annual meetings. Consideration was also given to the publication of the proceedings by Williams and Wilkins and Saunders, both of whom were contacted and indicated interest. Drs. Edeiken and Jacobson were selected to meet with each of these companies.

It was decided that Dr. Murray would be asked to write an editorial on the founding of the Society in one of the British Journals.

The first Newletter was addressed and mailed by Dr. Edeiken in the middle of June, 1973. In this Newsletter Dr. Edeiken reported the following:

1. He listed the members of the Steering Committee and the officers elected.
2. He informed the Founding Members that the Constitution and By-Laws were approved and that the Society has been incorporated in the State of Pennsylvania.
3. He discussed the purpose of the Society and informed the Founding Members that only one class of membership would prevail, but that an "Author's Club" would be formed in the Society, the purpose of the "Author's Club" being related to the encouragement of the members of the Society to contribute to the literature and not to establish exclusivity.
4. Dr. Edeiken indicated that the membership of the ISS would be by invitation only and would be limited to a total of 100 active members, Honorary Fellows or Scientists who had made outstanding contributions to skeletal radiology and related disciplines and who did not desire to be active. Inactive members would be designated from the active membership and would be those who had voluntarily retired from active practice or decreased their interest in skeletal radiology and had decided voluntarily to become inactive in the Society.
5. Drs. Reeder and Theors acted as the Ad Hoc Committee for establishing the first meeting of the Society in the Spring of 1974.
6. The operating rules for the Scientific Program (Closed Meeting) were listed.
7. The matter of social activities was addressed and Dr. Edeiken informed the Founding Members that a theatre-dinner party was planned for Saturday, March 23, 1974.
8. It was decided that the dues for the first year would be $ 75.00.
9. Dr. Edeiken would act as Program Director for the Refresher Course with members being charged $ 50.00 for this course and regular registrants $ 200.00 with a $ 100.00 fee for residents. The fee would include three lunches, coffee breaks and receptions.

A letter was sent to members of the "Author's Club" which was scheduled to meet on Friday, March 22, 1974, just before the regular meeting of the Society. It was planned at this meeting to show cases in which the diagnosis was in question or the case was extremely interesting, with the proposed presentations having interest for the entire Skeletal Society.

It was the decision of the Steering Committee that each member of the "Author's Club" would bring a minimum of three well prepared cases.

On July 25, 1973 letters were sent to a select group of individuals inviting them to be members of the "Author's Club" of the International Skeletal Society. This Club was being formed "to gather together those individuals who are outstanding in the field of skeletal radiology and also to stimulate the younger membership to fulfill the prerequisites of joining, which were authorship or co-authorship of a book or 12 articles on skeletal radiology". The first meeting was scheduled for 22 March, 1974, just preceding the regular meeting of the ISS. At least one eminent bone pathologist (it is hoped many more) would review the slides brought by the members of the "Author's Club" as necessary. The meeting was to last three hours.

Simultaneously, announcements went out concerning the first Annual Refresher Course of the ISS to be given March 25th through the 27th, 1974 at the Washington Hilton Hotel in Washington, D.C. The faculty consisted of Drs. Caffey, Cavanaugh, Dalinka, Edeiken, Feldman, Freiberger, Greenfield, Holt, Jacobson, Kaufmann, Kirkpatrick, Lodwick, Murray, Nelson, Neuhauser, Norman, Reeder, Silverman, Steinbach, Theros and Wilkinson.

A list of members of the "Author's Club" was prepared; forty-one members were included. The names selected for the "Author's Club" will not be listed because this organization was ultimately disbanded. The number of articles necessary was raised to 14. Atlases were excluded, as were Case Reports.

A letter was sent to the members of the "Author's Club" from Drs. Edeiken and Jacobson after the meeting in which those individuals who attended were thanked for "making the inaugural session so highly exciting and gratifying to all of us who were part of the Society".

This letter went on to state that considerable criticism had been raised and recommendations had been made that the "Author's Club" be abolished, since it appeared to be redundant and unnecessarily provocative to the rest of the membership of the ISS. The letter indicaed that "we are therefore canvassing the members of the "Author's Club" as to their attitudes regarding the desirability of retaining this small group within the International Skeletal Society". At the same time, Doctors Edeiken and Jacobson indicated that "for whatever it is worth, both of the undersigned believe that the "Author's Club" should be dissolved forthwith."

The vote was overwhelmingly in favor of abolishing the "Author's Club" and indeed it was abolished.

A second Newsletter was prepared by Dr. Edeiken and circulated in October, 1973 in which the decisions of the Steering Committee at its meeting in Montreal were included.

The issue of publishing a Journal as an official organ of the International Skeletal Society now received maximum attention at the beginning of November, 1973.

A Board of Editorial Consultants was now named. These included Doctors Pendergrass, Brady, Aegerter, Ackerman, Alexander, Cockshott, Dahlin, Dorfman, Fairbank, Freiberger, Gorlin, Gwinn, Hodes, Holt, Ivins, Jacobs, Johnson, Kaufmann, Keats, Kirkpatrick, Lodwick, Mankin, Martel, Meszaros, Middlemiss, Neuhauser, Olaf Norman, Poznanski, Reeder, Silverman, Sissons, Spjut, Spranger, Steinbach, Theros, Whalen, Wood and Heuck. It was decided officially to select Springer Verlag Inc. as the publisher of the Journal. It was also decided officially that Drs. Edeiken and Murray would be the Co-Chief Editors for the Manuscript Section of the Journal and Dr. Jacobson the Chief Editor for the Case Report Section. The Journal would be approximately 56 pages at the beginning. The suggested date of first publication was 1 July, 1975. Continued discussions between Springer Verlag, particularly, with its President, Dr. Heinz Götze were held. Dr. Edeiken did most of the negotiating concerning the business aspects of the Journal with Dr. Götze. The original correspondence between Dr. Götze, representing Springer Verlag on the one hand and Drs. Edeiken, Murray and Jacobson on the other, is available for review. After considerable discussion, a number of meetings and much correspondance (available in our files), Volume 1, Number 1 of the New Journal designated as SKELETAL RADIOLOGY – the Journal of the International Skeletal Society – was advertised to appear in 1976 and indeed, the first number, Volume 1 and Number 1 did appear early in 1976. The Editors-in-Chief were Drs. Edeiken, Jacobson and Murray and the Consulting Editors were those individuals named above.

A Publisher's letter appeared as an Editorial. The articles in the first issue were by Voegeli and Uehlinger on Arteriography in Bone Tumors, Myeloma Occurring with Paget Disease of Bone by C. H. G. Price; Hypophosphatemic Osteomalacia Secondary to Vascular Tumors of Bone and Soft Tissue by Drs. Renton and Shaw: Macrocranium and Macrencephaly in Neurofibromatosis by Drs. Holt and Kuhns; Geographic Differences in the Thickness of Cortical Bone – Comparison between a Welsh and Finnish Population by Dr. Virtama; Bone Scanning: A Review on Purpose and Method by Drs. Ell, Dash and Raymond; Craniodiaphyseal Dysplasia: Evolution over a Five-Year Period by Drs. Tucker, Lein and Antony.

Six Case Reports were published – 1 each by Drs. Uehlinger, Dalinka et al., Patchefsky, Alexander and Chapman and 2 by Dr. von Ronnen.

Volume 1, No. 2 included articles by: Alexander on the Effect of Growth Rate on the Strength of the Growth Plate-Shaft Junction; Patton on Differential Diagnosis of Inflammatory Spondylitis; Freedman, et al. on Nutritional and Metabolic Bone Disease in a Zoological Population: A Review of Radiologic Findings; Gehweiler, Jr et al. on Fractures of the Atlas Vertebra; Feigin, Strauss and James, Jr. on The Bone Marrow Scan in Experimental Osteomyelitis.

Eight Case Reports were published by Jacobs, Freiberger and Bullough on a single case; Dahlin, Siegelman and Dellon on a Case; Beabout et al. on a Case; Schreiber on a Case and Wilkinson and Kirkpatrick on a Case. It was initially decided to have four publications a year.

A verbal agreement was reached that the Case Report Section would occupy about $^1/_3$ of the number of pages of each issue of the Journal. The Journal began with six issues per year.

Many of the Case Reports appearing in our Journal are selected from the cases presented at the Closed Session each year. The mimeographed notes obtained from the Closed Sessions represent at this time a collection of a large number of cases, constituting a remarkable accumulation of case material, probably unsurpassed in the field of radiology and pathology of skeletal disorders. In judging the value of the presentations of the Case Reports, being assiduously recorded, mailed to members and a copy retained on permanent file, it should be stressed that the material present-ed each year at Closed Sessions is at the least uniformly good, but in many instances, unique and even awesome in scope.

The educational value of this annotated material, consisting as it does of a large number of one-of-a-kind disorders, is incalculable, considering the expertise of the individual members of the Society who present and discuss cases, which in most instances, have histological sections evaluated by the world's leading authorities in skeletal pathology. The opportunity for learning obviously is unique.

Thus are described the beginnings of the International Skeletal Society. Copies of programs since the first meeting in 1974 through 1985 are on file and available for those who would like to see them.

It has been a very rewarding experience. A single sentence voicing the belief that an International Society relating to the studies of diseases of the skeleton would be a good idea, nurtured by a visit to a meeting of the Fleischner Society, (dealing with diseases of the chest) and advanced by a third man who knew how to get things done, developed and blossomed into a major organization. The ISS encompasses currently, almost 250 members, including more than 30 outstanding bone pathologists, a number of superb clinical orthopaedists with almost $^3/_4$ of the membership consisting of outstanding skeletal radiologists. Of major importance, this organization has sired an official Journal in which all the members can take pride.

Before closing, it is important to emphasize that two individuals deserve heart-felt gratitude for their roles in establishing the Society and in helping in the formation of and finally the publication of the Journal. These individuals are Mrs. Rosalyn Levine, who was the secretary to one of us for many years and to whom grateful thanks are expressed for her very important role in devoting herself assiduously to the development of the Society and its Journal in its formative period. Similarly, gratitude is extended to Dr. Heinz Götze, the President of Springer Verlag, who because of his dedication to science and to the dissemination of scientific knowledge, made the Journal possible, giving it his personal imprimatur for excellence.

Finally, the undersigned feels it incumbent to state that of all his professional and even his social activities in a long and full life, nothing has afforded him more pleasure and gratification than to be a part of this great organization. It has not only been rewarding and hopefully important, but it has been genuinely enjoyable. Thus, grateful thanks are extended to all involved in this Society for making it possible for the under-signed to share in the privilege of being a part of this "labor of love".

Respectfully submitted,   Harold G. Jacobson, M.D., 1987

Index of Development

October 4, 1972
The initial organizational meeting was held in Washington D.C. during the Annual Meeting of the American Roentgen Ray Society.

Harold G. Jacobson, M.D. of New York outlined the purpose of this initial organizational meeting which was intended primarily to exchange ideas regarding the formation and establishment of a *radiologically oriented skeletal society*, international in scope, the major interest of which would be the dissemination of information pertaining to the skeleton.

Ronald O. Murray, M.D. of London indicated to the group that the ultimate success which might accrue from such an organization would have to depend upon a symbiotic alliance and inclusion of members in the allied fields of skeletal radiology such as orthopedics, pathology and physiology, to which all present agreed.

Jack Edeiken, M.D. of Philadelphia favored the concept of a small intimate and preferential group of members with rigorous prerequisites for membership, with the function and purpose of teaching and stimulating young radiologists to eventually seek membership in such a society.

The matter of a suitable name for this proposed skeletal organization was introduced and although some ideas were offered, it was decided that for the present the society would be referred to as "THE INTERNATIONAL SKELETAL SOCIETY".

Dr. med. Herbert Kaufmann of Berlin made the recommendation that a seven member *Steering Committee* also should be appointed to meet in the near future to work out details regarding governance, dues, membership, refresher courses etc.

November 28, 1972
Meeting of the *Steering Committee of the International Skeletal Society* in Chicago during the Annual Meeting of the Radiological Society of North America. Drs. Jack Edeiken, Harold G. Jacobson, Herbert Kaufmann, Gwilym Lodwick, Maurice Reeder and Elias G. Theros were present. Several parts of a tentative *Constitution* and *By-Laws* prepared by Jack Edeiken were introduced and read. Each member agreed to review the By-Laws.

February 15, 1973
Meeting of the *Steering Committee* of the International Skeletal Society at Thomas Jefferson University Hospital in Philadelphia, Pennsylvania. Jack Edeiken, John A. Kirkpatrick Jr., Harold G. Jacobson, Murray K. Dalinka, Maurice Reeder, Herbert Kaufmann, and Attorney Herbert R. Weiman were present. The By-Laws of the International Skeletal Society as prepared by Dr. Edeiken were essentially accurate and in good form. Mr. Weiman stated that minor additions and/or corrections would have to be included. It was indicated that a "main office" would have to be established. In as much as the

articles of incorporation are registered in the Commonwealth of Pennsylvania, the "main office" would have to be established in the State of Pennsylvania.

Jack Edeiken who will head the Program Committee introduced the matter of the *First Postgraduate Program* to be held from March 23–27, 1974 at the Washington Hilton in Washington D.C., USA.

November 29, 1973

Meeting of the *Steering Committee* of the International Skeletal Society in Chicago. Drs. Harold *G. Jacobson*, Elias G. Theros, Maurice Reeder, Gwilym Lodwick, Herbert Kaufmann, Jack Edeiken were present.

The Steering Committee agreed that the President and the President-Elect should serve two years. In the first two years Harold G. Jacobson should be Founding President. Each departing president will serve in the Steering Committee for an additional three years.

The Steering Committee approved in principal a journal to be published six times a year. In this journal will be published the cases presented at the Annual Meeting of the ISS and articles on skeletal radiology.

First Annual Meeting of the International Skeletal Society

March 22–27, 1974 in Washington D.C., USA
President: Harold G. Jacobson, M.D.
President-Elect: Ronald O. Murray, M.D.
Meeting of the Executive Committee for the first time. Drs. Harold G. Jacobson, Ronald O. Murray, and Jack Edeiken were present. The meeting opened with a long discussion concerning the various publishing houses, who had offered to publish the planned journal. It was decided to further explore Springer-Verlag.

Mike O'Connor of Williams & Wilkins Publ. of Baltimore, Md., USA would act as ISS Liaison with the travel agencies from the USA and the hotels in the London convention area.

The general meeting was opened by a few introductory remarks by Harold G. Jacobson, M.D. The minutes were read from the previous founders' meetings and of the Steering Committee meetings during the year 1973. They were approved.

A vote then was taken on the By-Laws and there was unanimous approval of them. The nominations of Harold G. Jacobson, M.D. for President, Ronald O. Murray, M.D. for President-Elect, and Jack Edeiken, M.D. for Secretary-Treasurer were approved. These officers were elected unanimously.

The first committees were appointed by Harold G. Jacobson as follows:
Chairman of Membership-Committee: Maurice Reeder, M.D., Honolulu
Chairman of Rules Committee: John A. Kirkpatrick Jr., M.D., Boston
Chairman of Auditing Committee: Gwilym Lodwick, M.D., Columbia, Missouri
Chairman of Program Committee: Howard M. Middlemiss, M.D., London, UK
No other committees were felt to be necessary at that time.

Second Annual Meeting of the International Skeletal Society

April 25–30, 1975 in London, UK
President: Harold G. Jacobson, M.D.
President-Elect: Ronald O. Murray, M.D.
Secretary-Treasurer: Jack Edeiken, M.D.
Chairman of Program Committee: Howard D. Middlemiss, M.D.
Meeting of the Executive Committee at the Royal National Orthopedic Hospital in London. Drs. Harold G. Jacobson, Ronald O. Murray, and Jack Edeiken were present.

The business meeting of the International Skeletal Society was held at the Royal National Orthopedic Hospital on April 25, 1975. After welcoming remarks by the President-Elect Ronald O. Murray, M.D. and the President Harold G. Jacobson, M.D. reports of various activities were given to the membership. The report of the chairman of the membership committee Maurice Reeder, M.D. showed 97 active members and 15 honorary members. 21 new members were voted into the ISS making, a total of 118 active members.

A report was given on the matter of the planned journal. Many meetings had been held with representatives of Springer-Verlag. A contractual agreement was signed which will require no money from the International Skeletal Society. The Editors-in-Chief are: Jack Edeiken, M.D. of Philadelphia in charge of manuscripts from the USA and Canada, Ronald O. Murray, M.D. of London in charge of manuscripts from the remainder of the world, and Harold G. Jacobson, M.D. of New York in charge of case reports. It will be a quarterly journal, one half of which will be dedicated to articles and the other half to case reports. There will be approximately 64 pages per issue. A consulting editorial board with a large international mix will be appointed. The first issue of the journal will come out in 1976. The first financial report of the International Skeletal Society was given by the Secretary-Treasurer Jack Edeiken, M.D. during this Annual Meeting.

April 11, 1976
Meeting of the Executive Committee of the ISS in Davos, Switzerland. Drs. Harold G. Jacobson, Ronald O. Murray, and Jack Edeiken were present.

Details of the journal were discussed. The major article for the first issue of the journal would be Dr. Colin Alexander's article.

The *Nominating Committee* was appointed by the President:
Chairman: Jack Edeiken, M.D.
Committee Members: Alex Norman, M.D., Lars Andren, M.D.
It was the unanimous opinion of the Executive Committee that Hubert A. Sissons, M.D. of London-New York should be nominated for President-Elect. Since the positions of President and Secretary-Treasurer were already filled, no further nominations were made.

Third Annual Meeting of the International Skeletal Society

September 10–15, 1976 in Montreal, Canada
President: Harold G. Jacobson, M.D.
President-Elect: Ronald O. Murray, M.D.

Secretary-Treasurer: Jack Edeiken, M.D.

Chairman of the Program Committee: William P. Cockshott, M.D.

The Executive Committee will consist of the President, the President-Elect, the Secretary-Treasurer, past Presidents, and Refresher Course chairperson. The Business Meeting was held on September 10, 1976 in Montreal, Canada. The chairman of the Nominating Committee Jack Edeiken, M.D. gave the report that Hubert A. Sissons, M.D. of New York was nominated for President-Elect.

Ronald O. Murray, M.D. donated a medallion to the ISS which had been made in London. Dr. Murray presented the medallion to the President Harold G. Jacobson, M.D. This medallion is to be held by the President during his term in office and is then passed to the next President. The President complimented William P. Cockshott, M.D. of Canada for the wonderful program that he had prepared.

Fourth Annual Meeting of the International Skeletal Society

September 2–7, 1977 in Amsterdam, Netherlands.

President: Ronald O. Murray, M.D.

President-Elect: Hubert A. Sissons, M.D.

Secretary-Treasurer: Jack Edeiken, M.D.

Programm Chairman: Jacob D. Mulder, M.D.

The meeting of the Executive Committee was held on September 2, 1977 in Amsterdam, Netherlands. Drs. Ronald O. Murray, Harold G. Jacobson, Jack Edeiken, Hubert A. Sissons and by special invitation Jacob D. Mulder were present. It was reported that the ISS needs an endowment of at least $ 100000.– to cover the expenses for one year.

The objectives of the ISS were established (1) to supply a forum for experts in skeletal diseases to inform each other, (2) to present a Refresher Course for postgraduates in radiology and other disciplines and (3) to publish a journal. After discussion with members of the Membership Committee it was decided that the ISS is primarily for radiologists. It was then agreed that 75% of the members should be radiologists; 12.5% could be pathologists and 12.5% could come from other disciplines. The business meeting was held on September 3, 1977. The ISS President Ronald O. Murray, M.D. had invited Prof. Clement Fauré from Paris and Dr. Claude Massare to the ISS meeting as guests. At this meeting Dr. Fauré was elected a member of the ISS which established another link to France. The report of Springer-Verlag stated that there were 699 subscriptions to date and back copies were being bought.

The President reported that the membership stood at 157 before the 1977 election. There were 100 radiologists, 14 pathologists, 17 orthopedic surgeons, and 26 members from other disciplines.

Fifth Annual Meeting of the International Skeletal Society

August 30 – September 3, 1978 in Boston, USA

President: Ronald O. Murray, M.D.

President-Elect: Hubert A. Sissons, M.D.

Secretary-Treasurer: Jack Edeiken, M.D.

Program Chairman: John A. Kirkpatrick Jr., M.D.

Chairman of Closed Meeting: Howard D. Dorfman, M.D.

The Executive Committee Meeting was held on August 30, 1978 in Boston. Drs. Ronald O. Murray, Harold G. Jacobson, Hubert A. Sissons, Jack Edeiken, John A. Kirkpatrick Jr., and Robert H. Wilkinson were present.

Dr. Murray read Dr. Akbar Bonakdarpour's letter and each point was carefully discussed by the Executive Committee. There were many good points in this letter concerning improvement in the programming of the convention, the make-up of the Program Committee and the type of presentations.

The journal "Skeletal Radiology" had reached a little less than 1000 subscriptions.

Harold G. Jacobson, M.D. nominated Hubert A. Sissons M.D. for President and John A. Kirkpatrick Jr. M.D. for President-Elect. This was passed by the membership.

William P. Cockshott, M.D. of Hamilton, Canada brought up the possibility of mini symposia in the future. This will be considered by the Program Committee.

John E. Madewell, M.D. of Houston and Harry K. Genant, M.D. of San Francisco expressed interest in a West Coast Meeting.

Sixth Annual Meeting of the International Skeletal Society

August 26–31, 1979 in Munich, West-Germany

President: Hubert A. Sissons, M.D.

President-Elect: John A. Kirkpatrick Jr., M.D.

Secretary-Treasurer: Jack Edeiken, M.D.

Refresher Course Chairman: Dr. med. Friedrich H.W. Heuck

Program Chairman of Closed Meeting: Howard D. Dorfman, M.D.

The Executive Committee Meeting was held on August 26, 1979 in Munich. Drs. Hubert A. Sissons, John A. Kirkpatrick Jr., Jack Edeiken, Harold G. Jacobson, Ronald O. Murray, Friedrich H.W. Heuck, and Howard D. Dorfman were present. Drs. Akbar Bonakdarpour of Philadelphia, Walter Bessler of Winterthur, Switzerland and Eric Voegeli of Lucerne, Switzerland were invited to participate.

Friedrich H.W. Heuck reported that there were 50 registrants from the USA and approximately 150 registrants from Europe. Four collegues – radiologists and pathologists from Eastern European Countries were invited to participate in the ISS Meeting.

A vote of thanks was given to Howard D. Dorfman and Akbar Bonakdarpour for the excellent planning and programming of the closed sessions, Jack Edeiken reported that on the basis of a favorable ruling from the International Revenue Service in 1974 the tax-exampt status of the International Skeletal Society had been approved. This was reaffirmed in January 1979 after an Internal Revenue Service audit.

New committees were established and the following chairpersons appointed.

Membership Committee: Lauren V. Ackerman, M.D.

Nominating Committee: Harold G. Jacobson, M.D.

Rules Committee: John A. Kirkpatrick Jr., M.D.

Auditing Committee: Alex Norman, M.D.

Refresher Course Committee: Harold G. Jacobson, M.D.

Seventh Annual Meeting of the International Skeletal Society

August 24–31, 1980 in Mexico City, Mexico
President: Hubert A. Sissons, M.D.
President-Elect: John A. Kirkpatrick Jr., M.D.
Secretary-Treasurer: Jack Edeiken, M.D.
Refresher Course Chairman: Harold G. Jacobson, M.D.
Program Chairman: Howard D. Dorfman, M.D.
The Executive Committee Meeting was held on August 24, 1980 in Mexico City. Drs. Hubert A. Sissons, John A. Kirkpatrick Jr., Jack Edeiken, Harold G. Jacobson, Ronald O. Murray, Howard D. Dorfman, Akbar Bonakdarpour, Lauren V. Ackerman, John C. Ivins, and Robert A. Wilkinson were present. It was suggested that a selection of mini symposia should be prepared before the end of this meeting.

The business meeting was held on August 26, 1980 in Mexico City and new officers of the ISS were elected. The report of the Nominating Committee was given by Harold G. Jacobson. He proposed Jack Edeiken, M.D. for President-Elect and Akbar Bonak-darpour, M.D. for Secretary-Treasurer. A motion to close the nominations was made by Harold G. Jacobson and seconded by Lauren V. Ackerman. Then Michael Bonfiglio made a motion to select the slate. This motion was seconded by John A. Ogden and was passed by the membership.

Another Meeting of the Executive Committee was held on August 29, 1980 and the thoughts of Akbar Bonakdarpour as new Secretary-Treasurer were brought out: his feeling of the position was outlined. He wanted total responsibility and transfer of all funds and minutes to his office in an orderly and immediate fashion. This was agreed by Jack Edeiken and all members of the Executive Committee.

Appointed chairpersons for the following committees were:
Membership Committee: Lauren V. Ackerman, M.D.
Nominating Committee: Dennis J. Stoker, M.D.
Rules Committee: Hubert A. Sissons, M.D.
Auditing Committee: Robert Freiberger, M.D.
Refresher Course Committee: Harold G. Jacobson, M.D.

Eighth Annual Meeting of the International Skeletal Society

September 21–27, 1981 in Madrid, Spain
President: John A. Kirkpatrick Jr., M.D.
President-Elect; Jack Edeiken, M.D.
Secretary-Treasurer: Akbar Bonakdarpour, M.D.
Refresher Course Chairman: Harold G. Jacobson, M.D.
Program-Chairman: Howard D. Dorfman, M.D.
The meeting of the Executive Committee was held on September 20, 1981 in Madrid. Drs. John A. Kirkpatrick Jr., Jack Edeiken, Akbar Bonakdarpour, Harold G. Jacobson, and Ronald O. Murray were present.

After proposal by Dr. Jacobson and unanimous approval by all members the Executive Committee established the "Founder's Lecture" in honor of well deserved members of the International Skeletal Society to be held annually during the meeting.

The first lecture will be in memory of the late Dr. John Caffey. The first distinguished lecturer will be Dr. Edward B. Neuhauser.

Dr. Ronald O. Murray wants to resign as Chief Editor of the journal "Skeletal Radiology". He stated that his decision was adamant and this was approved with regret. The Executive Committee proposed to replace him by Dr. Philip Jacobs. Dr. Jacobs accepted it as an interim position. Drs. Harold G. Jacobson, Ronald O. Murray, and Jack Edeiken donated their allowances to the International Skeletal Society. Each of the Editors-in-chief donated $ 1100.– for a total sum of $ 3300.–.

An additional meeting of the Executive Committee of the International Skeletal Society was held on December 14, 1981 in New York, N.Y. in Dr. Harold G. Jacobson's department. Those present were: Drs. John A. Kirkpatrick Jr., Jack Edeiken, Akbar Bonakdarpour, Harold G. Jacobson, Harry K. Genant, Hubert A. Sissons, and Robert Freiberger. After a general discussion of the next meeting in San Francisco the following chairpersons for committees were appointed:
Membership Committee: Lauren V. Ackerman, M.D.
Nominating Committee: Dennis J. Stoker, M.D.
Rules Committee: Hubert A. Sissons, M.D.
Auditing Committee: Robert Freiberger, M.D.
Refresher Course Committee: Harry K. Genant, M.D.

Ninth Annual Meeting of the International Skeletal Society

August 29 – September 4, 1982 in San Francisco, USA
President: John A. Kirkpatrick Jr., M.D.
President-Elect: Jack Edeiken, M.D.
Secretary-Treasurer: Akbar Bonakdarpour, M.D.
Refresher Course Chairman: Harry K. Genant, M.D.
Program Chairman: Howard D. Dorfman, M.D.
The Executive Committee Meeting was held on August 29, 1981 in San Francisco. Drs. John A. Kirkpatrick Jr., Jack Edeiken, Akbar Bonakdarpour, Harold G. Jacobson, Ronald O. Murray, Hubert A. Sissons, Robert Freiberger, and Harry K. Genant were present. After proposal of John A. Kirkpatrick Jr. to extend the membership of exceptional Past-Presidents in the Executive committee it was unanimously approved that Harold G. Jacobson and Ronald O. Murray may remain members for another year.

Murray K. Dalinka became the first Assistant Secretary and Walter Bessler became the first Assistant Treasurer of the ISS.

Jack Edeiken stated that he wanted to resign as the Chief Editor for North America. This was met with strong opposition by all members of the Executive Committee. A search committee headed by John C. Ivins was appointed to find an assistant Chief Editor. A new Editor-in-Chief for the journal "Skeletal Radiology" must be elected at the next ISS-Meeting. Ronald O. Murray accepted the position of interim European Editor-in-Chief. William M. Park, M.D. was proposed for the new Editor-in-Chief.

Hubert A. Sissons chairman of the Rules Committee gave a report on the reforms of the By-Laws.

The chairman of the Membership Committee Lauren V. Ackerman proposed 18 new members and pointed out that the criteria for selection of new members must remain very strict.

At the business meeting Dr. Dennis J. Stoker, chairman of the Nominating Committee, reported that Dr. med Friedrich H.W. Heuck had been nominated for President-Elect. This was responded to by applauds from the membership and was unanimously approved.

Appointed chairpersons for the following committees were:
Membership Committee: Amy Beth Goldman, M.D.
Nominating Committee: Harold G. Jacobson, M.D.
Rules Committee: Harry K. Genant, M.D.
Auditing Committee: David H. Baker, M.D.
Refresher Course Committee: Walter Bessler, M.D.
Ad Hoc Search Committee for a New Assistant Chief Editor: John C. Ivins, M.D.

Tenth Annual Meeting of the International Skeletal Society

October 2–8, 1983 in Geneva, Switzerland
President: Jack Edeiken, M.D.
President-Elect: Friedrich H.W. Heuck, Dr. med.
Secretary-Treasurer: Akbar Bonakdarpour, M.D.
Refresher Course Chairman: Walter Bessler, M.D.
Program Chairman: Howard D. Dorfman, M.D.
A Meeting of the Executive Committee was held on October 2, 1983.

Drs. Jack Edeiken, Akbar Bonakdarpour, Harold G. Jacobson, Ronald O. Murray, Walter Bessler, Robert Freiberger, John A. Kirkpatrick Jr., were present. Murray K. Dalinka was present by invitation. He was appointed as Assitant Secretary-Treasurer for the years 1983–1984. Drs. David Dahlin and Heinz Götze were elected as Honorary Members of the ISS. It was approved that all papers and case-presentations after presentation at the Closed Meeting or Refresher Course must be submitted to "Skeletal Radiology" first. At the Business Meeting the chairperson of the Membership Committee Amy Beth Goldman M.D., proposed 28 new members. She reported that an Ad Hoc Committee which includes Ronald O. Murray and Murray K. Dalinka had been appointed by the President to study the problems of admission of new members to the ISS. The Chairman of the Rules committee Harry K. Genant suggested several changes in the By-Laws which were approved by the membership. Theodore E. Keats, M.D. was recommended to become the new American Associate Editor-in-Chief and Dennis J. Stoker will be the Associate European Editor-in-Chief.

In 1983 the following members of the ISS passed away:
Crawford J. Campbell, M.D. of Boston, MA, USA
Sir J. Howard Middlemiss, M.D. of Bristol, UK
William M. Park, M.D. of Owestry, UK
Dr. med. Hanno Poppe of Göttingen, West-Germany
Appointed chairpersons for the following committees were:
Membership Committee: Amy Beth Goldman, M.D.
Nominating Committee: Michael Pitt, M.D.
Rules Committee: John K. Davidson, M.D.
Auditing Committee: Morrie Kricun, M.D.
Refresher Course Committee: Murray K. Dalinka, M.D.

Ad Hoc Committee to evaluate the time-in-office of the Editor-in-Chief: John C. Ivins, M.D.
Ad Hoc Committee to recommend guidelines for admission of new members: Amy Beth Goldman, M.D.

Eleventh Annual Meeting of the International Skeletal Society

September 9–15, 1984 in Philadelphia, USA
President: Jack Edeiken, M.D.
President-Elect: Friedrich H.W. Heuck, Dr. med.
Secretary-Treasurer: Akbar Bonakdarpour, M.D.
Refresher Course Chairman: Murray K. Dalinka, M.D.
Program Chairman: Howard D. Dorfman, M.D.
The Executive Committee Meeting was held on September 9, 1984. Drs. Jack Edeiken, Friedrich H.W. Heuck, Akbar Bonakdarpour, Murray K. Dalinka, Harold G. Jacobson, John A. Kirkpatrick Jr., Louis A. Gilula, Ronald O. Murray were present. Drs. Howard D. Dorfman, Walter Bessler, John K. Davidson attended the meeting as observers.

The report of the Nominating Committee was given by Michael Pitt, who proposed Howard D. Dorfman for President-Elect. Walter Bessler was nominated as a member-at-large in the Executive Committee.

Amy Beth Goldman chairperson of the Membership Committee recommended 21 new members.

Dennis J. Stoker proposed Drs. Iain Watt, Jacob D. Mulder and Hubert B.S. Kemp to be added as consulting Editors.

It was decided that during the Annual Meeting in Edinburgh a Memorial Lecture should be given for the late William M. Park.

The President-Elect Friedrich H.W. Heuck presented a very nicely inscribed silver-plated bell – styled like the "Liberty Bell" of Philadelphia – to the ISS to be used by the president and the chairpersons of the sessions to call the meetings to order.

Appointed chairpersons to the following committees were:
Membership Committee: Amy Beth Goldman, M.D.
Nominating Committee: John A. Kirkpatrick Jr., M.D.
Rules Committee: Walter Bessler, M.D.
Auditing Committee: Alex Norman, M.D.
Ad Hoc Committee to recommend Guidelines for Admission of new members: Amy Beth Goldman, M.D.
Editorial Committee: Harold G. Jacobson, M.D.

Twelfth Annual Meeting of the International Skeletal Society

September 29 – October 5, 1985 in Edinburgh, UK
President: Friedrich H.W. Heuck, Dr. med.
President-Elect: Howard D. Dorfman, M.D.
Secretary-Treasurer: Akbar Bonakdarpour, M.D.
Refresher Course Chairman: John K. Davidson, M.D.
Program Chairman: Hubert A. Sissons, M.D.

The Executive Committee Meeting was held on September, 29, 1985 in Edinburgh. The chairperson of the Membership Committee Amy Beth Goldman, M. D. reported, that 12 new members were admitted to the ISS, bringing the total number to 261 active members.

Murray K. Dalinka, M. D. was reappointed for another year as Assistant Secretary-Treasurer of the ISS. Donald Resnick, M. D. was elected member-at-large to the Executive Committee.

The members of the Executive Committee gave consent to the President's suggestion to draw up the designs for a "Founder's Medal" in gold, a "Medal of the ISS" in silver, and a "President's Medal" in bronze for the next year's meeting.

Upon the recommendation of the chairman of the Program Committee Hubert A. Sissons, M. D. the following format for future Closed Meetings has been adopted by the Executive Committee:

1. Time allotted to each case presentation will be limited to 10 minutes including discussion.
2. Time allotted to brief papers will be limited to 15 minutes including discussion.
3. Proposals for brief papers must include an abstract of about 150 words.
4. Each member will give no more than one presentation at the Closed Meeting.

New Committees and Chairpersons were appointed as follows:

Membership Committee: Amy Beth Goldman, M. D.
Nominating Committee: John A. Kirkpatrick Jr., M. D.
Rules Committee: Walter Bessler, M. D.
Auditing Committee: Alex Norman, M. D.
Refresher Course Committee: James W. Knickerbocker, M. D.
Program Chairman: Hubert A. Sissons, M. D.
Editorial Committee: Harold G. Jacobson, M. D.
Advisory Convention Planning Committee: Akbar Bonakdarpour, M. D.
Committee for Promotion of Refresher Courses outside of North America: Walter Bessler, M. D.

Thirteenth Annual Meeting of the International Skeletal Society

September 7 – 13, 1986 in Vancouver, Canada
President: Friedrich H. W. Heuck, Dr. med.
President-Elect: Howard D. Dorfman, M. D.
Secretary-Treasurer: Akbar Bonakdarpour, M. D.
Refresher Course Chairman: W. James Knickerbocker, M. D.
Program Chairman: Hubert A. Sissons, M. D.

The first Meeting of the Executive Committee was held on September 7, 1986 in Vancouver. Drs. Friedrich H.W. Heuck, Howard D. Dorfman, Akbar Bonakdarpour, Harold G. Jacobson, Jack Edeiken, W. James Knickerbocker, and Walter Bessler were present.

The chairperson of the Membership Committee Amy Beth Goldman, M. D. reported that 18 new members had been accepted. It was proposed to make Drs. William Enneking and N. Higginbotham honorary members. This was unanimously approved.

The chairman of the Nominating committee John A. Kirkpatrick Jr. proposed Akbar Bonakdarpour, M. D. for President-Elect, Murray K. Dalinka, M. D. for Secretary-

Treasurer, and Prof. Clement Fauré for member of the Executive Committee. They all were unanimously elected. It was decided to elect Donald Resnick, M.D. for Assistant Secretary and Barbara Weissman, M.D. for Assistant Treasurer.

The chairman of the Auditing Committee Alex Norman thanked Akbar Bonakdarpour for the diligence with which he persued the finances of the ISS. He stated that the ISS assets may be about $ 300000.– at this time.

The International Skeletal Society "Endowment Fund" was established and agreement was approved by the membership. The Board of Trustees consists of 7 permanent members as well as the President and the Secretary-Treasurer of the ISS. The permanent trustees are as follows:

Walter Bessler, M.D., Winterthur, Switzerland

Akbar Bonakdarpour, M.D., Philadelphia, Pa. USA

Howard D. Dorfman, M.D., New York, NY, USA

Jack Edeiken, M.D., Philadelphia, Pa., USA

Friedrich H.W. Heuck, Dr. med., Stuttgart, West-Germany

Harold G. Jacobson, M.D., New York, NY, USA

John A. Kirkpatrick, M.D., Boston, Mass., USA

The first meeting of the trustees of the ISS Endowment Fund was held on September 8, 1986 in Vancouver, Canada. All trustees were present. Murray K. Dalinka, M.D. the Secretary-Treasurer-Elect attended the meeting by invitation. Jack Edeiken, M.D. was elected as chairman of the Endowment Fund and Akbar Bonakdarpour, M.D. was elected as Secretary-Treasurer of the Trust Fund.

The winner of the best "Resident's Paper" was Duane Blatter, M.D. of Harvard University, Boston. The title of the paper was:

"31^P Magnetic Resonance Spectroscopy Induced Athritis in Rat." The paper will have to be published in "Skeletal Radiology".

The chairman of the Ad Hoc Committee for Founder's and Past President's Medals Friedrich H.W. Heuck gave report and presented samples for the

1. Founder's Gold Medal
2. International Skeletal Society Silver Medal
3. President's Medal in Bronze

    Financial support will be given by Siemens AG, West-Germany and by Agfa-Gevaert Inc. USA.

    Dr. Heuck also showed a sample of the Past-President's Medal.

    Dr. Akbar Bonakdarpour made a move to spend $ 1200.– for the Past-President's Medals.

This was unanimously approved.

The Guidelines for the Bestowing of the Gold-, Silver-, and Bronze-Medals were presented and approved by the Executive Committee.

At the end of his Presidency Dr. Friedrich H.W. Heuck donated to the ISS a nice Sterling Silver Chain, which contains all National Flags of the membership.

The following committees and chairpersons were appointed:

Membership Committee: Amy Beth Goldman, M.D.

Nominating Committee: Lee F. Rogers, M.D.

Rules Committee: Akbar Bonakdarpour, M.D.

Auditing Committee: Robert Freiberger, M.D.

Editorial Committee: Harold G. Jacobson, M.D.

Ad Hoc Committee for Future Planning: John A. Kirkpatrick Jr., M.D.

Fourteenth Annual Meeting of the International Skeletal Society

September 13–19, 1987 in Cannes, France
President: Howard D. Dorfman, M.D.
President-Elect: Akbar Bonakdarpour, M.D.
Secretary-Treasurer: Murray K. Dalinka, M.D.
Refresher Course Chairman: Clement Fauré, M.D.
Program Chairman: Hubert A. Sissons, M.D.
The Meeting of the Executive Committee was held on September 13, 1987 in Cannes, France.
Drs. Howard D. Dorfman, Akbar Bonakdarpour, Murray K. Dalinka, Harold G. Jacobson, Friedrich H.W. Heuck, and Donald Resnick were present.

The chairman of the Nominating Committee Lee F. Rogers, M.D. nominated Michael Bonfiglio, M.D. as a member-at-large of the Executive Committee for two years. This was unanimously approved.

The chairperson of the Membership Committee Amy Beth Goldman, M.D. reported that 24 new members had been accepted. It was reaffirmed that a member of the ISS can recommend only two individuals each year for membership in the International Skeletal Society.

It was indicated that there are 270 active members in the ISS from 19 countries. There are 20 honorary members and 6 inactive members. The business meeting was held on September 14, 1987.

Dr. Jack Edeiken presented the report of the Endowment Fund Committee. A working document is being developed and will be reviewed by the Executive Committee.

Dr. Friedrich H.W. Heuck presented details regarding the Founder's and Past-President's Medals. He indicated that 5 Gold-, 10 Silver-, and 10 Bronze-Medals had been approved by the Executive Committee at the cost of approximately $ 6000.–.

Dr. Louis Gilula reviewed briefly the work of the Convention Planning Committee.

At a meeting of the Executive Committee on September 18, 1987 the members unanimously agreed to refer the Endowment Trust Agreement to the Rules Committee for review and incorporation in the By-Laws.

Committees and Chairpersons were appointed as follows:
Membership Committee: Amy Beth Goldman, M.D.
Nominating Committee: Lee F. Rogers, M.D.
Rules Committee: Akbar Bonakdarpour, M.D.
Editorial Committee: Harold G. Jacobson, M.D.
Ad Hoc Committee for Future Planning: John A. Kirkpatrick Jr., M.D.
Ad Hoc Advisory committee for Convention Planning: Louis Gilula, M.D.
Ad Hoc Committee for Promotion of Refresher Courses outside North America: Walter Bessler, M.D.
Ad Hoc Awards Committee: Friedrich H.W. Heuck, Dr. med.
Ad Hoc Committee on Recruitment of Skeletal Radiologists: Daniel I. Rosenthal, M.D.

Fifteenth Annual Meeting of the International Skeletal Society

September 25 – October 1, 1988 in Sydney, Australia
President: Howard D. Dorfman, M.D.
President-Elect: Akbar Bonakdarpour, M.D.
Secretary-Treasurer: Murray K. Dalinka, M.D.
Refresher Course Chairperson: Janet McCredie, M.D.
Program Chairman: Hubert A. Sissons, M.D.
    Committees and Charipersons were appointed as follows:
Auditing Committee: Howard D. Dorfman, M.D.
Awards Committee: Friedrich W. Heuck, M.D.
Board of Trustees of the Endowment Fund. Jack Edeiken, M.D.
Editorial Committee: Jack Edeiken, M.D.; Theodore E. Keats, M.D., Co-Chair
Liaison Future Planning Committee: Andrew Poznansky, M.D.; Morrie E. Kricun, M.D., Co-Chair
Membership Committee: Harry K. Genant, M.D.; Amy Beth Goldman, M.D., Co-Chair
Nominating Committee: John A. Kirkpatrick Jr., M.D.
Program Committee: Peter G. Bullough, M.D.; Jack P. Lawson, M.D., Co-Chair
Refresher Course Committee: Robert Freiberger, M.D.; Alex Norman, M.D., Co-Chair
Rules Committee: Michael J. Pitt, M.D.
Ad Hoc Advisory Committee for Convention Planning: Louis A. Gilula, M.D., Murray K. Dalinka, Co-Chair
Ad Hoc Committee for Proceedings and Archives: Harold G. Jacobson, M.D.
Ad Hoc Committee for Promotion of Refresher Courses outside of North America: John K. Davidson, M.D.
Ad Hoc Committee on Recruitment of Skeletal Radiologists: Daniel I. Rosenthal, M.D.; Morrie E. Kricun, M.D., Co-Chair
Ad Hoc Nomenclature Committee: Hubert A. Sissons, M.D.; Jack Edeiken, M.D., Co-Chair

Sixteenth Annual Meeting of the International Skeletal Society

September 10 – 16, 1989 in New York, New York
President: Akbar Bonakdarpour, M.D.
President-Elect: Walter Bessler, M.D.
Secretary-Treasurer: Murray K. Dalinka, M.D.
Assistant Secretary: Donald Resnick, M.D.
Refresher Course Chairperson: Robert H. Freiberger, M.D.; Alex Norman, M.D., Co-Chair
    Committees and Chairpersons were appointed as follows:
Auditing Committee: Lawrence Bassette, M.D.
Awards Committee: Friedrich W. Heuck, M.D.
Board of Trustees of the Endowment Fund: Jack Edeiken, M.D.
Closed Program Committee: Peter G. Bullough, M.D.; Jack P. Lawson, M.D., Co-Chair
Committee for Fellowship-Accreditation of Musculoskeletal Radiology: Donald Resnick, M.D.
Committee for Promotion of Refresher Courses outside of North America: John K. Davidson, M.D.
Convention Planning Committee: Louis A. Gilula, M.D.; Donald Resnick, M.D., Co-Chair

Corinne Farrel Prize Committee: Frieda Feldman, M.D.
Editorial Committee: Jack Edeiken, M.D.; Theodore E. Keats, M.D., Co-Chair
Liaison Future Planning Committee: Andrew Poznansky, M.D.; Morrie E. Kricun, M.D.
Membership Committee: Harry G. Genant, M.D.; Amy Beth Goldman, M.D., Co-Chair
Nominating Committee: John A. Kirkpatrick, M.D.
Refresher Course Committee: Friedrich W. Heuck, M.D.
Rules Committee: Michael J. Pitt, M.D.
Ad Hoc Committee for Proceedings and Archives: Harold G. Jacobson, M.D.
Ad Hoc Committee on Recruitment of Skeletal Radiologist in the USA: Daniel J. Rosenthal, M.D.; Morrie E. Kricun, M.D., Co-Chair
Ad Hoc Nomenclature Committee: Hubert A. Sissons, M.D.; Jack Edeiken, M.D., Co-Chair

Seventeenth Annual Meeting of the International Skeletal Society

September 9–15, 1990 in Salzburg, Austria
President: Akbar Bonakdarpour, M.D.
President-Elect: Walter Bessler, M.D.
Secretary: Murray K. Dalinka, M.D.
Refresher Course Chairperson: Friedrich H.W. Heuck, Dr. med.
   Committees and Chairpersons were appointed as follows:
Auditing Committee: Lawrence Bassette, M.D.
Awards Committee: Friedrich W. Heuck, M.D.
Board of Trustees of the Endowment Fund: Jack Edeiken, M.D.
Closed Program Committee: Peter G. Bullough, M.D.; Jack P. Lawson, M.D., Co-Chair
Committee for Fellowship-Accreditation of Musculoskeletal Radiology: Donald Resnick, M.D.
Committee for Promotion of Refresher Courses outside of North America: Holger Pettersson, M.D.
Convention Planning Committee: Louis A. Gilula, M.D.; Donald Resnick, M.D., Co-Chair
Corinne Farrel Prize Committee: Frieda Feldman, M.D.
Editorial Committee: Jack Edeiken, M.D.; Dennis J. Stoker, Jr., M.D., Co-Chair
Liaison Future Planning Committee: Morrie E. Kricun, M.D., Michael Bonfiglio, M.D., Co-Chair
Membership Committee: Harry G. Genant, M.D.; Amy Beth Goldman, M.D., Co-Chair
Nominating Committee: John A. Kirkpatrick, M.D.
Refresher Course Committee: Donald Resnick, M.D.
Representative to the ACR: Lee F. Rogers, M.D.
Rules Committee: Akbar Bonakdarpour, M.D.
Ad Hoc Committee for Proceedings and Archives: Harold G. Jacobson, M.D.
Ad Hoc Committee on Recruitment of Skeletal Radiologist in the USA: Daniel J. Rosenthal, M.D.; Morrie E. Kricun, M.D., Co-Chair
Ad Hoc Nomenclature Committee: Krishnan K. Unni, M.D.; Theodore E. Keats, M.D., Co-Chair

Eighteenth Annual Meeting of the International Skeletal Society

September 22–28, 1991 in San Diego, California
President: Walter Bessler, M.D.
President-Elect: Andrew Poznanski, M.D.
Secretary: Murray K. Dalinka, M.D.
Treasurer: Donald Resnick, M.D.
Refresher Course Chairperson: Donald Resnick, M.D.
   Committees and Chairpersons were appointed as follows:
Auditing Committee: Lawrence Bassette, M.D.
Awards Committee: Friedrich W. Heuck, M.D.
Board of Trustees of the Endowment Fund: Jack Edeiken, M.D.
Closed Program Committee: Peter G. Bullough, M.D.; Jack P. Lawson, M.D., Co-Chair
Committee for Fellowship-Accreditation of Musculoskeletal Radiology: Donald Resnick, M.D.
Committee for Promotion of Refresher Courses outside of North America: Holger Pettersson, M.D.
Convention Planning Committee: Louis A. Gilula, M.D.; Donald Resnick, M.D., Co-Chair
Corinne Farrel Prize Committee: Frieda Feldman, M.D.
Editorial Committee: Jack Edeiken, M.D.; Dennis J. Stoker, Jr., Co-Chair
Liaison Future Planning Committee: Morrie E. Kricun, M.D.; Michael Bonfiglio, M.D., Co-Chair
Membership Committee: Harry G. Genant, M.D.; Amy Beth Goldman, M.D., Co-Chair
Nominating Committee: John A. Kirkpatrick, M.D.
Refresher Course Committee: Donald Resnick, M.D.
Representative to the ACR: Lee F. Rogers, M.D.
Rules Committee: Akbar Bonakdarpour, M.D.
Ad Hoc Committee for Proceedings and Archives: Harold G. Jacobson, M.D.
Ad Hoc Committee on Recruitment of Skeletal Radiologist in the USA: Daniel J. Rosenthal, M.D.; Morrie E. Kricun, M.D., Co-Chair
Ad Hoc Nomenclature Committee: Krishnan K, Unni, M.D.; Theodore E. Keats, M.D., Co-Chair

Nineteenth Annual Meeting of the International Skeletal Society

August 23–29, 1992 in Stockholm, Sweden
President: Walter Bessler, M.D.
President-Elect: Andrew Poznanski, M.D.
Secretary: Murray K. Dalinka, M.D.
Treasurer: Donald Resnick, M.D.
Refresher Course Chairperson: Holger Pettersson, M.D.; Donald Resnick, M.D., Co-Chair
   Committees and Chairpersons were appointed as follows:
Auditing Committee: John H. Harris, Jr., M.D.
Awards Committee: Walter Bessler, M.D.
Board of Trustees of the Endowment Fund: Jack Edeiken, M.D.
Closed Program Committee: Peter G. Bullough, M.D.; Jack P. Lawson, M.D., Co-Chair
Committee for Promotion of Refresher Courses outside of North America: Holger T.A. Pettersson, M.D.

Convention Planning Committee: Louis A. Gilula, M.D.; William P. Cockshott, M.D., Co-Chair
Corinne Farrel Prize Committee: Judy Adams, M.D.
Committee for Evaluation of Research Grants: Harry K. Genant, M.D.
Editorial Committee: Theodore E. Keats, M.D.; Dennis J. Stoker, M.D., Co-Chair
Liaison Planning Committee: B.J. Manaster, M.D.; Morrie E. Kricun, M.D., Co-Chair
Membership Committee: Harry K. Genant, M.D.
Nomenclature Committee: Krishnan K. Unni, M.D.; Donald P. Speer, M.D., Co-Chair
Nominating Committee: Amy B. Goldman, M.D.
Refresher Course Committee: William P. Cockshott, M.D.; Donald Resnick, M.D., Co-Chair
Ad Hoc Proceedings Committee: Harold Jacobson, M.D.

Twentieth Annual Meeting of the International Skeletal Society

August 15–21, 1993 in Toronto, Ontario, Canada
President: Andrew Poznanski, M.D.
President-Elect: Murray K. Dalinka, M.D.
Secretary: Donald Resnick, M.D.
Treasurer: Michael J. Pitt, M.D.
Refresher Course Chairperson: W. Peter Cockshott, M.D.
    Committees and Chairpersons were appointed as follows:
Auditing Committee: John H. Harris, Jr., M.D.
Awards Committee: Walter Bessler, M.D.
Board of Trustees of the Endowment Fund: Jack Edeiken, M.D.
Closed Program Committee: Peter G. Bullough, M.D.; Jack P. Lawson, M.D., Co-Chair
Committee for Evaluation of Research Grants: Harry K. Genant, M.D.
Committee for Promotion of Refresher Courses outside of North America: Holger T. A. Pettersson, M.D.
Convention Planning Committee: Louis A. Gilula, M.D.
Corinne Farrel Prize Committee: Judy Adams, M.D.
Editorial Committee: Theodore E. Keats, M.D., Co-Chair; Dennis J. Stoker, M.D., Co-Chair
Liaison Planning Committee: Iain Watt, M.D., Co-Chair; Morrie E. Kricun, M.D., Co-Chair
Membership Committee: Harry K. Genant, M.D.
Nomenclature Committee: Krishnan K. Unni, M.D., Co-Chair; Donald P. Speer, M.D., Co-Chair
Nominating Committee: Amy B. Goldman, M.D.
Refresher Course Committee: Herbert Kaufman, Co-Chair, M.D.; Donald Resnick, M.D., Co-Chair, Dietrich H. Banzer, M.D., Co-Chair
Ad Hoc Proceedings Committee: Harold Jacobson, M.D.

Twenty First Annual Meeting of the International Skeletal Society

August 13–20, 1994 in Berlin, Germany
President: Andrew Poznanski, M.D.
President-Elect: Murray K. Dalinka, M.D.
Secretary: Donald Resnick, M.D.
Treasurer: Michael J. Pitt, M.D.
Refresher Course Chairperson: Herbert J. Kaufmann, M.D.; Dietrich H. Banzer, M.D., Co-Chair
    Committees and Chairpersons were appointed as follows:
Historian: Morrie E. Kricun, M.D.
Auditing Committee: John H. Harris, Jr., M.D.
Awards Committee: Holger T. A. Pettersson, M.D.
Board of Trustees of the Endowment Fund: Walter Bessler, M.D.
Closed Program Committee: Peter G. Bullough, M.D., Co-Chair; Jeremy Kaye, M.D., Co-Chair
Committee for Evaluation of Research Grants: Harry K. Genant, M.D.
Committee for Promotion of Refresher Courses outside of North America: Walter Bessler, M.D.
Convention Planning Committee: Louis A. Gilula, M.D.
Corinne Farrel Prize Committee: Amy Beth Goldman, M.D.
Editorial Committee: Theodore E. Keats, M.D., Chief Editor; Dennis J. Stoker, M.D., Chief Editor; Jeremy Kaye, M.D., Chief Editor
Editorial Search Committee: Donald Resnick, M.D.
Liaison Planning Committee: Robert Dussault, M.D., Co-Chair; Clyde Helms, M.D., Co-Chair
Membership Committee: Jeremy Kaye, M.D.
Nomenclature Committee: Krishnan K. Unni, M.D.
Nominating Committee: Helene Pavlov, M.D.
Refresher Course Committee: B. Gil Brogdon, M.D.
Rules Committee: Akbar Bonakdarpour, M.D.
Ad Hoc Proceedings Committee: Frieda Feldman, M.D.

Twenty Second Annual Meeting of the International Skeletal Society

October 14–21, 1995 in New Orleans, Louisiana
President: Murray K. Dalinka, M.D.
President-Elect: Holger T. A. Pettersson, M.D.
Secretary: Donald Resnick, M.D.
Treasurer: Michael Pitt, M.D.
Refresher Course Chairperson: B. Gil Brogdon, M.D.
    Committees and Chairpersons were appointed as follows:
Historian: Morrie E. Kricun, M.D.
Auditing Committee: John H. Harris, Jr., M.D.
Awards Committee: Holger T. A. Pettersson, M.D.
Board of Trustees of the Endowment Fund: Walter Bessler, M.D.
Closed Program Committee: Leonard Kahn, M.D., Co-Chair; Jeremy Kaye, M.D., Co-Chair

Committee for Evaluation of Research Grants: Harry K. Genant, M.D.
Committee for Promotion of Refresher Courses outside of North America: Walter Bessler, M.D.
Convention Planning Committee: Louis A. Gilula, M.D.
Corinne Farrel Prize Committee: Amy Beth Goldman, M.D.
Editorial Committee: Theodore E. Keats, M.D., Chief Editor; Dennis J. Stoker, M.D., Chief Editor; Jeremy Kaye, M.D., Chief Editor
Editorial Search Committee (American): Donald Resnick, M.D.
Editorial Search Committee (European): Bryan Preston, M.D.
Liaison Planning Committee: Robert Dussault, M.D., Co-Chair; Clyde Helms, M.D., Co-Chair
Membership Committee: Jeremy Kaye, M.D.
Nomenclature Committee: Krishnan K. Unni, M.D.
Nominating Committee: Helene Pavlov, M.D.
Refresher Course Committee: Alain Chevrot, M.D., Co-Chair; Daniel Vanel, M.D., Co-Chair; Jean-Denis Laredo, M.D., Co-Chair
Rules Committee: Akbar Bonakdarpour, M.D.
Ad Hoc Proceedings Committee: Frieda Feldman, M.D.

Twenty Third Annual Meeting of the International Skeletal Society

August 18–23, 1996 in Paris, France
President: Murray K. Dalinka, M.D.
President-Elect: Holger T. A. Pettersson
Secretary: Donald Resnick, M.D.
Treasurer: Michael Pitt, M.D.
Refresher Course Chairpersons: Alain Chevrot, M.D., Daniel Vannel, M.D., Jean-Denis Laredo, M.D.
    Committees and Chairpersons were appointed as follows:
Historian: Morrie E. Kricun, M.D.
Auditing Committee: Richard H. Gold, M.D.
Awards Committee: Donald Resnick, M.D.
Board of Trustees of the Endowment Fund: Howard Dorfman, M.D.
Closed Program Committee: Leonard Kahn, M.D.; Javier Beltran, M.D., Co-Chair
Committee for Evaluation of Research Grants: Robert Dussault, M.D.
Committee for Promotion of Refresher Courses outside of North America: Walter Bessler, M.D.
Convention Planning Committee: Louis A. Gilula, M.D.
Corinne Farrel Prize Committee: Frieda Feldman, M.D.
Editorial Committee: Jeremy Kaye, M.D.
Liaison Planning Committee: Clyde Helms, M.D.; Amy Beth Goldman, M.D., Co-Chair
Membership Committee: Ian McCall, M.D.
Nominating Committee: Helene Pavlov, M.D.
Nomenclature Committee: K. Krishnan Unni, M.D.
Refresher Course Committee: Jeremy Kaye, M.D.
Rules Committee: Akbar Bonakdarpour, M.D.

September 10–13, 1997 in Santa Fe, New Mexico
President: Holger T. A. Pettersson, M.D.
President-Elect: Donald L. Resnick, M.D.
Secretary: Harry K. Genant, M.D.
Treasurer: Michael J. Pitt, M.D.
Refresher Course Chairperson: Jeremy J. Kaye, M.D.
     Committees and Chairpersons were appointed as follows:
Historian: Morrie E. Kricun, M.D.
Auditing Committee: Richard H. Gold, M.D.
Awards Committee: Donald Resnick, M.D.
Board of Trustees of the Endowment Fund: Howard Dorfman, M.D.
Closed Program Committee: Leonard Kahn, M.D.; Javier Beltran, M.D., Co-Chair
Committee for Evaluation of Future Structure and Format of ISS Meetings: Harry K. Genant, M.D.; Javier Beltran, M.D., Co-Chair
Committee for Evaluation of Research Grants: Robert Dussault, M.D.
Committee for Promotion of Refresher Courses outside of North America: Walter Bessler, M.D.
Convention Planning Committee: Louis A. Gilula, M.D.
Corinne Farrel Prize Committee: Frieda Feldman, M.D.
Editorial Committee: Jeremy Kaye, M.D.
Liaison Planning Committee: Clyde Helms, M.D.; Amy Beth Goldman, M.D., Co-Chair
Membership Committee: Iain McCall, M.D.
Nomenclature Committee: K. Krishnan Unni, M.D.
Nominating Committee: Helene Pavlov, M.D.
Refresher Course Committee: B. Gil Brogdon, M.D.
Rules Committee: Akbar Bonakdarpour, M.D.

By-Laws of the International Skeletal Society

(Effective September 30, 1985)

Article I

Name

Section 1 This organization shall be known as
The International Skeletal Society (ISS).

Article II

Objects of the Society

Section 1 to advance the science and art of skeletal radiology through an educational non-profit society of radiologists and individuals in related fields of medicine and science.

Section 2 to bring together radiologists and individuals in related fields to improve the understanding, research and teaching of skeletal radiology, and to promote closer fellowship and exchange of ideas.

Section 3 to provide meetings for the reading and discussion of papers and dissemination of knowledge.

Section 4 to provide continuing education through refresher courses.

Section 5 to publish a journal that will be the official organ of the Society.

Article III

Membership

Section 1 membership in the Society shall be restricted to radiologists with a substantial interest in the practice, teaching or research in skeletal radiology, who are certified by the American Board of Radiology or its foreign equivalent and to MD's, DO's, DVM's or PhD scientists working in related fields.

Section 2 the categories of membership shall be:
(1) Active members;   (2) Honorary members;
(3) Inactive members.

Active Members: Radiologists with a substantial interest in the practice, teaching or research in skeletal radiology, and physicians or scientists working in related fields.

Honorary Members: Physicians or scientists who have made outstanding contributions to skeletal radiology or related disciplines. Honorary members shall be elected by the Executive Committee.

Inactive-Members: Shall be designated from among the active membership and shall be those who have retired from active practice. Application for inactive status must be made in writing, to the Secretary. Inactive members shall be exempt from dues.

Section 3 membership should be sustained by attending no less than one meeting in four years. If a member has missed four successive meetings he will be notified by the Secretary, and if he does not attend the subsequent meeting, his membership may be terminated by the Executive Committee.

Article IV

Officers

Section 1 officers of the Society shall be the President, President-elect, Secretary and Treasurer. One member may be elected Secretary and Treasurer or one member may be elected as Secretary and another as Treasurer. The term of office shall be two (2) years for President and President-elect, and three (3) years for the Secretary, Treasurer, or Secretary-Treasurer. Each officer shall be an active member in good standing.

Section 2 the President shall be presiding officer of the Society, Chairperson of the Executive Committee, and a member ex-officio of all committees. He shall perform all the duties which custom and parliamentary practice commonly associate with the office of President. His term of office as President shall begin at the adjournment of the annual meeting during which he was installed as President. The President shall serve on the Executive Committee for two (2) years after his term of office expires.

Section 3 the President-elect shall succeed the President. If the President is unable to act, he shall perform the duties of the President. The President-elect shall be a member of the Executive Committee.

Section 4 the Secretary shall perform the duties of the President if both the President and President-elect are unavailable to act. He shall be a member of the Executive Committee and a member ex-officio of all other committees except the Nominating Committee.

the Secretary shall keep or cause to be kept a correct and permanent record of the proceedings of the Society. He shall keep a current alphabetical list of the members specifying their current addresses, year of election and classification of their membership. He shall conduct correspodence, notify applicants for membership in the Society of their acceptance within thirty (30) days of the annual meeting, and perform all other duties that usually and customarily pertain to the office of Secretary. He shall provide safe keeping for all records and transactions of the Society which possess historical value. Not later than three (3) months after each annual meeting of the Society, he shall cause to be printed and distributed to each member of the Society a transcript of the minutes of the annual meeting, which shall include the reports of all officers and committees.

Section 5 Assistant Secretary (or Assistant Secretary-Treasurer). The Executive Committee may appoint, on the recommendation of the Secretary, an Assistant Secretary (or Assistant Secretary-Treasurer). This appointment will be for a term of one (1) year, but will be renewable. The Assistant Secretary may attend meetings of the Executive Committee, but will not be a member of that body.

Section 6 the Treasurer shall collect and be accountable for all funds of the Society and shall disperse from the treasury such funds only upon order of the Executive Committee, if the amount exceeds two thousand dollars or as modified in the future by the Executive Committee. He shall keep the complete and permanent record of the financial transactions of the Society. He shall make a full financial report and present a budget for the following year at the annual meeting of the Society, which shall be incorporated in the minutes of the meeting. The Treasurer shall be a member of the Executive Committee.

Section 7 Assistant Treasurer. The Executive Committee may appoint, on the recommendation of the Treasurer, an Assistant Treasurer. The appointment will be for a term of one (1) year, but will be renewable. The Assistant Treasurer may attend the meeting of the Executive Committee, but will not be a member of that body.

Article V

Committees

Section 1 standing committees of the Society shall be as follows: Executive Committee, Program Committee, Refresher Course Committee, Auditing Committee, Nominating Committee, Membership Committee, Rules Committee, Editorial Committee, Awards Committee, Liaison-Future Planning Committee, Convention Planning Committee, and Committee for the Promotion of the Refresher Course outside of North America. Committee appointments, including the chairperson, shall be made by the President, in consultation with the Executive Committee, unless otherwise provided for in the By-Laws. Actions of all committees shall be reported in the membership and are subject to review and approval unless otherwise provided for in the By-Laws.

Section 2 the Executive Committee shall consist of the President, the President-elect, Secretary, Treasurer, immediate Past President, five Members-at-large, two of whom shall not be radiologists, and others (see Article IV, Section 2).

Section 2 the Executive Committee shall consist of the President, the President-elect, Secretary, Treasurer, immediate Past President, five Members-at-large, two of whom shall not be radiologists, and others (see Article IV, Section 2). The Officers shall each serve for a period of two (2) years; the Members-at-large shall each serve for a period of two years and shall not be eligible for consecutive reappointment; the Secretary, Treasurer, or Secretary-Treasurer shall serve for a period of three (3) years. The Refresher Course Chairperson will serve as co-opted member of the Committee for the current year. The President shall be the chairperson of the Executive Committee. The Executive Committee shall be empowered to carry out the business of the Society between meetings of the membership and to manage the funds and expenditures of the Society. No money or other valuable property of the Society shall be expended or otherwise disbursed without the sanction of the majority of the Executive Committee, unless ordered by a three-fourths vote of the members present voting at the annual meeting. It shall require a three-fourths vote of the members present to reject any recommendation of the Executive Committee relative to the finances of the Society. The Executive Committee shall fix the time and place of meetings, as well as the apportionment of the time and nature of the various portions of the meetings. Dues for the ensuing year which shall be consistent with the operational needs of the Society shall be fixed by the Executive Committee. Changes in dues must be ratified by vote of the membership. The Refresher Course fee shall be set each year by the Executive Committee and shall be consistent with the operational expenses of the course. Surplus funds shall be applied to the general treasury funds. The Executive Committee shall have general supervision of the affairs of the Society not otherwise provided for.

Section 3 the Program Committee shall consist of the Secretary and Treasurer plus three active members, each of whom shall serve for two years. A chairperson will be appointed; exceptionally, the tenure of appointment may be extended at the discretion of the president. In addition to these, the President may appoint one or more active members to serve for one year in order to help with the arrangements for a particular meeting. It shall be the duty of the Committee to determine the character and scope of the scientific proceedings of the Membership Meeting of the Society at each annual meeting. It shall have the right to accept or reject papers for presentation at the meeting and shall exercise proper control over the format, time allotments, including discussion, and the arrangement of the presentations. The Secretary must receive the program from the Program Chairman at a reasonable time prior to the annual meeting. A program shall be mailed to each member of the Society at least two weeks prior to the meeting.

Section 4 the Refresher Course Committee shall consist of the Secretary and Treasurer, the President-Elect and three active members, each of the latter shall serve for three (3) years. These should include the immediate past, the present and the succeeding person responsible for local organization of the refresher course. A chairperson will be appointed. In addition to these the President may appoint one or more active members to serve for one year in order to help with the arrangements for a particular meeting. A refresher course of at least two to three days may be given each year following the annual meeting. It shall be the duty of the Refresher Course Committee to determine the character and scope of the courses and exercise control over the format, time allotments, including discussion, and arrangements for presentations. The Secretary must receive the program from the Refresher Course Committee eight (8) months before the course. The Refresher Course Committee shall make all arrangements for rooms, projection equipment, tickets, packet and registration and reservations for meeting areas.

Section 5   the Auditing Committee shall consist of three active members appointed by the President for a two (2) year period and one of whom shall be chairperson. The Auditing Committee shall audit the accounts of the Treasurer at least once a year. A CPA may be hired by this Committee. The results of the audit shall be reported to the membership each year.

Section 6   members of the Nominating Committee shall serve for two (2) years. They shall consist of the President, the Chairperson of the Rules Committee and three active members appointed by the Executive Committee from the membership at large, one of whom shall not be a radiologist. One of the latter members so appointed shall be designated by the Executive Committee to serve as Chairperson. This Committee shall perform its duties in accordance with the provision of Article IX of these By-Laws.

Section 7   the Membership Committee shall consist of seven active members, one of whom shall be chairperson, each of whom shall serve for two (2) years. It shall be the responsibility of the Membership Committee to assure satisfactory balance of membership in the Society between radiologist and other scientists, such that the Society shall maintain a primary interest in the radiology of skeletal diseases. The Membership Committee shall review all applications for membership in accordance with the provisions of Articles III and X of these By-Laws to insure that they fulfill the requirements for membership in the appropriate category.

Section 8   the Rules Committee shall consist of three active members, one of whom shall be chairperson, each of whom shall serve for two (2) years. The Rules Committee shall be responsible for the By-Laws and may be called upon to interpret By-Laws when questions arise. It shall on order of the Executive Committee prepare and submit amendments to the By-Laws, edit and present to the members any amendments proposed by members of the Society, and may on its own motion preface and present to the members any amendments which it deems necessary. It shall receive all resolutions introduced by members; it may reword them or combine those having the same intent to prepare for presentation. It shall present such amendments to the members accompanied by the recommendation of the Committee.

Section 9   the members of the Editorial Committee shall consist of the Chief Editors, Emeritus Chief Editors, Assistant Chief Editors, President, President-Elect, Secretary, Treasurer and three members of the Editorial Board. The Chairperson of the Editorial Committee will be appointed by the President for a term of two years with the approval of the Executive Committee.

the three members of the Editorial Board will be proposed by the President to the Editorial Committee and after approval of the Editorial Committee the president will propose them for the approval of the Executive Committee.

there will be three Chief Editors; one North American Chief Editor, one non-American Chief Editor whose native language is English and one Case Report Chief Editor.

the Chief Editors shall serve for two years and their appointment can be extended annually by the Executive Committee. Each chief editor may have an assistant chief editor with a basic tenure of two years but subject to reappointment annually by the Executive Committee.

Section 10   the Awards Committee shall consist of the President, President-Elect, and five active members. Each of the latter shall be appointed for an overlapping term of up to five years with the possibility of reappointment.

Awards shall take the following form:

1. *The Founders' Medal*
   This Founders' medal is presented in honor of the founders of the International Skeletal Society and its Presidents, Harold G. Jacobson, Ronald O. Murray, and Jack Edeiken, that they may be preserved in memory for future generations.

   This gold medal honors those who not only distinguished themselves through their outstanding dedication to the International Skeletal Society but have further distinguished themselves by excellence in their field of science. It should be awarded to not more than one person each year.

2. *The Medal of the International Skeletal Society*
   This silver medal is presented to persons who have actively supported the endeavors of the International Skeletal Society. The prospective recipient of this award therefore need not be a member or an honorary member of the International Skeletal Society.

3. *The President's Medal*
   This bronze medal is intended for members of the International Skeletal Society in special recogniton of their outstanding scientific achievements on an international level and who have as yet not completed their 45th year of age. It may be awarded on an annual basis, and accompanied by a monetary award.

The names of the recipient(s) of the Medal(s) shall be published in *SKELETAL RADIOLOGY*.

Section 11   all other necessary committees and representatives not specifically mentioned previously shall be appointed by the President.

Section 12   where committee appointments are for more than one year, the principle of overlapping tenure should be applied when possible.

Section 13   a historian shall be appointed by the Executive Committee to serve for a period of four years which may be renewable on a yearly basis thereafter.

Section 14   The Liaison – Planning Committee shall consist of a chairperson and at least 12 other members, all appointed by the President for an overlapping term of three years. Committee composition should reflect a cross-section of the membership regarding the medical specialty, nationality, and experience. This committee, serving as a liaison between the general membership and Executive Committee, shall initiate and/or receive and evaluate suggestions from the general membership or Executive Committee pertinent to the improvement and function of the society which might be more appropriately discussed in a smaller forum than in the open meeting. The committee will be advisory to the Executive Committee and will transmit recommendations and committee proceedings to the Executive Committee.

Section 15   the Convention Planning Committee shall consist of a chairperson appointed by the President for a two (2) year term, the Secretary, the Treasurer or the Secretary-Treasurer, the President-Elect, the chairperson of the immediate past and the tentative chairpersons of the next three refresher courses. The Secretary-Treasurer or the Treasurer of the International Skeletal Society will be co-chairperson of the committee. The Convention Planning Committee will act as an advisory committee to the officers and the Executive Committee of the International Skeletal Society for planning the future meetings of the society. It will oversee, review, and advise the convention manager. This committee will not have the power to make definitive decisions without approval of the Treasurer or Secretary-Treasurer of the International Skeletal Society. All members of the committee will be active members of the society.

Section 16   the Committee for the Promotion of the Refresher Course outside of North America shall consist of at least twelve active members, each of whom shall serve for two years. The chairperson and members of the committee will be appointed by the President. In addition, the President may appoint one or more active members to serve for one year in order to help with the promotion of a particular meeting. The responsibility of the committee will be the commercial promotion of the refresher course outside of North America. The chairperson of this committee should directly coordinate activities with the Secretary or Secretary-Treasurer of the International Skeletal Society.

Article VI

Meetings

Section 1   the Society shall meet annually and such meetings shall consist of business and scientific sessions. This may be followed by a two or three day refresher course.

Section 2   a quorum for conducting business at the annual meeting for election of officers shall be 25 % of the United States active membership when voting in the U.S., or 20 % of active membership when the meeting is in other countries.

Article VII

International Skeletal Society Endowment Fund

A trust fund shall be established to further the philanthropic and scientific aims of the Society, as determined by the executive committee and the membership.

The trust fund shall be set up and operated as set out in the amended agreement between the International Skeletal Society and the Endowment Fund.

Article VIII

Procedures

Section 1   the fiscal year shall begin on the first of June and shall end on the thirty first of May.

Section 2   in the absence of contrary statements in the By-Laws, Robert's Rules of Order shall govern procedure.

Section 3   order of business:

    (1) call to order
    (2) reading of minutes
    (3) business arising from minutes
    (4) Secretary's report
    (5) Treasurer's report
    (6) report of committees
    (7) unfinished business
    (8) report of Membership Committee
    (9) election of members
  (10) new business
  (11) report of Nominating Committee
  (12) election of officers
  (13) installation of officers
  (14) appointment of committees
  (15) adjournment

Article IX

Elections

Section 1   officers of this Society shall be elected at the annual meeting to serve for a period as indicated in the By-Laws.

Section 2   the procedure for election of officers of this Society shall be as follows: The Nominating Committee shall nominate one candidate for each of the offices of the Society (President, President-Elect, Secretary, Treasurer) and for the five Members-at-large to serve on the Executive Committee. Having obtained the candidate's consent, they shall report the names to the Society at the annual meeting. The President shall give opportunity for other nominations to be made from the floor, after which all nominations shall be closed.

Section 3   in all cases where more than one person shall be nominated for the same office, votes shall be cast by secret ballot.

Section 4   in case of a tie ballot, the presiding officer shall declare the election for the position void. Additional nominations shall be called for before another vote is taken. If more than two candidates are nominated and there is a tie between two of these candidates, then the candidate with the lesser number of votes shall be dropped and the election performed again.

Article X

Procedures for Election of Membership

Section 1   application for membership in the Society may be made by radiologists with a substantial interest in the practice, teaching or research in skeletal radiology, who are certified by the American Board of Radiology or its foreign equivalent and by MD's, DO's, DVM's or PhD scientists working in related fields.

Section 2   applications must be made, in writing to the Secretary of the Society, and must be accompanied by the curriculum vitae of the applicant and a list of his or her publications in skeletal radiology or related fields. Supporting letters from two active members of the Society should be sent directly to the Secretary.

Section 3   those applications received six (6) months in advance of the annual meeting of the Society will be considered by the Membership Committee, who will make recommendations to the Executive Committee. The names of persons whose recommendations are endorsed by the Executive Committee will be proposed for election as members of the Society by the membership at the annual meeting.

Section 4   a list of approved candidates shall be presented at the annual meeting for approval by the Society. A two-thirds vote of the attending voting active members shall be necessary for election. All those elected shall be members of the Society immediately following the vote.

Article XI

Membership Dues and Fees

Section 1   the dues of this Society shall be due and payable on July 1st. Dues so paid shall cover the fiscal year beginning on that date. Subject to the approval of the membership, the dues shall be set annually by the Executive Committee and shall be consistent with the needs of the Society.

Section 2   the dues shall be delinquent on December 31 of each year and delinquent members shall be notified by that date. Failure to pay the dues shall result in dropping of the delinquent member from the Society unless there are extenuating circumstances.

Article XII

Balloting

Section 1   voting at meetings shall be in the usual manner of other balloting except as otherwise specified in the By-Laws.

Section 2   if the Executive Committee so decides, a mail ballot may be conducted if it seems desirable. Such votes shall have the same effect as those at any meeting.

Article XIII

Amendments

Section 1   these By-Laws may be amended in any annual business meeting of the Society by two-thirds vote of the active members present. Notice of the proposed amendments shall be circulated with the agenda for the meeting at which the vote is to be taken.

Article XIV

Dissolution

Section 1   in the event of the dissolution of the Society, all real assets and remaining monies shall be donated to the American College of Radiology, the Radiological Society of North America, and the American Roentgen Ray Society.

Guidelines for Bestowing of Medals

Article 1

The Founders' Medal is presented in honor of the initiators of the International Skeletal Society and its former Presidents, Harold Jacobson, Ronald O. Murray and Jack Edeiken, that they may be preserved in memory for future generations.

This gold medal honors those who not only distinguished themselves through their outstanding dedication to the International Skeletal Society but, beyond this, have on an international scale, further distinguished themselves by conspicuous excellence in their field of science.

Article 1 A

Two other categories of awards are as follows:

The Medal of the International Skeletal Society
This silver medal may be bestowed on persons who have actively supported the endeavors of the International Skeletal Society. The prospective recipient of this award therefore need not be a member or an honorary member of the International Skeletal Society.

The President's Medal
This bronze medal is intended for members of the International Skeletal Society in special recognition of their outstanding scientific achievements on an international level and who have as yet not completed their 45th year of age. In connection with this award, a monetary grant will be afforded to the awardee to aid his/her research endeavors.

Article 2

The Founder's Medal in Gold to deserving candidates in recognition of their scientific achievements should be conferred to no more than one person each year. The committee, however, is not strictly bound to this time cycle.

The conferral of the Medal of the International Skeletal Society in Silver is not restricted to any particular time cycle.

The President's Medal in Bronze may be conferred on an annual basis. This time span, however, may be greater if no suitable candidate is nominated by the Awards Committee.

The conferral of these medals is made without legal recourse.

Article 3

The members of the Awards committee shall be comprised of current members of the
Executive Committee of the International Skeletal Society.

The selection of a candidate should, if possible, be the result of an unanimous vote.
If unanimous accord is lacking, a two-thirds majority vote resulting from the first
ballot shall determine the outcome. The electoral process shall be strictly confidential.

Article 4

In connection with the honor awarded by the International Skeletal Society, the
recipient of a Medal shall receive a document bearing his name and the reasons for his
selection. This document shall bear the signature of the President of the International
Skeletal Society, together with the date and place of presentation.

The Awards Committee is obliged to compose an appropriate text or to delegate this
to a committee member. The text should be approved by the Executive Committee.

Article 5

The President of the International Skeletal Society shall, during the next meeting of the
International Skeletal Society following the selection, introduce the nominee(s) by
reading the text of the documents and present the medal(s).

The names of the recipient(s) of the Medal(s) shall be published in *Skeletal
Radiology*.

Recipients of ISS Medals

Founders' Medal (Gold)

		ISS Meeting
1989	David C. Dahlin, M.D.	New York
1990	Gwilym S. Lodwick, M.D.	Salzburg
1991	John A. Kirkpatrick Jr., M.D.	San Diego
1992	Mario Campanacci, M.D.	Stockholm
1993	William Martel, M.D.	Toronto
1994	Akbar Bonakdarpour, M.D.	Berlin
1995	Friedrich H.W. Heuck, M.D.	New Orleans
1996	Alex Norman, M.D.	Paris
1997	Andrew Poznanski, M.D.	Santa Fe
1998	Murray K. Dalinka, M.D.	Dublin

Medal of the International Skeletal Society (Silver)

		ISS Meeting
1989	John McGlynn	New York
1990	Heinz Götze, M.D.	Salzburg
1991		San Diego
1992	John K. Davidson, M.D.	Stockholm
1993	Dennis J. Stoker, M.D.	Toronto
1994	Peter G. Bullough, M.D.	Berlin
1995	Theodore E. Keats, M.D.	New Orleans
1996		Paris
1997	Wolfgang Remagen, M.D.	Santa Fe
1998	Louis Gilula, M.D.	Dublin

President's Medal (Bronze)

		ISS Meeting
1989	David J. Sartoris, M.D.	New York
1990	Jean-Denis Laredo, M.D.	Salzburg
1991	Klaus Bohndorf, M.D.	San Diego
1992	Daniel Vanel, M.D.	Stockholm
1993	Phoebe A. Kaplan, M.D.	Toronto
1994	J. Bruce Kneeland, M.D.	Berlin
1995	Marnix T. van Holsbeeck, M.D.	New Orleans
1996	Lynne Steinbach, M.D.	Paris
1997	Mark Murphey, M.D.	Santa Fe

Recipients of Founders' Lectures

In Honor of	Lecturer	ISS Meeting
1981 John Caffey, M.D.	Edward B.D. Neuhauser, M.D.	Madrid
1982 Ronald O. Murray, M.D.	Alexander R. Margulis, M.D.	San Francisco
1983 E. Uehlinger, M.D.	Lauren V. Ackerman, M.D.	Geneva
1984 Howard Middlemiss, M.D.	William P. Cockshott, M.D.	Philadelphia
1985 J.R. Van Ronnen, M.D.	David Dahlin, M.D.	Edinburgh
1986 Ernest Aegerter, M.D.	John A. Kirkpatrick Jr., M.D.	Vancouver
1987 Clement C. Fauré, M.D.	Andrew K. Poznanski, M.D.	Cannes
1988 Hubert A. Sissons, M.D.	Jack Edeiken, M.D.	Sydney
1989 Harold G. Jacobson, M.D.	Murray K. Dalinka, M.D.	New York
1990 Friedrich H.W. Heuck, M.D.	Harry K. Genant, M.D.	Salzburg
1991 Jack Edeiken, M.D.	Michael J. Pitt, M.D.	San Diego
1992 Akbar Bonakdarpour, M.D.	Donald Resnick, M.D.	Stockholm
1993 Howard D. Dorfman, M.D.	Jack P. Lawson, M.D.	Toronto
1994 Prof. Dr. Walter T. Bessler	Amy Beth Goldman, M.D.	Berlin
1995 Robert H. Freiberger, M.D.	Jeremy J. Kaye, M.D.	New Orleans
1996		Paris
1997 Andrew K. Poznanski, M.D.	Ramiro Hernandez, M.D.	Santa Fe
1998 Murray K. Dalinka, M.D.	Morrie E. Kricun, M.D.	Dublin

Founder's Lectures

The First Founders' Lectures was in memory of John Caffey, M.D., by Edward B.D. Neuhauser, M.D.: "The Split Notochord Syndrome and Its Skeletal Manifestations." September 26, 1981, Madrid, Spain.

The Second Founders' Lecture was in honor of Ronald O. Murray, M.D., by Alexander R. Margulis, M.D.: "The Golden Era of Radiology." September 1, 1982, San Francisco, California.

The Third Founders' Lecture was in memory of Professor E. Uehlinger by Lauren V. Ackerman, M.D.: "Environment and Cancer: Experiences in South Africa, Mainland China and Vietnam." October 5, 1983, Geneva, Switzerland.

The Fourth Founders' Lecture was in memory of Sir J. Howard Middlemiss, M.D., by William P. Cockshott, M.D.: "Tropical Disorders Affecting Bone." September 12, 1984, Philadelphia, Pennsylvania.

The Fifth Founders' Lecture was in honor of J.R. Von Ronnen, M.D., by David Dahlin, M.D.: "Newer Entities in the Field of Bone Tumors." October 2, 1985, Edinburgh, Scotland.

The Sixth Founders' Lecture in honor of Ernest E. Aegerter, M.D., by John A. Kirkpatrick, Jr., M.D.: "Metabolic Bone Disease in Neonates and Infants." September 10, 1986, Vancouver, Canada.

The Seventh Founders' Lecture in honor of Prof. Clement Fauré, M.D. by Andrew Poznanski, M.D.: "Radiologic Approach to the Pediatric Hip." September 16, 1987, Cannes, France.

The Eigth Founders' Lecture in honor of Professor Hubert A. Sissons, M.D. by Jack Edeiken, M.D.: "Many Faces of Osteosarcoma and New Treatment Response." September 28, 1988, Sydney, Australia.

The Ninth Founders' Lecture in honor of Harold G. Jacobson, M.D., by Murray K. Dalinka, M.D.: "Modern Techniques of Joint Imaging." September 13, 1989, New York, New York.

The Tenth Founders' Lecture in honor of Friedrich H.W. Heuck, M.D., by Harry K. Genant, M.D.: "Osteoporosis: Advanced Diagnostic Assessment." September 12, 1990, Salzburg, Austria.

The Eleventh Founders' Lecture in honor of Jack Edeiken, M.D., by Michael J. Pitt, M.D.: "Rickets and Osteomalacia." September 25, 1991, San Diego, California.

The Twelfth Founders' Lecture in honor of Akbar Bonakdarpour, M.D. by Donald Resnick, M.D.: "MRI of Articular Abnormalities." August 26, 1992, Stockholm, Sweden.

The Thirteenth Founders' Lecture in honor of Howard Dorfman, M.D. by Jack P. Lawson, M.D.: "Painful Normal Variants of Bone." August 18, 1993, Toronto, Ontario, Canada.

The Fourteenth Founders' Lecture in honor of Walter Bessler, M.D. by Amy Beth
Goldman M.D.: "Skeletal Surface Lesions with an Osteoid-Osseous Matrix." August
17, 1994, Berlin, Germany.
The Fifthteenth Founders' Lecture in honor of Robert Freiberger, M.D. by Jeremy J.
Kaye, M.D.: "Tumors and Tumor-like Conditions in and around Joints." October 18,
1995, New Orleans, Louisiana.
The Sixteenth Founders' Lecture in honor of Andrew K. Poznanski, M.D. by Ramiro
Hernandez, M.D.: "Bone Marrow MRI in Children." September 10, 1997*, Santa Fe,
New Mexico.
The Seventeenth Founders' Lecture in honor of Murray K. Dalinka, M.D. by Morrie E.
Kricun, M.D.: "MR of the Marrow: Age Related Considerations and Responses to
Disease." September 8, 1998, Dublin, Ireland.

---

* No Founders' Lecture was given in 1996.

Past Presidents of the ISS

Harold G. Jacobson, M.D.	1974–76
Ronald O. Murray, M.D.*	1976–78
Hubert A. Sissons, M.D.	1978–80
John A. Kirkpatrick, Jr., M.D.*	1980–82
Jack Edeiken, M.D.	1982–84
Friedrich H.W. Heuck, Dr. med.	1984–86
Howard D. Dorfman, M.D.	1986–88
Akbar Bonakdarpour, M.D.	1988–90
Walter Bessler, M.D.	1990–92
Andrew Poznanski, M.D.	1992–94
Murray K. Dalinka, M.D.	1994–96
Holger Pettersson, M.D.	1996–98

* Deceased.

ISS Meeting Sites

1974	Washington	USA
1975	London	England
1976	Montreal	Canada
1977	Amsterdam	The Netherlands
1978	Boston	USA
1979	Munich	Germany
1980	Mexico City	Mexico
1981	Madrid	Spain
1982	San Francisco	USA
1983	Geneva	Switzerland
1984	Philadelphia	USA
1985	Edinburgh	Scotland
1986	Vancouver	Canada
1987	Cannes	France
1988	Sydney	Australia
1989	New York	USA
1990	Salzburg	Austria
1991	San Diego	USA
1992	Stockholm	Sweden
1993	Toronto	Canada
1994	Berlin	Germany
1995	New Orleans	USA
1996	Paris	France
1997	Santa Fe	USA
1998	Dublin	Ireland
1999	Seattle	USA
2000	Barcelona	Spain

Membership by Specialities*

Radiologists	268
Pathologists	73
Orthopaedic Surgeons	52
Rheumatologists	6
Plastic Surgeon	1
Physician	1
Oncologist	1
Pediatrician	1
Not Known	21
Other	3
Total number of active members (not including honorary members)	427
Honorary members	20

* As of October 1997.

Membership by Countries*

Argentina	2	Italy	9
Australia	7	Japan	22
Austria	4	Korea	5
Belgium	3	Netherlands	4
Brazil	1	Norway	1
Canada	12	Oman	1
Chile	1	Poland	1
China	7	Slovenia	1
Czech Republic	4	South Africa	1
Denmark	2	Spain	5
Finland	3	Sweden	15
France	15	Switzerland	9
Germany	20	Turkey	1
Hungary	2	United Kingdom	26
India	1	United States	238
Israel	3	Yugoslavia	1

* As of October, 1997 and not including Honorary Members.

List of Members

ABDELWAHAB, IBRAHIM FIKRY M.D.

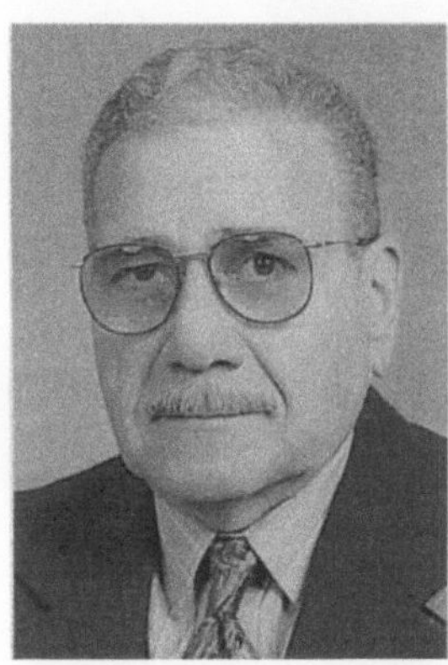

Academic Title: Adjunct Clinical
Professor of Radiology

Position at Affiliation: Musculoskeletal
Radiologist

Business Address:
New York Medical College
Department of Radiology
Valhalla, NY 10595
U.S.A.
212-241-4007 (work)
212-427-8137 (fax)

Home Address:
70-25 Yellowstone Boulevard
Apartment 24D
Forest Hills, NY 11375
U.S.A.
718-261-3526 (home)

Specialty/Certification: Radiology, 1975

Education:
1954 – Alexandria School of Medicine,
Alexandria Univ. Alexandria, Egypt
(MB, B.CH)
1954–1955 – Alexandria University
Hospitals (internship) Alexandria, Egypt
1955–1957 – Alexandria School of
Medicine (residency) Alexandria, Egypt
1974–1975 – Mount Sinai Hospital
(fellowship) New York, NY

ISS Member 1989

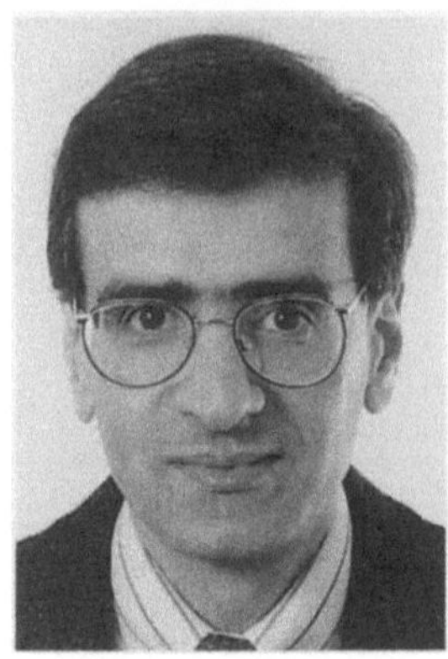

Academic Title: Associate Professor

Position at Affiliation: Director, Anatomic Pathology

Business Address:
University Hospitals of Cleveland/Case Western
Reserve University
Institute of Pathology
2085 Adelbert Road
Cleveland, OH 44122
U.S.A.
216-844-1807 (work)
216-844-1810 (fax)

Home Address:
21300 W. Byron Road
Shaker Heights, OH 44106
U.S.A.
216-561-3233 (home)

Specialty: Cytology

Education:
1972–79 – American College of Beirut, Lebanon (MD)
1979–83 – Anatomic Path,
CWRU Institute of Pathology, Cleveland OH (residency)
1983–84 – Pathology, Univ. Texas System Cancer Center
M.D. Anderson Hospital and Tumor Inst., Houston, TX (fellowship)

ISS Member 1995

Spouse: Randa

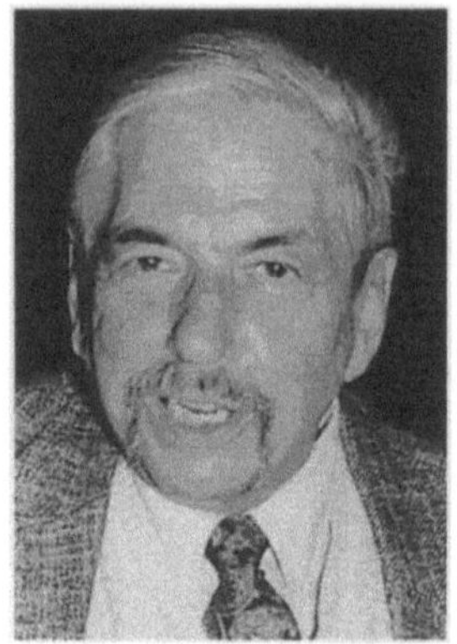

Birthdate: March 24, 1916

Academic Title: Clinical Professor Emeritus

Position at Affiliation: Stanford University Hospital Staff; Fairmont Contract Radiologist

Business Address:
Stanford University Medical School
Stanford, CA
U.S.A.
Fairmont County Hospital
U.S.A.
510-667-3226 (work)
510-483-7325 (fax)

Home Address:
21635 Knoll Way
Castro Valley, CA 94546-6851
U.S.A.
510-357-3289 (home)

Specialty/Certification: Radiology, 1948

Education:
1936 – University of Pennsylvania (college)
1940 – University of Pennsylvania (M.D.)
1942 – City Hospital, New York (residency)

ISS Member 1980

Spouse: Anne S.

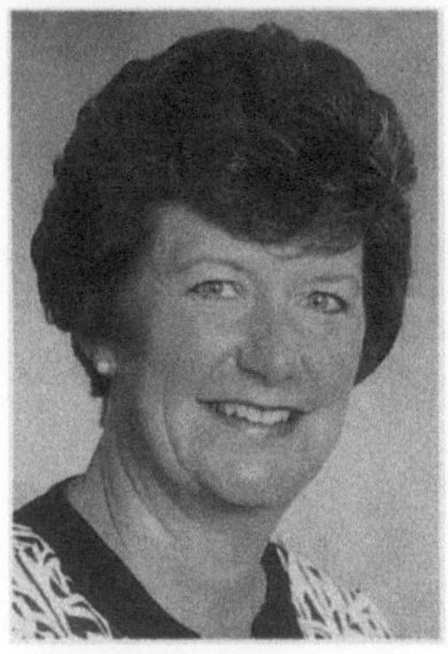

Birthdate: May 16, 1945

Academic Title: Professor

Position at Affiliation: Head of Department

Business Address:
University of Manchester
Department of Diagnostic Radiology
Stopford Building
Oxford Road
Manchester M13 9PT
England
44-161-275-5114 (work)
44-161-275-5594 (fax)

Home Address:
Fairholm Hawley Lane, Hale Barns
Altrincham, Cheshire, WA15 ODR
England
44-161-904-0234 (home)
44-161-904-0234 (fax)

Specialty/Certification: Radiology
1968; 1975; 1988

Education:
Graduate of University of London
University College Hospital
Radiology training – Manchester

ISS Member 1986

ISS Committees:
Corinne Farrell Prize Committee, Member 1991 to date, Chairman, 1993 – 95

Spouse: Prof. Peter H. Adams

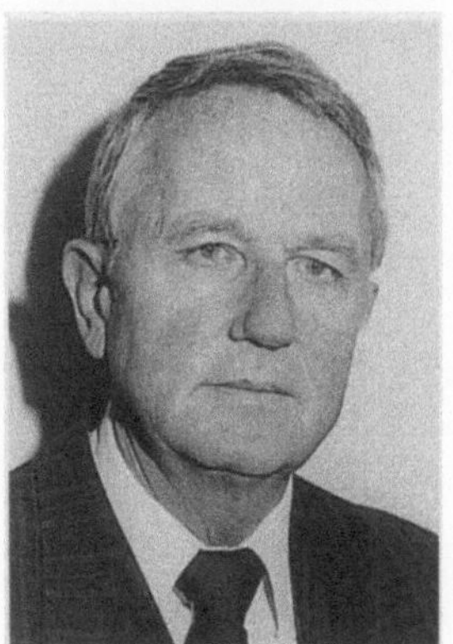

Birthdate: December 13, 1937

Academic Title: Professor Dr. Med. M.D.

Position at Affiliation: Head of the Reference Center of Bone Diseases

Business Address:
Institute of Pathology
(Ludwig-Aschoff-Haus)
University of Freiburg i. Br.
Alberstrasse 19
Germany
40-761-203-6741 (work)
40-761-203-6790 (fax)

Home Address:
Scheffelstr. 24
D-79194 Gundelfingen
Germany
40-761-58 18 89 (home)

Specialty: Pathology

ISS Member 1977

ISS Committees:
Nomenclature Committee
Membership Committee

Spouse: Dr. Maria Adler

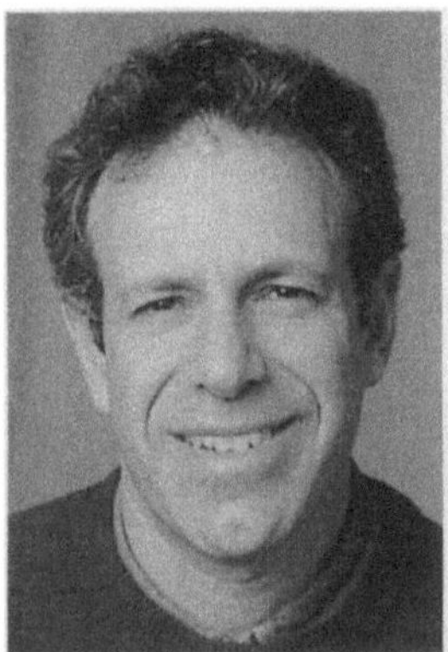

Birthdate: November 11, 1950

Academic Title: Associate Professor

Position at Affiliation: Director, Musculoskeletal Division

Business Address:
University of Michigan
Department of Radiology, 810502
1500 East Medical Center Drive
Ann Arbor, MI 4810
U.S.A.
313-936-8864 (work)
313-936-7948 (fax)
ronaldler@umich.edu (e-mail)

Home Address:
3440 Vintage Valley
Ann Arbor, MI 4810
U.S.A.
313-996-2611 (home)

Specialty: Radiology

Education:
1973 – CCNY (B.S. Physics)
1977 – University of Michigan (Ph.D., Nuclear engineering)
1984 – Wayne State University (M.D.)

ISS Member: 1996

Spouse: Judith

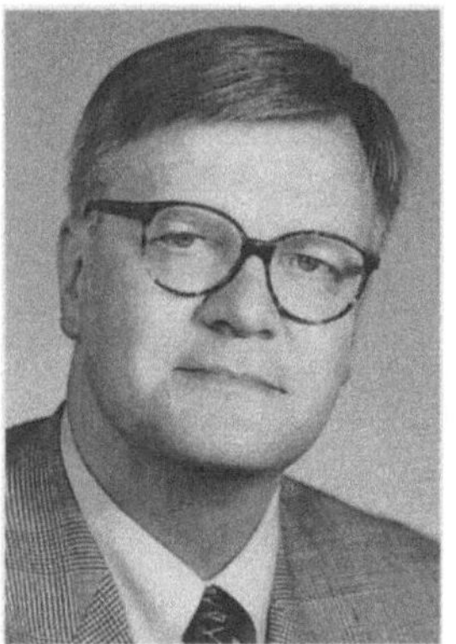

Position at Affiliation: Chief Radiologist

Business Address:
Division of Radiology
Military Central Hospital
Mannerheimintie 164
FIN-00300 Helsinki
Finland
358-09-16-15-611 (work)
358-09-16-15-792 (fax)

Home Address:
Rentukkatie 6 B1
FIN-01350 Vantaa
Finland
358-09-837-316 (home)

Specialty: Radiology

Education:
1976 – University of Helsinki (MD)
1982 – University of Helsinki (Specialist in Radiology)
1985 – University of Helsinki (Ph.D)

ISS Member 1989

Spouse: Marjut Raiskio

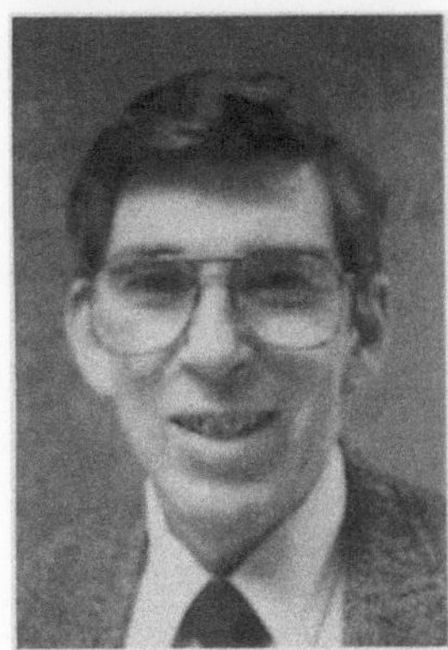

Business Address:
Diagnostic Radiology Department
22 South Greene Street
Baltimore, MD 21201-1595
U.S.A.
301-328-3477 (work)
301-328-8783 (fax)
301-294-2210 (home)

Specialty: Radiology

ISS Member 1972

Spouse: Joyce

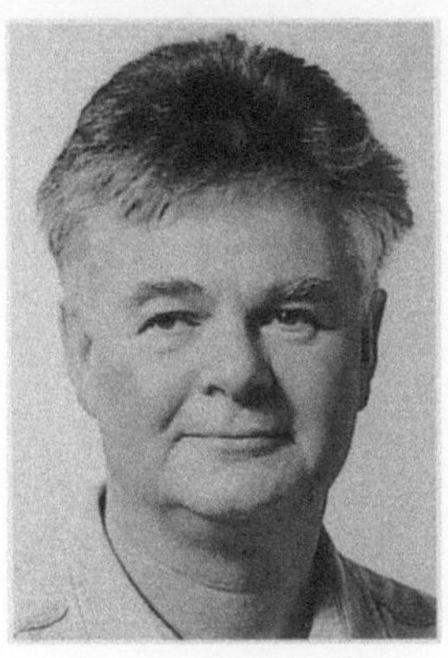

Birthdate: May 19, 1940

Academic Title: Professor

Position at Affiliation: Head of Staff

Business Address:
Regionsykemuset Trondheim
N-7006 Trondheim
Norway
73-998772 (work)
73-997855 (fax)

Home Address:
Åsvangvn. 28, N-7048
Tronoheim
Norway
73-940743 (home)

Specialty/Certification: Radiology, 1979

Education:
1966 – Oslo University (MD)
1969 – Trondheim (Radiology)
1970–72 – Orthopedic surgery
1973–96 – Radiology residency
1991 – Ph.D.

ISS Member 1994

Spouse: May Brith

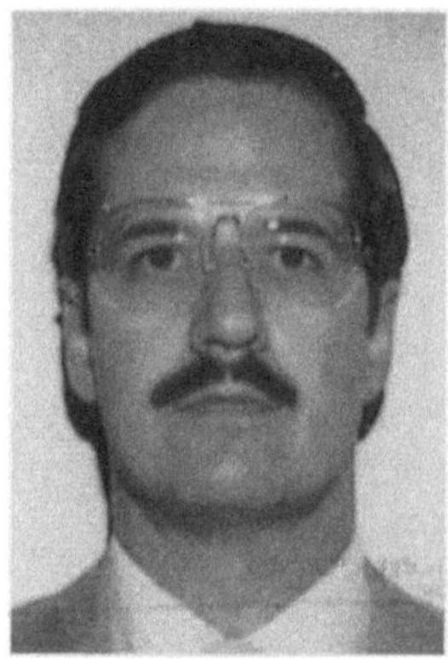

Academic Title: Clinical Associate Professor (University of Chicago)

Position at Affiliation: Chair, Radiology Department

Business Address:
Mercy Hosp. & Med. Center
Stevenson Exp. at King Drive
Chicago, IL 60616
U.S.A.
312-567-2712 (work)
312-567-2616 (fax)

Home Address:
5807 S. Harpe Avenue
Chicago, IL 60637-1842
U.S.A.
312-643-1312 (home)

Specialty/Certification: Radiology, 1974; Nuclear Medicine, 1975

Education:
1966 – Princeton Univ., Princeton, NJ (AB)
1970 – Harvard Medical School, Boston, MA (MD)
1970–74 – University Chicago Hospitals (Diagnostic Radiology)
1974–75 – University Chicago Hospitals (Nuclear Medicine)

ISS Member 1983

Spouse: Gretchen

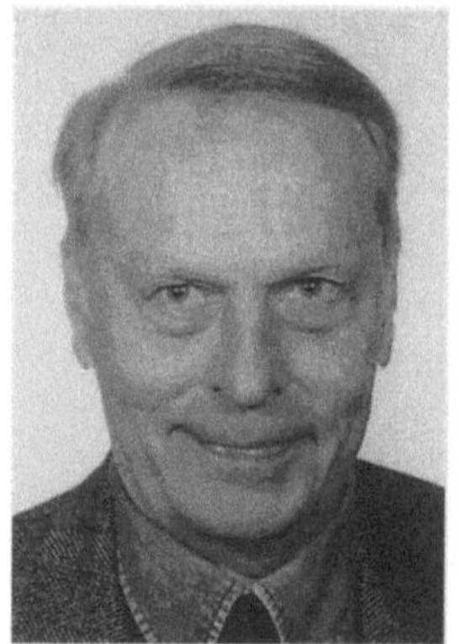

Birthdate: September 17, 1926

Academic Title: Professor

Position at Affiliation: Professor Emeritus

Business Address:
Department of Pathology
Sahlgren University Hospital
S-413 45 Göteborg
Sweden
31/60 19 78 (work)
31/82 71 94 (fax)

Home Address:
Västerbergsgatan 6
431 69 Möldal
Sweden
31/82 92 02 (home)

Specialty: Pathology

Education:
1954 – M.D.
1959 – Ph.D.

ISS Member 1981

ISS Committees:
Membership Committee

Spouse: Anne-Marie

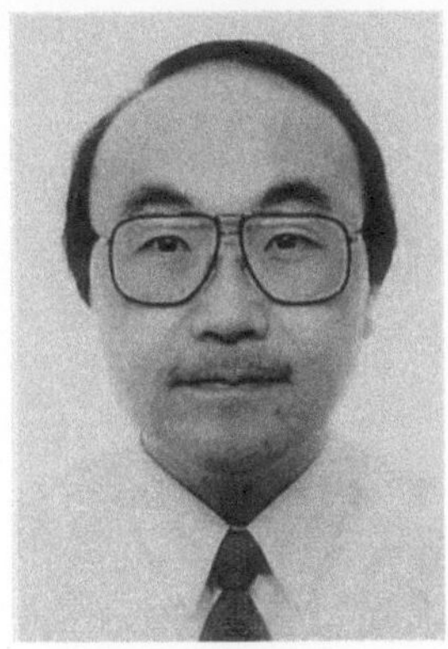

Birthdate: March 15, 1954

Academic Title: Associate Professor

Business Address:
Diagnostic Radiology
Gunma University Hospital
3-39-22 Showa-Machi
Maebashi 371
Japan
81-27-220-8610 (work)
81-27-220-8409 (fax)
junaoki@sb.gunma-u.ac.jp (e-mail)

Home Address:
301-1 Sekine-Machi
Maebashi 371
Japan
81-27-232-5344 (home and fax)

Specialty: Radiology

Education:
1979 – Kyoto University School of Medicine (M.D.)
1987 – Kyoto University (Ph.D.)
1987 – 89 – Armed Forces Institute of Pathology-Radiologic Pathology (fellow)

ISS Member 1994

Spouse: Hiroko

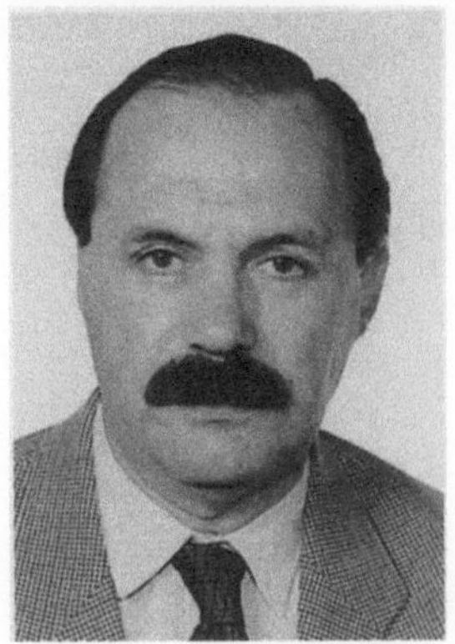

Birthdate: February 22, 1950

Position at Affiliation: Chief of Section

Business Address:
c./Callosa de Ensarriá 12
46007 Valencia
Spain
96 380 70 00 (work)
96 380 72 08 (fax)

Home Address:
c/o Dr. Sanchis Sivera N° 18
46008 – Valencia
Spain
3849053 (home)

Specialty/Certification: Radiology, 1977

Education:
Facultad de Medicina Valencia
Hospital La Fe

ISS Member 1992

Spouse: Maria Pilar

ARKUN, EMINE REMIDE M.D.

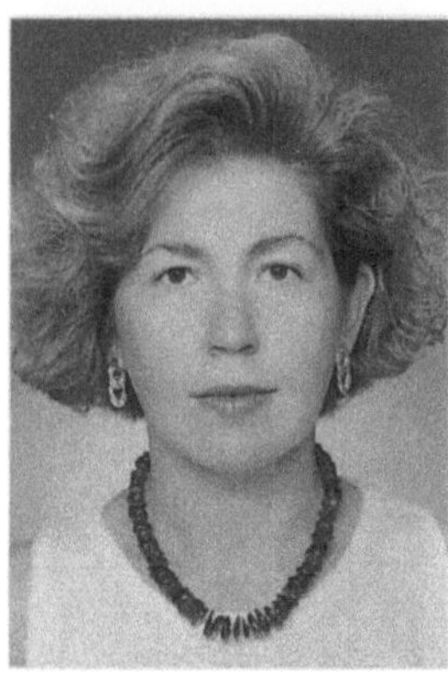

Birthdate: July 8, 1956

Academic Title: Professor

Position at Affiliation: Attending Radiologist

Business Address:
Ege University
School of Medicine
Department of Radiology
Bornova 35100
Izmir
Turkey
90-232-388-13-90 (work)
90-232-342-00-01 (fax)

Home Address:
111 Sokak 11/6 Göztepe
35290 Izmir
Turkey
90-232-285-82-43 (home)

Specialty/Certification: Radiology, 1985

Education:
1979 – Ege University (M.D.)
1985 – Ege University (Radiology)

ISS Member 1995

ATHANASOU, NICHOLAS A. PH.D., MBBS, MRCP, FRC (PATH)

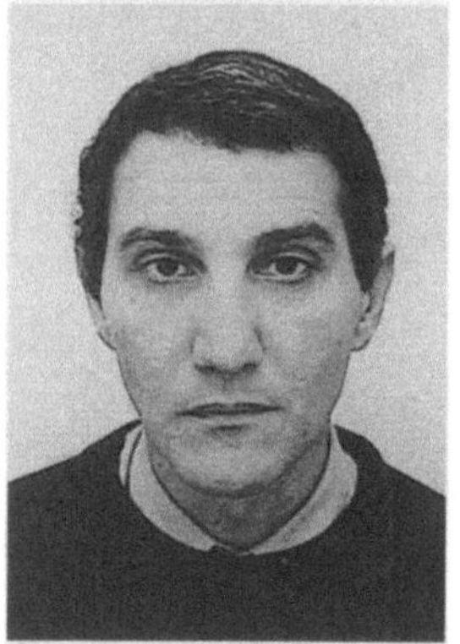

Birthdate: April 26, 1953

Academic Title: Dr.

Position at Affiliation: Consultant Pathologist; Reader in Orthopaedic Pathology, University of Oxford

Business Address:
Nuffield Orthopaedic Centre
Department of Pathology
Oxford, OX3 7LD
United Kingdom
1865 227619 (work)
1865 742348 (fax)

Home Address:
Greystones
Charlton NR Banbury O17 3DR
United Kingdom
1295 811347 (home)

Specialty: Pathology

Education:
Sydney University – MB; BS
St. Bartholomew's Medical College, University of London (Ph.D.)

ISS Member: 1990

Spouse: Linda Hulls

AYALA, ALBERTO G. M.D.

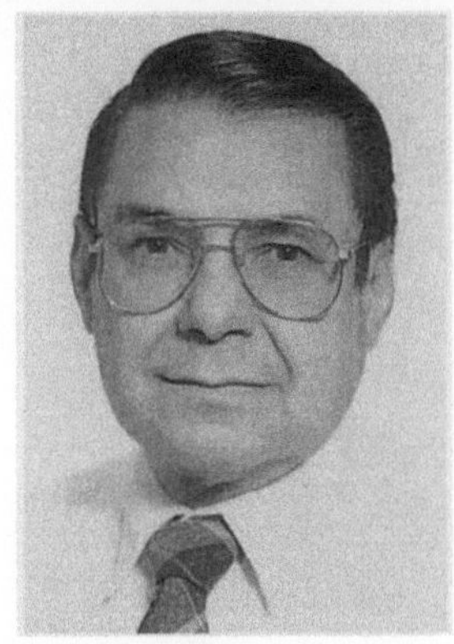

Birthdate: March 24, 1937

Academic Title: Professor of Pathology

Position at Affiliation: Division Chairman, Department of Pathology (ad-interim)

Business Address:
UTMDACC-Pathology-Box 85
1515 Holcombe Boulevard
Houston, TX 77030
U.S.A.
713-792-3151 (work)
713-794-1695 (fax)
alberto_ayala@path.mdacc.tme.edu
(e-mail)

Home Address:
9406 Albury
Houston, TX 77096
U.S.A.
713-771-1747 (home)

Specialty/Certification: Anatomic Pathology, 1980 recertified 1997

Education:
1954–1960 – Univ. of Nuevo Leon
(Medical School); Faculty of Medicine
1960–61 – St. Joseph's Hospital,
St. Joseph, MO (internship)
1962 – Medical School,
Final Examination
1963–67 – Univ. of Texas Medical
Branch, Galveston, TX (residency)
1967 – M.D. Anderson Cancer Center
(Pathology fellowship)

ISS Member 1985

ISS Committees:
Consulting Editorial Board of Skeletal
Radiology

Spouse: Mary

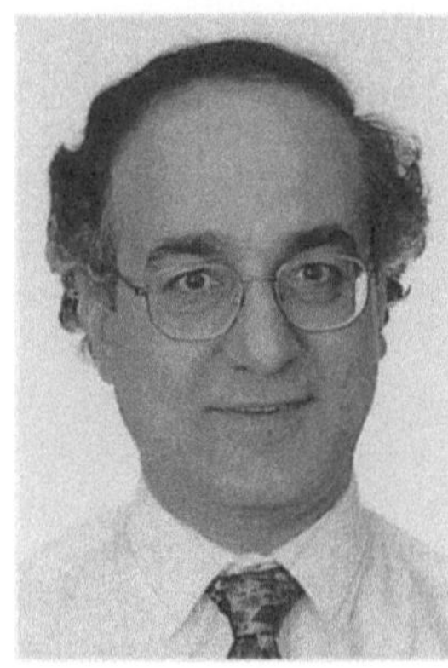

Academic Title: Professor of Radiology

Position at Affiliation: Assistant Director

Business Address:
Montreal Children's Hospital
2300 Tupper Street
Montreal, Quebec H3H 1P3
Canada
514-934-4450 (work)
514-934-4347 (fax)
mazomi @ mch.mcgill.ca (e-mail)

Home Address:
6899 Schweitzer Road
Cote St. Luc
P. Quebec H4W IL2
Canada
514-488-2488 (home)

Specialty/Certification: Radiology, 1974

Education:
1962–68 – Faculty of Medicine,
Alexandria Univ., Egypt
1970–72 – Sherbrooke Univ., P.Q.
Canada, (Diagnostic Radiology)
1972–74 – McGill University, Montreal,
P.Q., Canada (Diagnostic Radiology)

ISS Member 1989

Spouse: Nicole

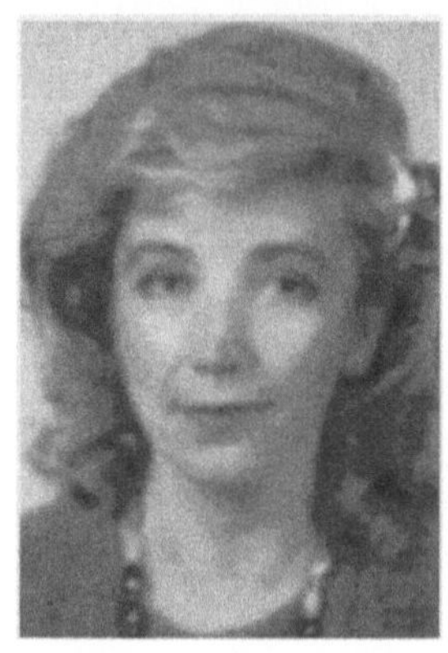

Business Address:
USL 28 Ospedale M. Malpighi
Servizio di Anatomia Ed
Isotologia Patologia
Via Albertoni 15
40138 Bologna
Italy

ISS Member 1988

BAHK, YONG-WHEE M.D., PH.D.

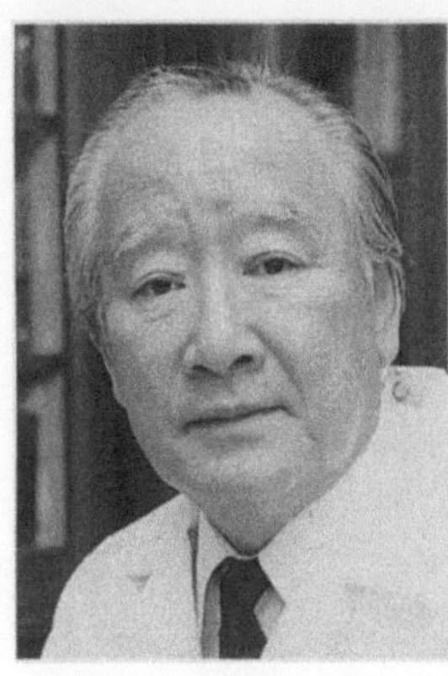

Academic Title: Professor Emeritus (CUMC)

Position at Affiliation: Advisor

Business Address:
Samsung Cheil General Hospital
Mookjong Dong
Seoul
Korea
82-2-262-7369 (work)
82-2-277-8598 (fax)

Home Address:
201-24 Dong-Gyo-Dong, Mapo-Ku
Seoul 121-200
Korea
82-2-337-0839 (home)

Specialty: Radiology

Education:
Chonnam National University Medical School (M.D.)
Catholic University Graduate School (Ph.D.)
1959 – 60 – Boston City Hospital (Radiology residency)

ISS Member 1992

Spouse: Yeon-Soo Cho

BANZER, DIETRICH H. M.D.

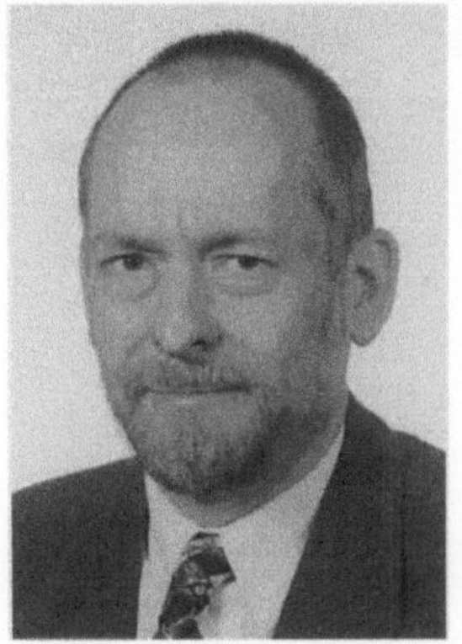

Academic Title: Docent of Radiology

Position at Affiliation: Head of Radiology Department

Business Address:
Behring Municipal Hospital
Teaching Hospital, Free University Berlin
Radiology Department
Gimpelsteig 3-5, D-14165 Berlin
Germany
49-30-8102-1319 (work)
49-30-8102-1741 (fax)
banzer@berlin.snafu.de (e-mail)

Home Address:
Heerstrasse 75
D-14055 Berlin
Germany
49-30-305-3897 (home)
49-30-30810125 (fax)

Specialty/Certification: Radiology, 1973

Education:
Free University Berlin, Medical School
Medical High School Hannover
Hosp. University California Davis
Hosp. University of Pennsylvania, Philadelphia, PA

ISS Member 1990

ISS Committees:
Co-Chairman ISS course in Berlin, 1994

Spouse: Lieselotte

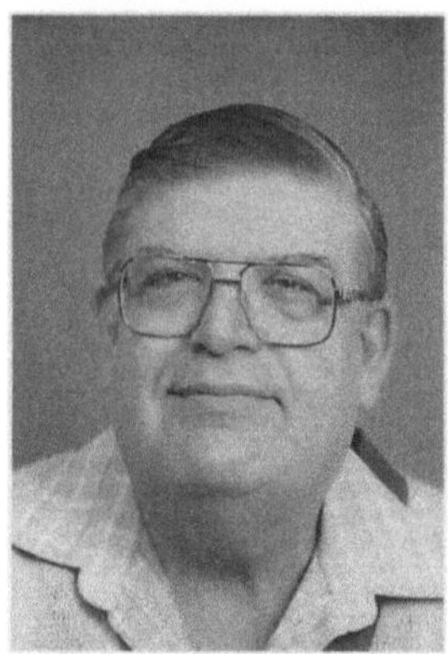

Academic Title: Professor of Radiology

Position at Affiliation: Chairman, Department of Radiology

Business Address:
Hadassah University Hospital
Ein Kerem
POB 12000
Jerusalem,
Israel 91120
972-2-776901 (work)
972-2-437531 (fax)

Home Address:
2 Akiva Street Raanana
Israel 43262
972-9-915422 (home)
972-9-422961 (fax)

Specialty/Certification: Radiology, 1970

Education:
1962 – Hadassah & Hebrew University (M.D.)
1965 – 70 –·Soroka Med. Center, Beer Sheva (Radiology training)
1973 – 75 – Montreal Children's Hosp. McGill (fellowship in Pediatric Rad.)

ISS Member 1995

Spouse: Gila

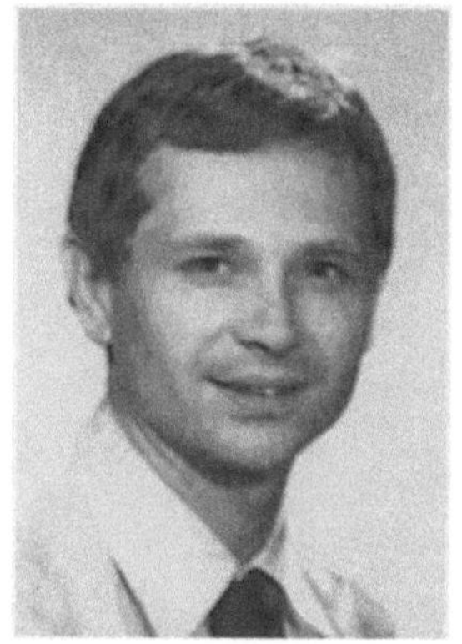

Business Address:
U.C.L.A. School of Medicine
Department of Radiological Sciences
10833 Le Conte Avenue
Los Angeles, CA 90024-1721
U.S.A.
310-650-5985 (home)
310-206-9608 (work)
310-825-3205 or 310-794-1428 (fax)

Specialty: Radiology

ISS Member 1983

Birthdate: October 5, 1950

Position at Affiliation: Staff, Departments of Anatomic Pathology and Orthopaedic Surgery

Business Address:
Department of Anatomic Pathology L25
Cleveland Clinic Foundation
500 Euclid Avenue
Cleveland, OH 44195-5138
U.S.A.
216-444-6830 (work)
216-445-6967 (fax)
osteoclast@aol.com (e-mail)

Home Address:
3158 Falmouth Road
Shaker Heights, OH 44142
U.S.A.
216-991-0632 (home)

Specialty: Anatomic and Clinical Pathology

Education:
University of Colorado – (Organismic Biology)
University of Nebraska – (Graduate College) (Ph.D.)
University of Nebraska College of Medicine – (M.D.)
John Hopkins – (internship-residency in Anatomic & Clinical Pathology)

ISS Member 1991

Spouse: Paula

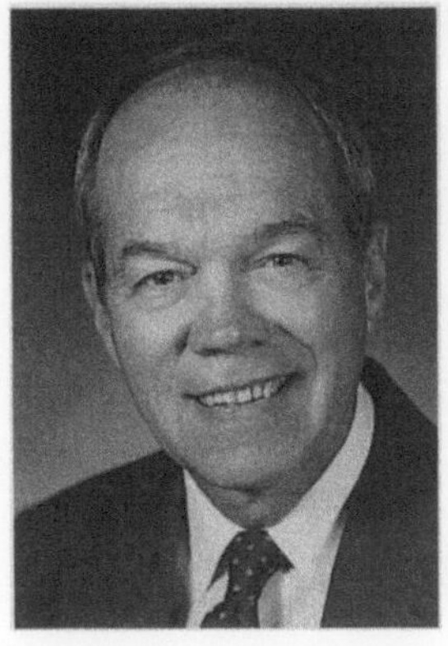

Birthdate: March 30, 1932

Academic Title: Professor of Radiology

Position at Affiliation: Consultant

Business Address:
Mayo Clinic
200 First Street S.W.
Rochester, MN 55905
U.S.A.
507-284-3632 (work)
507-284-9245 (fax)

Home Address:
1406 30th Street, S.W.
Rochester, MN 55902
U.S.A.
507-288-4779 (home)

Specialty: Radiology

Education:
1950–54 – Depauw University in Greencastle, IN (college)
1954–58 – Northwestern University, Chicago, IL (medical school)
1962–65 – Mayo Graduate School, Rochester, MN (residency)

ISS Member 1973

Spouse: Jeanne

BEAUREGARD, C. GERMAIN M.D.

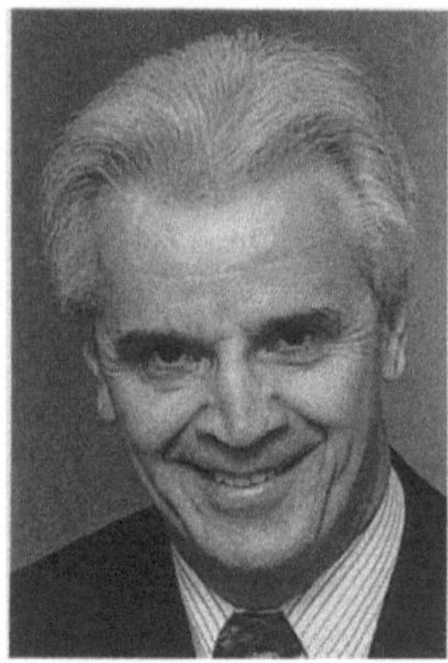

Birthdate: February 22, 1937

Academic Title: Assistant Professor

Position at Affiliation: Staff Radiologist

Business Address:
Radiologie Laënnec Inc.
1100, Avenue Beaumont
bureau 104
Ville Mont-Royal, Québec, H3P 3H5
Canada
514-738-7877 (work)
514-738-4659 (fax)

Home Address:
241, Le Baron
Boucherville
Québec J4B 2E3
Canada
514-655-2976 (home)

Specialty: Radiology

Education:
Universite de Montreal
AFIP, Washington, DC
UCSD, San Diego, CA
Hopital Cochin, Paris, France

ISS Member Founding member

ISS Committees:
Scientific Committee, 1992-93
Nomenclature Committee, 1994
Future Meeting Committee, 1991-92
Editorial Board, Skeletal Radiology –
1995

Spouse: Evelyn

BECKER, MELVIN H. M.D.

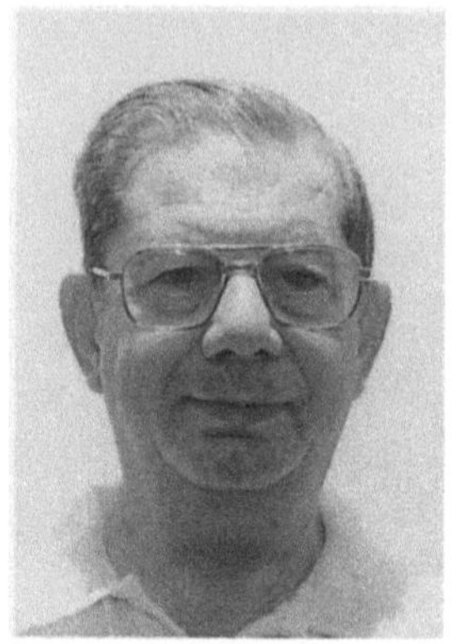

Birthdate: August 27, 1924

Academic Title: Professor of Radiology

Position at Affiliation: Professor and
Attending Radiologist

Business Address:
New York University Medical Center
550 First Avenue
New York, NY 10016, U.S.A.
212-263-6469 and 212-238-7514 (work)

Home Address:
160 Chestnut Road
Manhasset, NY 11030, U.S.A.
516-627-1685 (home)

Specialty/Certification: Radiology, 1954

Education:
1944 – Washington University, St. Louis,
MO (B.A.)
1948 – Univ. of Missouri Medical School
(B.S. in Medicine)
1950 – Washington University School of
Medicine, St.Louis, MO (M.D.)
1950–51 – Medical College of Alabama
(internship)
1951–54 – University of Michigan
(residency in Radiology)

ISS Member Founding member

ISS Committees:
Auditing Committee
Program Committee when meeting in
New York
Liason Committee – 1996
Grants Committee – 1996 –

Spouse: Rhoda

BEGGS, IAN MB, CHB, FRCR

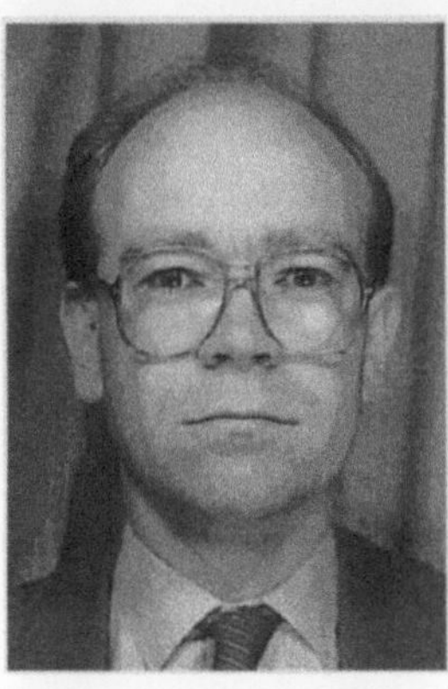

Academic Title: Dr.

Position at Affiliation: Consultant Radiologist

Business Address:
Royal Infirmary, Lauriston Place
Department of Clinical Radiology
Edinburgh EH3 9YW
United Kingdom
44 131 536 4713 (work)
44 131 536 4640 (fax)

Home Address:
35 Morton Hall Road
Edinburgh EH9 2HN
United Kingdom
44 131 668 3135 (home)

Specialty/Certification: Radiology, 1979

Education:
University of Glasgow
University of Edinburgh

ISS Member: 1996

Spouse: Jean

BEIGHTON, PETER H. M.D., PH.D., FRCP, DCH

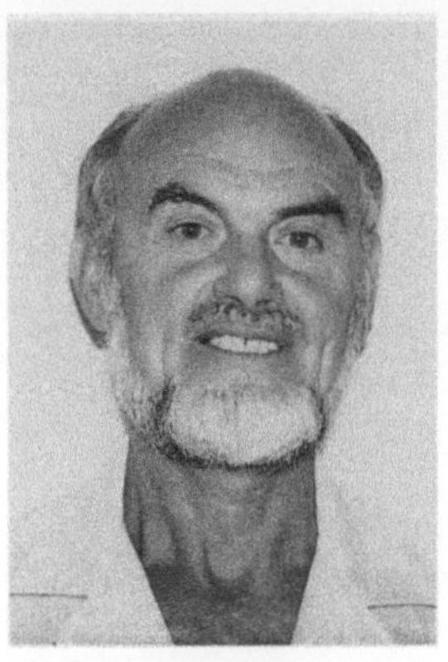

Academic Title: Professor

Position at Affiliation: Department Head

Business Address:
Department of Human Genetics, Medical School,
Observatory, Cape Town 7925
South Africa
021-47-406-6297 (work)
021-47703 (fax)
pb@anat.uct.ac.za (e-mail)

Home Address:
16 Garton Road
Rundebosch
Cape Town 7700
South Africa
021-689-8087 (home)

Specialty/Certification: Genetics, 1957

Education:
1957 – St. Mary's Hospital, University of London
1962–68 – St. Thomas Hospital (M.D.)
1968–69 – Johns Hopkins, Baltimore, MD (Research fellowship in genetics)

ISS Member 1980

Spouse: Greta

BELTRAN, JAVIER M.D.

Birthdate: July 1, 1946

Academic Title: Professor of Radiology

Position at Affiliation: Chairman,
Radiology Department

Business Address:
Hospital for Joint Diseases
Department of Radiology
305 East 17th Street
New York, NY 10003
U.S.A.
212-598-5374 (work)
212-598-6125 (fax)
jbeltran46@msn.com (e-mail)

Home Address:
25 E. 9th Street
New York, NY 10003
U.S.A.
212-533-5432 (home)

Specialty/Certification: Radiology, 1976

Education:
University of Barcelona (M.D.)
Ohio State University

ISS Member 1989

ISS Committees:
Closed Meeting Committee, 1995, 1996
Co-Chairman Closed Meeting, 1997

Spouse: Andrea

BELUFFI, GIAMPIERO E.V. M.D.

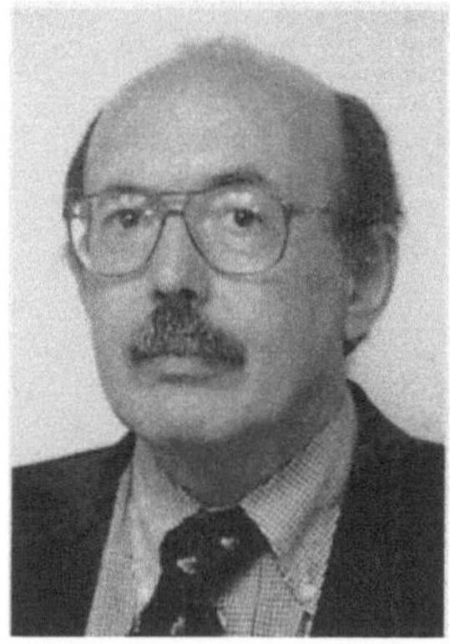

Birthdate: April 28, 1960

Academic Title: Professore a Contratto

Position at Affiliation: Staff Radiologist

Business Address:
Servizio Radiodiagnostica
Modulo Operativo Radiologia Pediatrica
IRCCS Policlinico S. Matteo
Piazzale Golgi, 2
I-27100 Pavia PV
Italy
39-382-502838 (work)
39-382-528597 (fax)

Home Address:
via G. Franchi Maggi, 5
I-27100 Pavia PV
Italy
39-382-23764 (home)

Specialty/Certification: Radiology, 1968

Education:
1966 – University of Pavia Medical
School (M.D.)
1968 – University of Pavia Radiology
Specialization School

ISS Member 1988

Spouse: Margherita

Business Address:
Babies Hospital
Columbia University Medical Center
3959 Broadway
New York, NY 10032
U.S.A.

Specialty: Radiology

ISS Member 1984

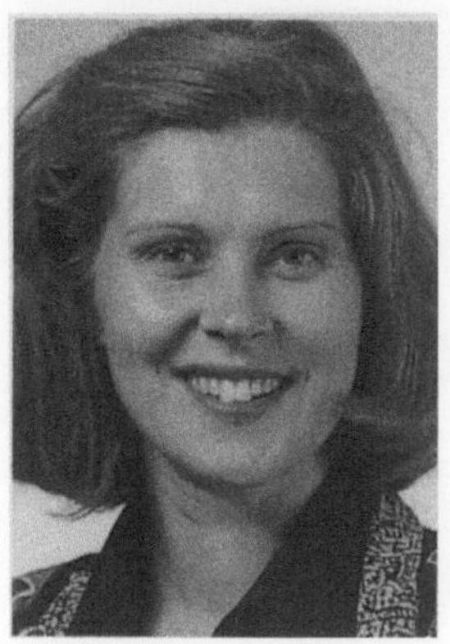

Birthdate: August 18, 1953

Academic Title: Assistant Professor

Position at Affiliation: Chief, Musculo-skeletal Radiology Section

Business Address:
Department of Radiology
Stanford University Medical Center
300 Pasteur Drive
Stanford, CA 94305-5105
U.S.A.
415-725-8018 (work)
415-725-7296 (fax)
gabrielle.bergman@forsythe.stanford.edu (e-mail)

Home Address:
940 Cottrell Way
Stanford, CA 94305-1012
U.S.A.
415-493-2357 (home)

Specialty/Certification: Radiology (USA), 1985; Radiology (Sweden), 1989

Education:
University of Lund, Sweden (M.D.)
University of Lund, Sweden (internship)
New York University, New York, NY (internship)
1984–85 – New York University, New York, NY (fellowship)
1985–87 – University of California San Diego, San Diego, CA (fellowship)

ISS Member 1990

Spouse: Mattias

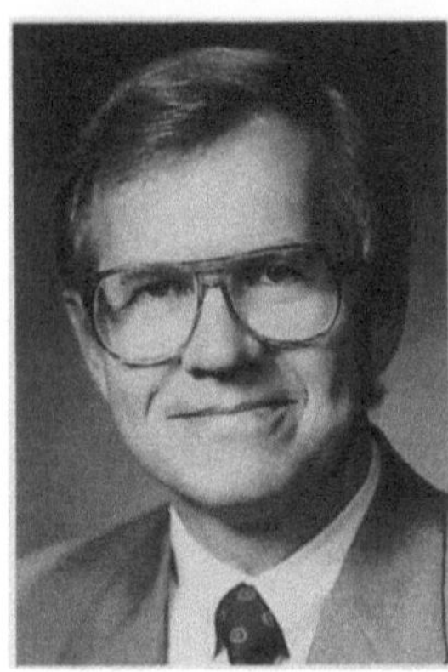

Birthdate: September 10, 1945

Academic Title: Professor of Diagnostic Radiology

Position at Affiliation: Chair, Department of Diagnostic Radiology

Business Address:
Department of Radiology
Mayo Clinic
4500 San Pablo Road
Jacksonville, FL 32224
U.S.A.
904-953-2149 (work)
904-953-2883 (fax)
berquist.thomas@mayo.edu (e-mail)

Home Address:
2312 Clubview Court
Ponte Vedra Beach, FL 32082
U.S.A.
904-285-1069 (home)

Specialty/Certification: Radiology, 1975

Education:
1971 – Washington University School
of Medicine, St. Louis, MO (M.D.)
1971–72 – Mayo Graduate School,
Rochester, MN (internship)
1972–75 – Mayo Graduate School,
Rochester, MN (Radiology residency)

ISS Member 1984

Spouse: Kay

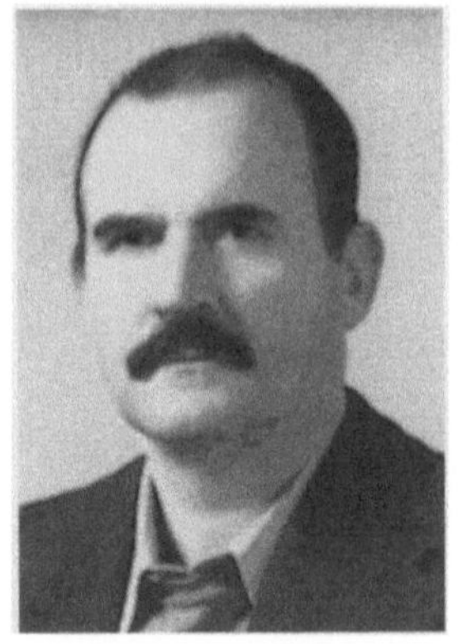

Business Address:
Ospedale Provinciale Specializzato
M. Malpighi Hospital
Isologia Patologica
Via Albertoni 15
40128 Bologna
Italy

ISS Member 1981

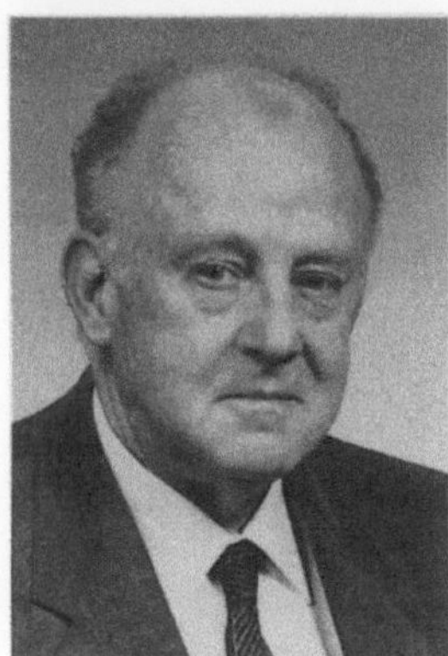

Academic Title: Professor Dr. Med.

Position at Affiliation: Consultant Radiologist

Business Address:
Retired
Former Chief of the Department of Radiology
Kantonsspital Winterthur
Department of Radiology
University of Zürich
Switzerland

Home Address:
Rosentalstrasse 81
CH-8400 Wintherthur
Switzerland
41 52 2134722 (home)
41 52 2134722 (fax)
41 12-78-2755 (fax) (c/o Dr. Heidi Bessler)

Specialty/Certification: Radiology, 1955; Nuclear Medicine, 1956

Education:
1950–55 – University of Zürich, Dept. of Radiology, Univ. Hosp. Zürich
Gymnasium Zürich
Universities Zürich and Lausanne

ISS Member 1977

Offices Held in ISS and Dates of Service:
President, 1991–92

ISS Medals and Awards:
Founders Lecture, Berlin, 1994

ISS Committees:
Executive Committee 1985–86, 1988–95
Trustee Endowment Fund 1988–96, Chairman 1992–95
Member of 12 other committees since 1982

Spouse: Dr. Heidi Bessler

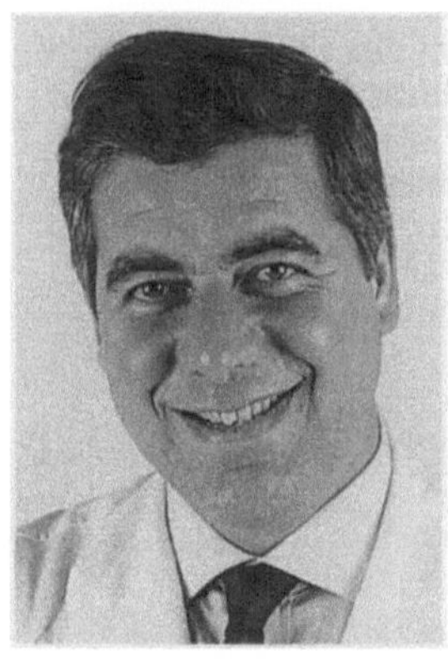

Birthdate: January 31, 1958

Academic Title: Assistant Professor

Position at Affiliation: Chief, Musculo-skeletal Section

Business Address:
E.O. Ospedale Galliera
Dpt. of Radiology
Via Volta 4
16100 Genova
Italy
39-10-5632375 (work)
39-10-5632669 (fax)

Home Address:
Corso Paganini 1/5
16125 Genova
Italy
39-10-2471134 (home)
39-10-2467479 (fax)
bianchi@tn.village.it (e-mail)

Specialty/Certification: Rheumatology, 1986; Radiology, 1990

Education:
1982 – University of Genoa – School of Medicine

ISS Member 1995

Spouse: Maria Pia Zamorani

Business Address:
Benvenutolaan 3
2253 AH Voorschoten
The Netherlands
17-177924 (home)
71-262993 (work)
71-142508 (fax)

ISS Member 1989

Spouse: Els

BLOOM, RONALD A. M.D.

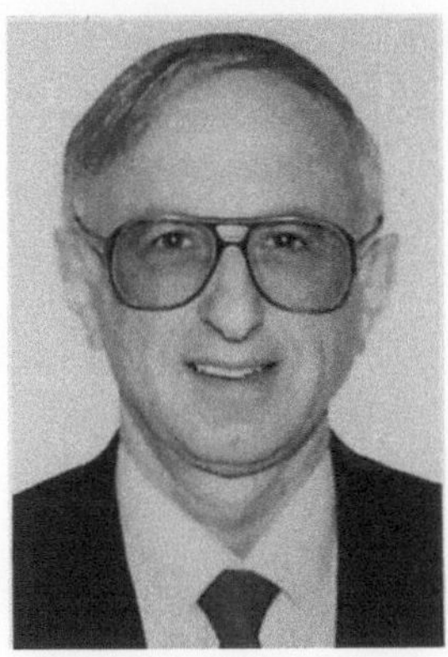

Birthdate: March 2, 1939

Academic Title: Associate Professor

Position at Affiliation: Radiologist

Business Address:
Department of Radiology
Hadassah University Hospital
Ein Kerem
Jerusalem
Israel
972-2-6777393 (work)

Home Address:
48 Uziel Street
Bayit Vegan
Jerusalem
Israel
972-2-6411-594 (fax)
972-2-6411-594 (home)
ronbloom@cc.huji.ac.il (e-mail)

Specialty: Radiology

Education:
St. Bartholomews Hospital Medical
School, London
Kings College Hospital, London

ISS Member 1985

ISS Committees:
Promotion of Overseas Conferences

Spouse: Doris

BOHNDORF, KLAUS M.D.

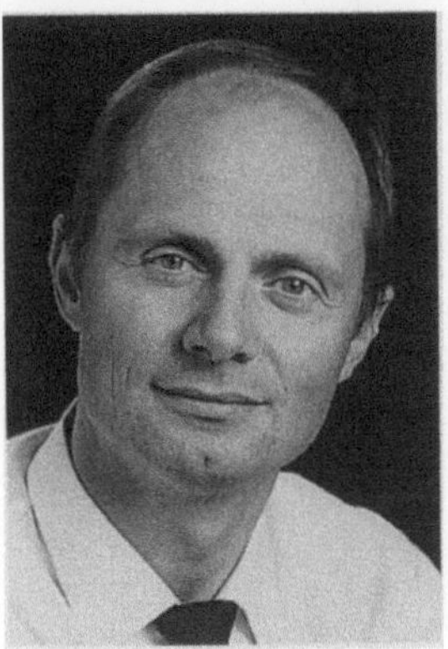

Birthdate: June 7, 1949

Academic Title: Professor of Radiology

Position at Affiliation: Director

Business Address:
Klinik fuer Diagnostische Radiologie
Med Neuroradiologie
Zentralklinikum Augsburg
Stenglinstrasse
86156 Augsburg,
Germany
49-821-4002441 (work)
49-821-4003312 (fax)

Home Address:
Steppacherstrasse 13
86356 Neusass
Germany
49-821-481346 (home)

Specialty/Certification: Radiology, 1986

Education:
1969–76 – University of Wuerzburg,
Kiel, Medical School
1979–86 – St. Georg Hospital Hamburg,
University of Cologne (training in
Radiology)

ISS Member 1989
ISS Medals and Awards:
President's Medal, San Diego, 1991

ISS Committees:
Editorial Board, Skeletal Radiology

Spouse: Susanne

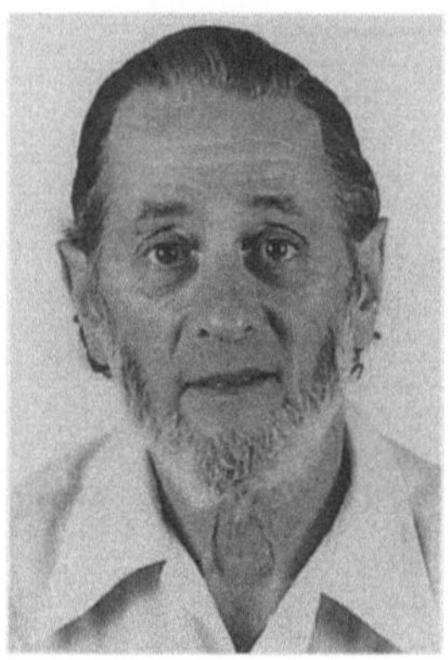

Birthdate: May 1, 1934

Academic Title: Professor

Position at Affiliation: Professor of Radiology

Business Address:
Department of Radiology
Bowman Gray School of Medicine
Medical Center Blvd.
Winston-Salem, NC 27157-1088
U.S.A.
910-748-2478 (work)
910-748-2029 (fax)

Home Address:
3254 Paddington Lane
Winston-Salem, NC 27106-5432
U.S.A.
910-768-4179 (home)

Specialty: Radiology

ISS Member Founding member

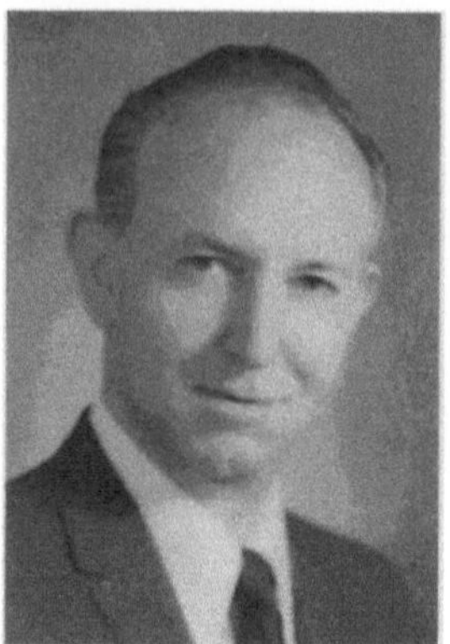

Birthdate: March 23, 1929

Academic Title: Professor

Position at Affiliation: Musculoskeletal Radiologist

Business Address:
Department of Diagnostic Imaging
Temple University Hospital
3401 North Broad Street
Philadelphia, PA 19140, U.S.A.
215-707-4220 (work)
215-707-4464 (fax)
abonakda@nimbus.ocis.temple.edu (e-mail)

Home Address:
4015 Briar Lane
Lafayette Hill, PA 19444, U.S.A.
610-825-0207 (home)

Specialty/Certification: Radiology, 1961

Education:
Tehran Univesity (M.D.)
Temple University (M.S. Radiology)

ISS Member 1973

Offices Held in ISS and Dates of Service:
Secretary-Treasurer, 1980 – 86
President Elect, 1986 – 88
President, 1988 – 90

ISS Medals and Awards:
Founders' Lecture, Stockholm, 1992
Founders' Gold Medal, Berlin, 1994

ISS Committees:
Served on every committee

Business Address:
3411 Warden Drive
Philadelphia, PA 19129
U.S.A.

Specialty: Pediatric Radiology

ISS Member 1975

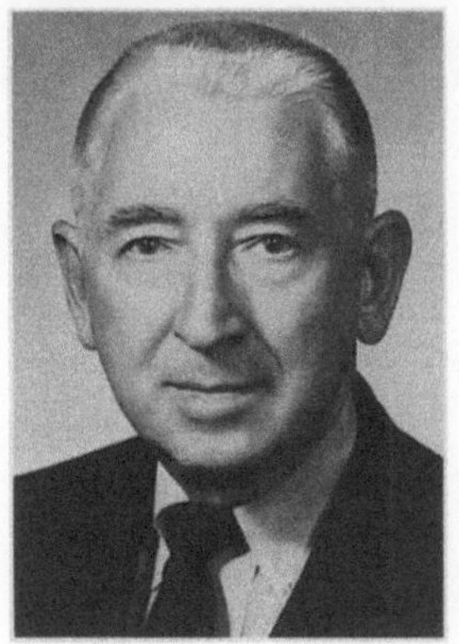

Birthdate: October 25, 1925

Academic Title: Professor of Radiology

Position at Affiliation: Professor

Business Address:
Allegheny University Hospitals, Center City
Broad and Vine Street, M.S. 200
Philadelphia, PA 19102-1192
U.S.A.
215-762-8419 (work)
215-762-8523 (fax)

Home Address:
226 West Washington Square, #3522
Philadelphia, PA 19106
U.S.A.
215-922-5854 (home)

Specialty/Certification: Radiology, 1956

Education:
1946 – George Washington University,
Washington, DC (BA)
1948 – George Washington University,
Washington, DC (M.D.)
1953–55 – Jefferson Medical College
Hospital, Philadelphia, PA (residency)
1955–56 – Hospital of the Univ. of PA,
Philadelphia, PA (residency)

ISS Member Founding member

BRAUNSTEIN, ETHAN M. M.D.

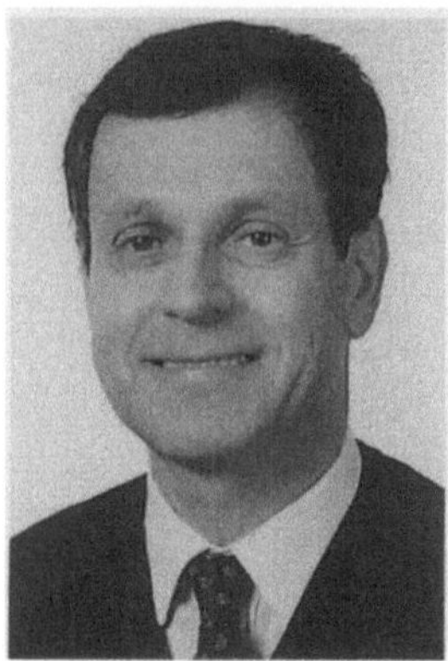

Birthdate: June 16, 1945

Academic Title: Professor of Radiology

Position at Affiliation: Professor of Radiology; Adjunct Professor of Anthropology

Business Address:
Indiana University Medical Center
Department of Radiology
550 N. University Blvd.
Indianapolis, IN 46202-5253
U.S.A.
317-274-4348 (work)
317-274-1848 (fax)
ebraun@xray.indyrad.iupui.edu (e-mail)

Home Address:
5026 Beaumont Way South
Indianapolis, IN 46202-5253
U.S.A.
317-845-9961 (home)

Specialty/Certification: Radiology, 1976

Education:
Dartmouth College
Northwestern University Medical School (M.D.)
University of Chicago (internship)
Harbor General Hospital, Torrance, CA (Radiology residency)
Cedars Sinai Medical Center, Los Angeles, CA (Radiology residency)

ISS Member 1982

ISS Committees:
Editorial Committee
Membership Committee
Liaison Committee for Future Planning

Spouse: Susan White, M.D.

BRILL, PAULA M.D.

Business Address:
Department of Radiology
The New York Hospital
Cornell Medical Center
New York, NY 10021
U.S.A.
212-746-2554 (work)
212-288-1451 (home)
212-746-8645 (fax)

Specialty: Radiology

ISS Member 1991

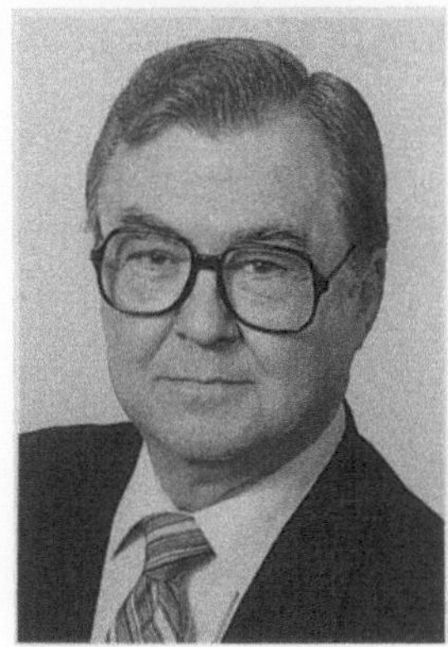

Birthdate: January 22, 1929

Academic Title: University Distinguished Professor Emeritus of Radiology

Position at Affiliation: University Distinguished Professor Emeritus of Radiology

Business Address:
University of South Alabama Medical Center
2451 Fillingim Street
Mobile, AL 36617
U.S.A.
334-471-7868 (work)
334-471-7882 (fax)
vbrown@usmail.usouthal.edu (e-mail)

Home Address:
61 Ridgelawn Drive E.
Mobile, AL 36608
U.S.A.
334-344-3069 (home)

Specialty/Certification: Radiology, 1956

Education:
1951 – University of Arkansas (B.S., BS.M)
1952 – University of Arkansas, School of Medicine (M.D.)
1952–55 – University of Arkansas (Radiology internship & residency)
1955–56 – Bowman Gray (Radiology residency)

ISS Member 1986

ISS Committees:
1993 – present, Refresher Course Committee
1994–95 – Executive Committee
1993 – present – Refresher Course Committee
1994–95 – Chairman, Refresher Course Committee
1996 – present – Convention Planning Committee
1995 – Host for Annual Meeting, New Orleans
1997 – Host for Annual Meeting, Dublin 1998

Spouse: Babs

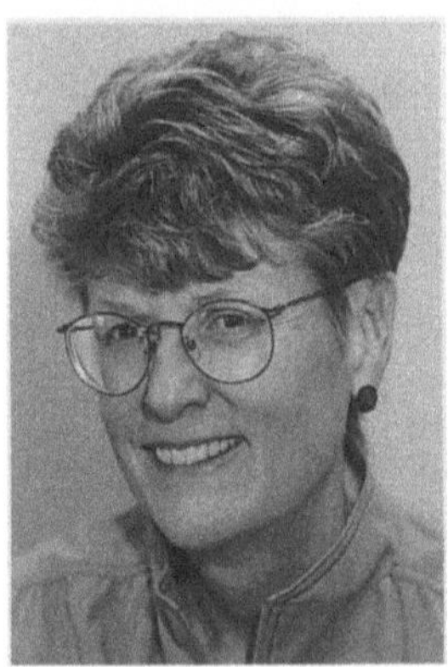

Academic Title: Professor

Position at Affiliation: Professor and Chair

Business Address:
Eastern Virginia Medical School
Department of Radiology
825 Fairfax Avenue, Suite 541
Norfolk, VA 23507-1912
U.S.A.
757-446-8990/8992 (work)
757-446-8441 (fax)
ACB@mccoy.evms.edu (e-mail)

Home Address:
1000 West Princess Anne Road
Norfolk, VA 23507-1220
U.S.A.
757-622-2563 (home)
757-622-4759 (fax)

Specialty/Certification: Radiology, 1974

Education:
Smith College (B.A.)
Columbia University (M.D.)
University of Virginia (internship, residency and fellowship in Radiology)

ISS Member 1978

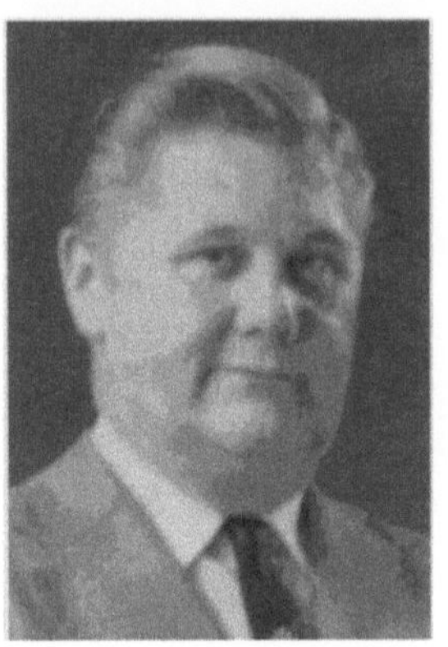

Business Address:
Faculty of Health Sciences
McMaster University, Rm. 2F10
1200 Main Street, West
Hamilton, Ontario L8N 3Z5
Canada
416-521-2100 ext. 6411 (work)
416-627-9896 (home)
416-521-0048 (fax)

ISS Member 1981

Spouse: Margaret Marion

BUCKWALTER, JOSEPH A. IV, M.D.

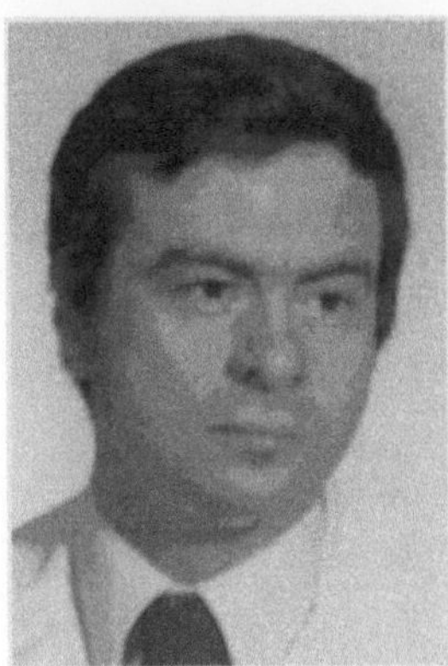

Business Address:
University of Iowa Hospitals and Clinics
Department of Orthopaedic Surgery
1201 Carver Pavillion
Iowa City, IA 52242
U.S.A.
319-356-1616.

Specialty: Orthpaedic Surgery

ISS Member 1985

BUIRSKI, GRAHAM MBBS, MRCP (UK), FRCR, FRACR

Business Address:
Taft Diagnostic Imaging
195 Blackburn Road
Blackburn, Victoria
Australia
015 365 377 (work)
03-9882 5980 (fax)

Home Address:
22, The Ridge
Canterbury
Victoria 3126
Australia
03-9882 0376 (home)

Specialty/Certification: Radiology, 1974; 1984

ISS Member 1991

Spouse: Freida Mary

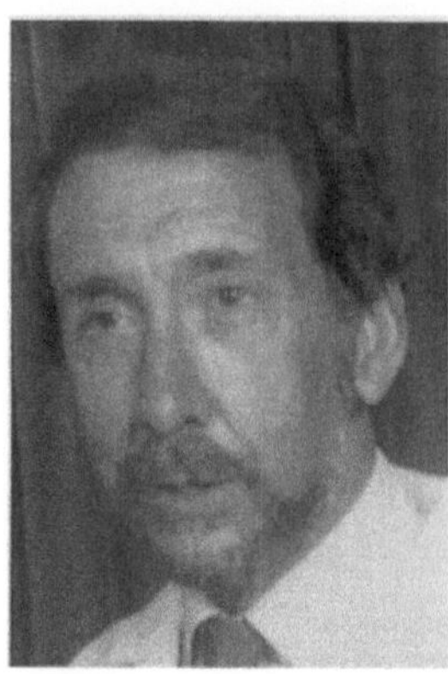

Academic Title: Professor of Pathology,
Correll University Medical
College

Position at Affiliation: Director of
Laboratory Medicine

Business Address:
Department of Orthopaedic Pathology
The Hospital for Special Surgery
535 E. 70th Street, Rm. 244B
New York, NY 10021
U.S.A.
212-606-1341 (work)
212-606-1910 (fax)

Home Address:
320 E. 57th Street 9B
New York, NY 10022
U.S.A.
212-752-2054 (home)

Specialty: Pathology

Education:
1956 – Liverpool University Medical
School

ISS Member 1978

Business Address:
Woodhouse Farm
York Road
Leeds 15, LS154NW
West Yorkshire
England

ISS Member Founding member

ISS Medals and Awards:
Medal of the ISS (Silver), Berlin, 1994

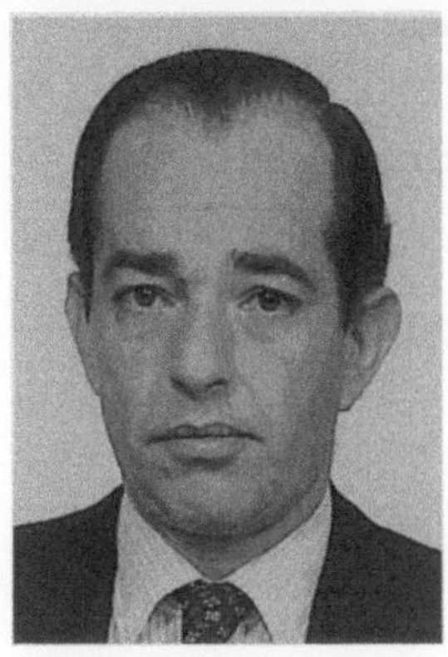

Birthdate: April 8, 1942
Academic Title: M.D.
Position at Affiliation: Jefe de Patologia osteoarticular
Business Address: Jefe De Patologia Osteoarticular ·
"Hospital Ramon Y Cajal"
Carretera De Colmenar Viejo, Km9.100
28034 Madrid
Spain
34-1-738 10 97 (work)
34-1-738 10 97 (fax)
mcalvo@telprof.eurociber.es (e-mail)
Home Address:
San Pablo, 4
28230-Las Rozas
Madrid
Spain
34-1-637 24 47 (home)
34-1-637 59 53 (fax)
Specialty/Certification: Pathology, 1973
Education:
1962–65 – Salamanca University
(medical school)
1966–68 – Madrid University
(medical school)
1969–74 – Hospital La Paz
(Pathology department)
ISS Member 1981
ISS Committees:
Committee for Promotion of Courses
outside North America, 1986–93
Spouse: Felicity

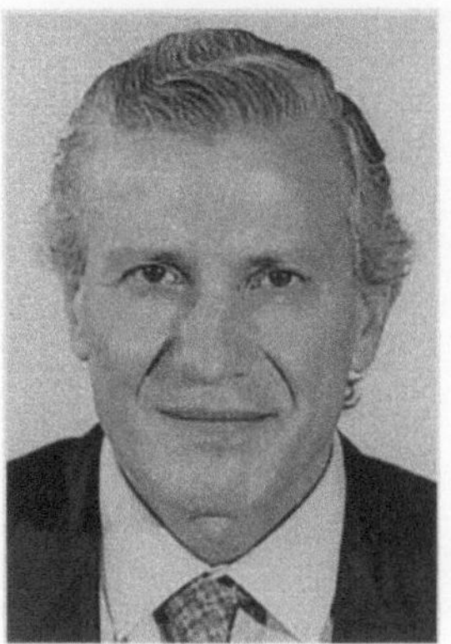

Birthdate: January 13, 1932

Academic Title: Professor of Orthopaedics

Business Address:
Clinica Ortopedica Dell 'Universita'
Instituto Ortopedico Rizzoli
via G.C. Pupilli, 1
40136 Bologna
Italy
39 51-582388 (work)
39 51-331710 (fax)

Home Address:
Via Levi Civita 2
40100 Bologna
Italy
39 51 6447612 (home)
39 51-6446984 (fax)

Specialty/Certification: Orthopaedic Surgery, 1960

ISS Member 1975

ISS Medals and Awards:
Founders' Gold Medal, Stockholm, 1992

Spouse: Giuliana

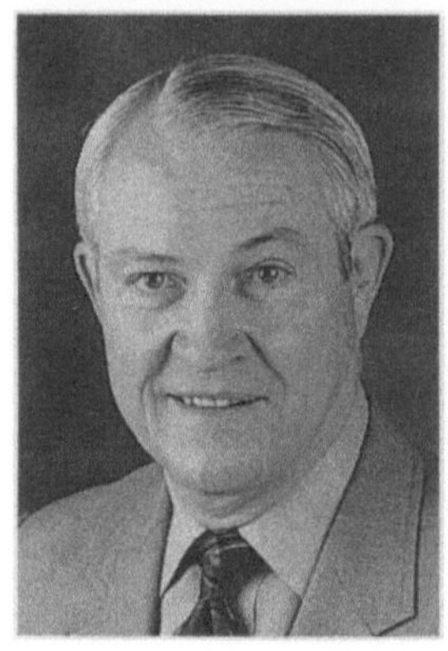

Birthdate: July 23, 1934

Academic Title: Clinical Professor

Position at Affiliation: Director,
Pediatric Radiology

Business Address:
Arnold Palmer Hospital for Children
and Women
92 West Miller Street
Orlando, FL 32806
U.S.A.
407-649-6909 (work)
407-872-7739 (fax)

Home Address:
1873 Wind Willow Road
Orlando, FL 32809
U.S.A.
407-826-0278 (home)

Specialty/Certification: Pediatrics 1964,
Radiology 1968, Pediatric
Radiology CAQ 1994

Education:
University of Minnesota (B.A., B.S.)
University of Minnesota (M.D.)
1960–62 – Pediatric residency
1965–68 – Radiology residency
1971–72 – Pediatric Radiology fellowship

ISS Member 1991

Spouse: Mary

Business Address:
First Orthopaedic Clinic of University &
Bone Tumor
Center of the Rizzoli Institute
Bologna
Italy

ISS Member 1991

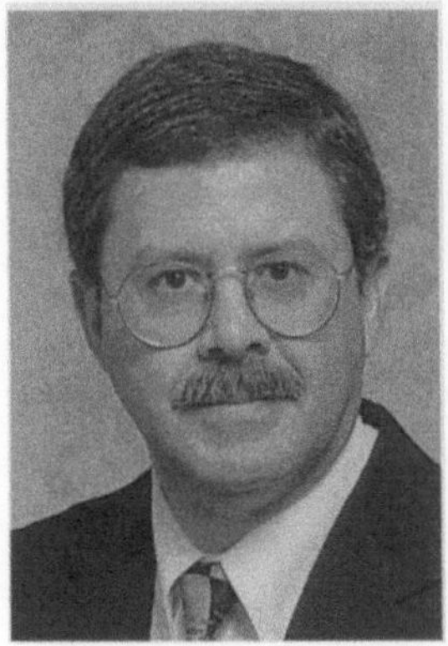

Birthdate: May 11, 1946

Academic Title: Professor of Radiology, Orthopaedic Surgery and Medicine (Rheumatology)

Position at Affiliation: Chief, Diagnostic Radiology

Business Address:
Medical College of Wisconsin
Radiology – Froedtert Memorial Luth. Hosp.
9200 W. Wisconsin Avenue
Milwaukee, WI 53226
U.S.A.
414-777-3750 (work)
414-259-9290 (fax)

Home Address:
4095 Stonewood Court
Brookfield, WI 53045
U.S.A.
414-781-7336 (home)

Specialty/Certification: Radiology, 1976

Education:
1968 – Harvard College (AB)
1972 – Harvard Medical School (MD)
Peter Brent Brigham Hospital, Boston (internship in Internal Medicine and residency in Diagnostic Radiology)

ISS Member 1982

Spouse: Nancy

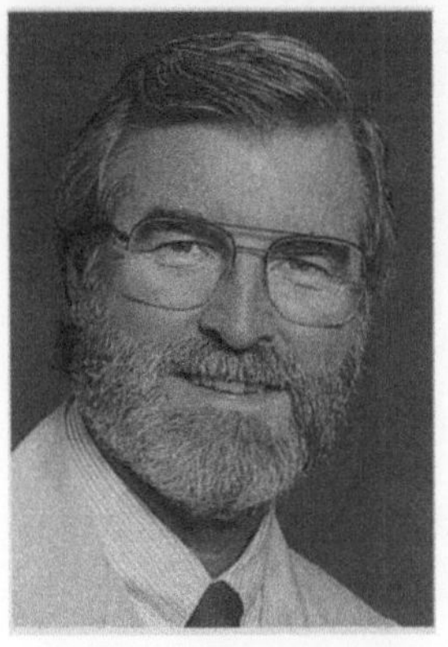

Birthdate: July 5, 1933

Academic Title: Professor

Position at Affiliation: Orthopaedic Surgeon

Business Address:
680 North Lake Shore Drive
Suite 1208
Chicago, IL 60611
U.S.A.
312-951-9099 (work)
312-951-9198 (fax)
n-carroll@nwu.edu (e-mail)

Home Address:
526 West Grant Peace
Chicago, IL 60614
U.S.A.
773-472-7618 (home)
773-472-7618 touch 526 (fax)

Specialty/Certification: Orthopaedic Surgery, 1967

Education:1955 – University of New Brunswick (B.S., B.Sc.)
1960 – Dalhouse University (M.D.)
1967 – University of Toronto (FRCSC)

ISS Member 1991

Spouse: Heather

CASSAR-PULLICINO, VICTOR N. M.D.

Business Address:
Dept. of Diagnostic Imaging
The Robert Jones and Agnes Hunt Hospital
Owestry, Shropshire SY10 7AG
United Kingdom
44-0691-655311 x 3546 (work)
44-0691-670649 (fax)

Specialty: Radiology

ISS Member 1994

CATTO, MARY ELIZABETH M.D. FRC PATH

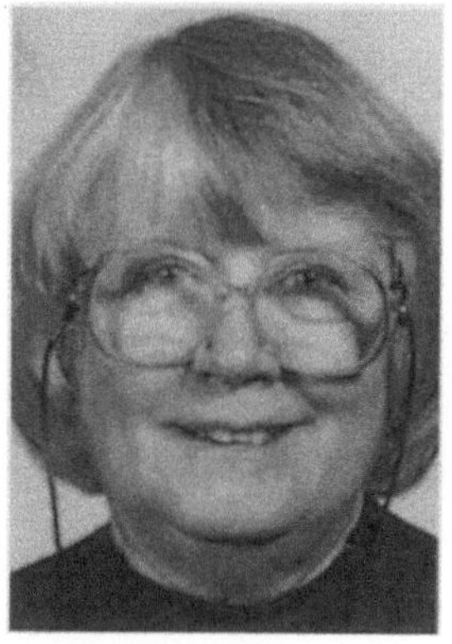

Business Address:
Pathology Department
Western Infirmary
Glasgow G11 6NT
Scotland
United Kingdom
0141-211-2062 or 2055 (work)
0141-337-2494 (fax)

Home Address:
20, Victoria Crescent Road
Glasgow G12 9DD
Scotland
United Kingdom
0141-334-5891 (home)

Specialty: Pathology

Education:
University of Glasgow

ISS Member 1977

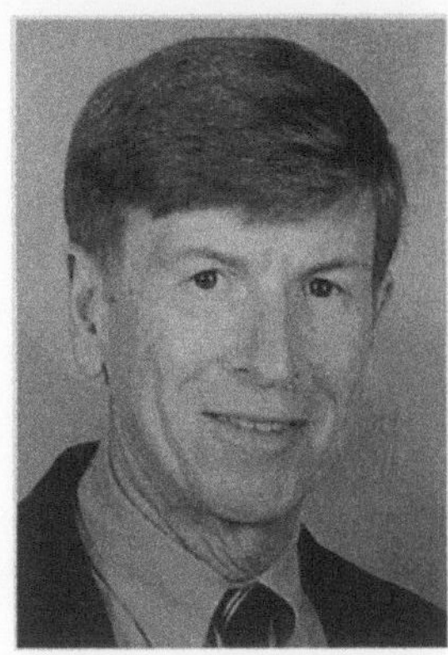

Position at Affiliation: Staff Radiologist

Business Address:
Bethesda Memorial Hospital
2815 South Seacrest Boulevard
Boynton Beach, FL 33435
U.S.A.
407-737-7733 ext. 4574 (work)
407-375-8778 (fax)

Home Address:
4134 Shelldrake Lane
Boynton Beach, FL 33436
U.S.A.
407-736-8151 (home)

Specialty/Certification: Radiology, 1968

Education:
1959 – Seton Hall University (B.A.)
1963 – UMDNJ-New Jersey Med. School
(M.D.)
1964–67 – Fitzsimons General Hosp.,
Denver, CO (residency)

ISS Member Founding member

Business Address:
Department of Radiology
Catholic University Hospital
Marcoleta 347
Santiago, Chile

Specialty: Radiology

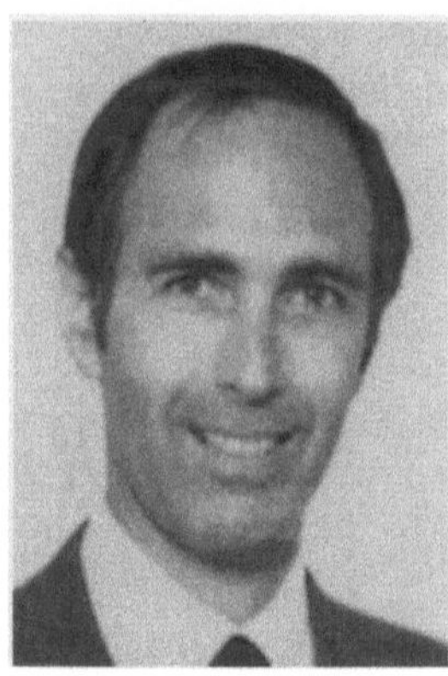

Birthdate: January 4, 1945

Position at Affiliation: Medical Director

Business Address:
Oracle Imaging Services, Inc.
28364 S. Western Avenue
Suite 507
Rancho Palos Verdes, CA 90275
U.S.A.
310-833-2233 (work)
310-833-2213 (fax)
nchafetz@pop.net (e-mail)

Home Address:
30527 Palos Verdes Drive East
Rancho Palos Verdes, CA 90275
U.S.A.
310-521-9123 (home)
310-521-9214 (fax)

Specialty/Certification: Radiology, 1977

Education:
Cornell University (B.A.)
University of North Carolina (M.D.)
University of Florida (internship)
University of North Carolina
(Radiology)
University of California San Diego
(Imaging fellowship)
University of California San Francisco
(Imaging fellowship)

ISS Member 1982

Spouse: Karin

Business Address: Chief, Musculoskeletal Radiology
Brooke Army Medical Center
Department of Radiology
3851 Roger Brooke Drive
San Antonio, TX 78234
U.S.A.
210-916 -4218 (work)
210-916-5193 (fax)
71212.703@compuserve.com (e-mail)

Home Address:
166-G Elizabeth Road
San Antonio, TX 78209
U.S.A.
210-824-4652 (home)
210-829-5246 (fax)

Specialty/Certification: Radiology, 1989

Education:
University of Chicago (B.A.)
Ohio State University (M.D.)
Ohio State University (MS Radiology)
University of California, San Diego
(Osteoradiology fellowship)

ISS Member 1995

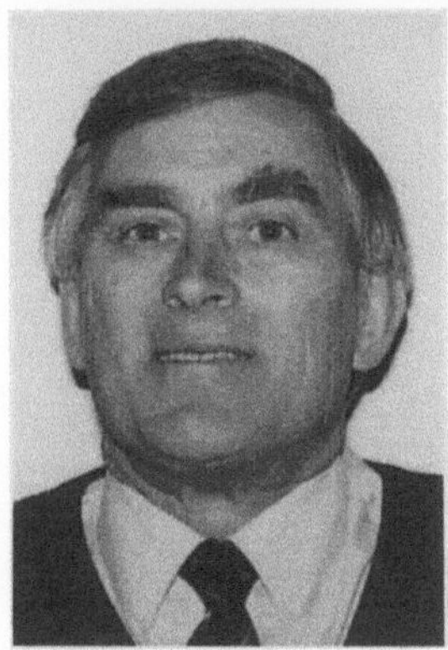

Birthdate: May 30, 1932

Academic Title: Dr.

Position at Affiliation: Visiting Radiologist

Business Address:
Royal North Shore Hospital
Sydney
Australia

Home Address:
P.O. Box 238
Cremorne
N.S.W. 2090
Australia
(02) 9909 3415 (home)
(047) 82 3381 (fax)

Specialty/Certification: Radiology, 1960

Education:
1949-54 – Sydney University

ISS Member 1983

ISS Committees:
Co-organizer ISS meeting, Sydney, 1988
Member ISS Executive Committee,
1993–95

Spouse: Hildegard

Business Address:
Department of Radiology
The Middlesex Hospital
Mortimer Street
London W1N 8AA
England

ISS Member Founding member

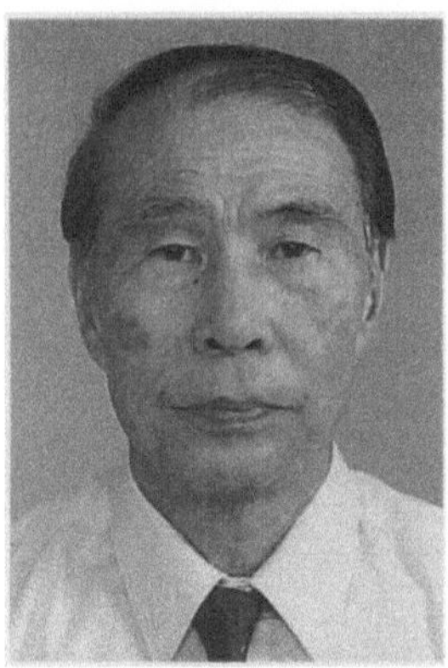

Academic Title: Professor

Position at Affiliation: Professor

Business Address:
MRI Section, Department of Radiology
No. Affiliated Hospital/China Medical
University
36 Sanhaojie St.
Shenyang 110003, Liaoning Province
Peoples Republic of China
24-3846292 (work)
24-3892617 (fax)

Home Address:
Apt. 3 Unit 2 #501
Lane 150, Zhong-Shan Rd.
Shenyang 110001, Liaoning Province
Peoples Republic of China
24-3853826 (home)

Specialty: Radiology

Education:
1942–49 – Hsiang-Ya (Yale-in-China)
Medical College
1949–50 – Hsiang-Ya Medical College
(residency)
1950–55 – China Medical University
(residency)

ISS Member 1988

Spouse: Liu Yu-tang, M.D.

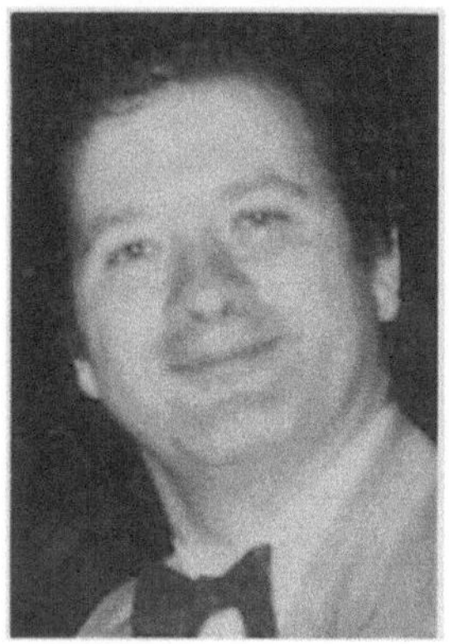

Birthdate: October 31, 1940

Academic Title: Professor

Position at Affiliation: Chief of Department

Business Address:
Hopital Cochin
27, Rue du Faubourg-Saint Jacques
75674 Paris
France Cedex 14
33-1-42-34-17-68 (work)
33-1-43-20-26-80 (fax)
alain.chevrot@cch.ap-hop-paris.fr

Home Address:
19 Rue Campagne Premiere
75014 Paris
France
33-1-43-20-26-80 (home)

Specialty: Radiology

ISS Member 1986

ISS Committees:
Chairman, Committee for Planning the
Paris Meeting, 1996

Chew, Felix S. M.D.

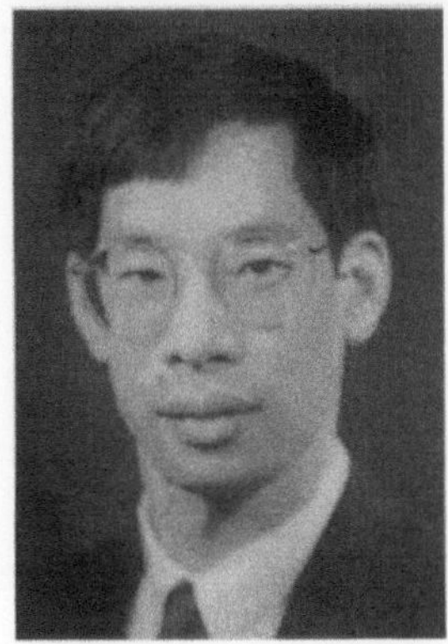

Birthdate: October 11, 1954

Academic Title: Associate Professor

Position at Affiliation: Associate Radiologist

Business Address:
Harvard Medical School and
Massachusetts General Hospital
32 Fruit Street
Boston, MA 02114
U.S.A.
617-726-6801 (work)
617-726-5282 (fax)
chew@helix.mgh.harvard.edu (e-mail)

Home Address:
21 Amberwood Drive
Winchester, MA 01890
U.S.A.
617-729-3904 (home)

Specialty/Certification: Radiology, 1987

Education:
1975 – Princeton University (A.B.)
1979 – University of Florida (M.D.)
1983–87 SUNY Health Science Center at
Syracuse (residency)
1995 – Harvard University (EdM)

ISS Member 1995

Spouse: Annemarie

Chhem, Rethy K. M.D.

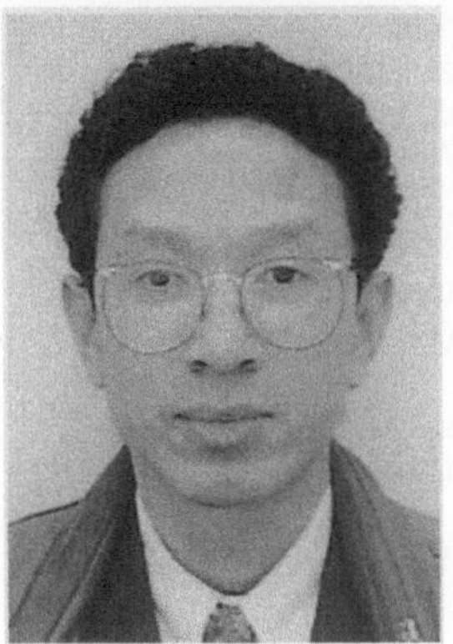

Academic Title: Associate Professor

Position at Affiliation: Director,
Musculoskeletal Imaging Division

Business Address:
Montreal General Hospital McGill
University
1650 Cedar Avenue
Montreal 43G 1A4, QC
Canada
514-934-8003 (work)
514-934-8263 (fax)
chhem@radiology.mgh.mcgill.ca
(e-mail)

Home Address:
580 Lazard Avenue
Town of Mount Royal
H3R1P7, QC
Canada
514-344-8369 (home)

Specialty: Radiology

Education:
University of Paris, Paris, France (M.D.)

ISS Member 1995

Spouse: Yanny

Business Address:
Medical College of Virginia
Dept. of Radiology
Box 6515 MCV Station
Richmond, VA 24017
U.S.A.
804-786-5203 (work)
804-371-6066 (fax)

Home Address:
804-741-1975 (home)

ISS Member 1992

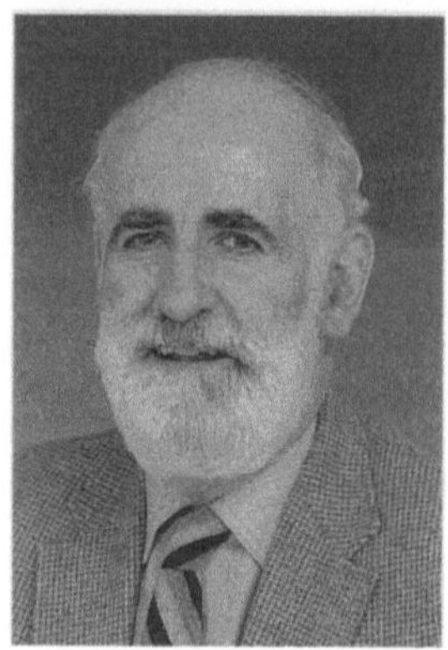

Birthdate: August 9, 1930

Academic Title: Professor

Position at Affiliation: Professor of
Radiology and Orthopaedic Surgery

Business Address:
University of Missouri School of
Medicine
1 Hospital Drive
Columbia, Missouri 65212
U.S.A.
573-882-8183 (work)
573-884-4729 (fax)
fcopeoi@mail.coin.missouri.edu

Home Address:
908 Martin Drive
Columbia, MO 65203
U.S.A.
573-445-8121 (home)

Specialty/Certification: Radiology, 1979

Education:
1954 – University of Liverpool, England
(M.B., Ch.B.)
1965 – University of Edinburgh
(MRCP Ed)
1969 – University Edinburgh
(D.M.R.(D))

ISS Member 1990

Spouse: Frances

CREMIN, BRYAN M.D.

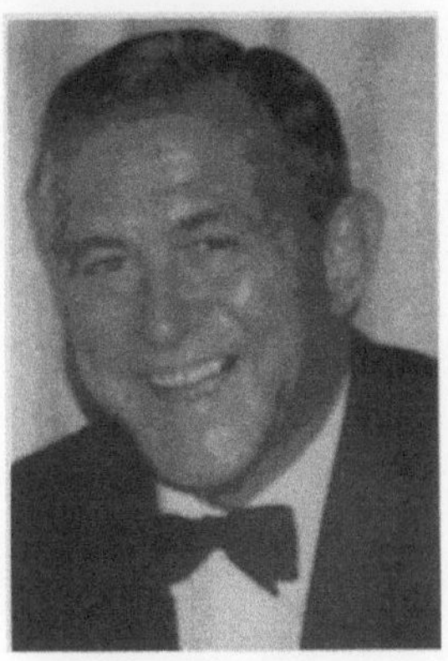

Business Address:
Department of Radiology
Red Cross Children's Hospital
Cape Town 7700
South Africa
685 2336 (work)
794 5243 (home)

Specialty: Radiology

ISS Member 1972

CRUES, JOHN V. M.S., M.D.

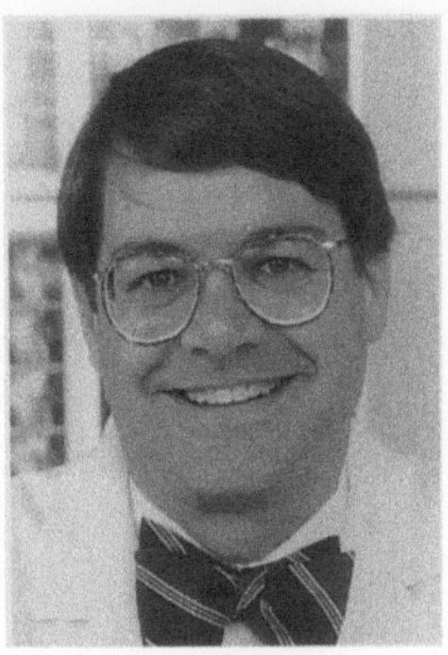

Position at Affiliation: Medical Director

Business Address:
Radnet Management, Inc.
1516 Cotner Avenue
Los Angeles, CA 90025
U.S.A.
310-445-5666 (work)
310-478-5810 (fax)

Home Address:
2663 Centinela #305
Santa Monica, CA
U.S.A.
310-450-1787 (home)
310-450-1787 (fax)

Specialty: Radiology

Education:
Harvard College (M.S.)
University of Illinois Graduate (M.D.)
Harvard Medical School (internship)
Cedar Sinai (residency in Diagnostic
Radiology)

ISS Member 1993

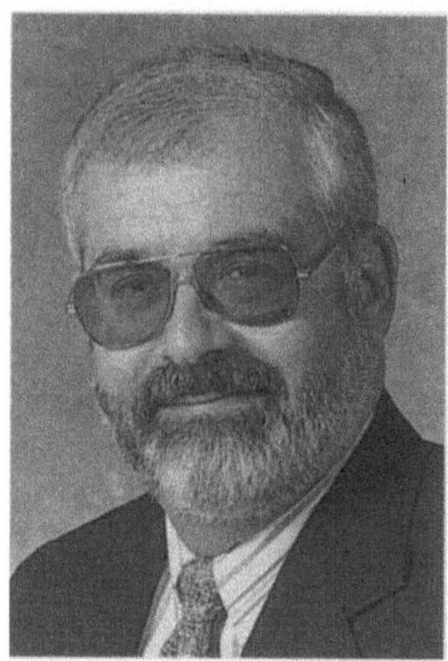

Birthdate: August 20, 1941

Academic Title: Professor

Position at Affiliation: Professor of Radiologic Sciences

Business Address:
Allegheny General Hospital
Department of Radiology
320 East North Avenue
Pittsburgh, PA 15212
U.S.A.
(412) 359-4111 (work)
(412) 323-8310 (fax)
Alvdaf@aol.com (e-mail)

Home Address:
858 Osage Road
Pittsburgh, PA 15243-1057
U.S.A.
(412) 344-0557 (home)

Specialty/Certification: Radiology, 1974

Education:
1963 – Albany College of Pharmacy, Albany, NY (B.S.)
1967 – State University of New York at Buffalo, Buffalo, NY (M.D.)
1970 – 73 Duke University Medical Center, Durham, NC (residency)

ISS Member 1982

ISS Committees:
Audit Committee

Spouse: Alva

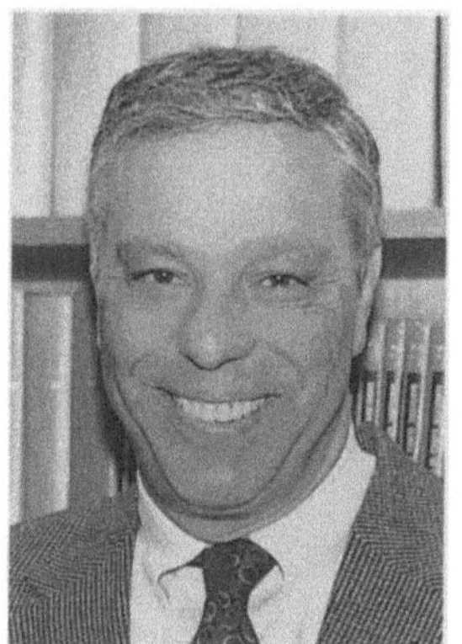

Birthdate: May 13, 1938

Academic Title: Professor of Radiology and Orthopedic Surgery

Position at Affiliation: Chief Musculo-skeletal Radiology

Business Address:
Department of Radiology
University of Pennsylvania Medical Center
3400 Spruce Street
Philadelphia, PA 19104
U.S.A.
215-662-3019 (work)
215-662-7011 (fax)
dalinka@oasis.rad.upenn.edu (e-mail)

Home Address:
318 South 21st Street
Philadelphia, PA 19103
U.S.A.
215-732-3875 (home)

Specialty/Certification: Radiology, 1969

Education:
1956 – 60 – University of Michigan (B.S.)
1960 – 64 – University of Michigan School of Medicine (M.D.)
1964 – 65 – Pennsylvania Hospital, Philadelphia, PA (rotating intern)
1965 – 68 – Montefiore Hospital, Bronx, NY (resident in Radiology)

ISS Member Founding member

Offices Held in ISS and Dates of Service:
Assistant Secretary-Treasurer 1983–86
Secretary-Treasurer 1986–90
Secretary 1990–92
President-Elect 1992–94
President 1994–96

ISS Awards and Medals:
Founders' Medal, Dublin, 1998
Founders' Lecture, Dublin, 1998

ISS Committee:
Executive Committee
Board of Trustees of the Endowment
Fund
Closed Program Committee

Spouse: Janice Kolber

DANIEL, WILLIAM W. JR., M.D.

Business Address:
University of Alabama
Department of Radiology
619 South 19th Street
Birmingham, Alabama 35233
U.S.A.

Specialty: Radiology

ISS Member 1990

DANZIG, LARRY A. M.D.

Academic Title: Associate Clinical
Professor Orthopaedic Surgery

Position at Affiliation: Associate
Professor Orthopaedic Surgery

Business Address:
UCSD Medical School
La Jolla, CA
U.S.A.
714-558-7365 (work)
714-541-0722 (fax)

Home Address:
9 Pt. Lora Drive
Corona del Mar, CA 92625
U.S.A.
714-640-0370 (home)

Specialty/Certification: Orthopaedic
Surgery, 1975

Education:
1965 – Rutgers University (B. A.)
1969 – SUNY Upstate Medical Center,
Syracuse
1969–75 – internship surgery, resident
surgery, resident Orthopaedic Surgery

ISS Member 1990

Spouse: Valerie

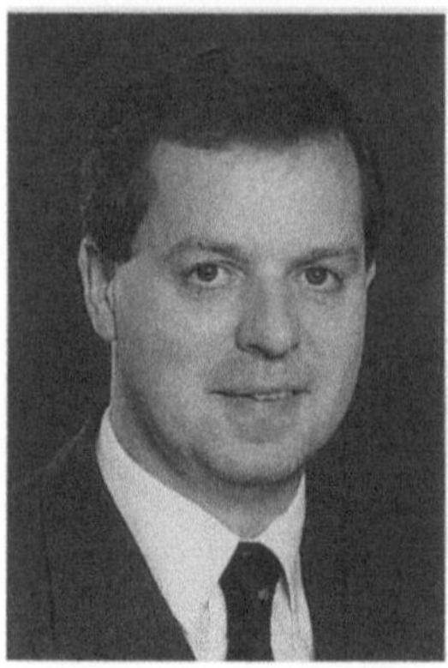

Birthdate: November 12, 1954

Academic Title: Dr.

Position at Affiliation: Clinical Director

Business Address:
MRI Centre
Royal Orthopaedic Hospital
Birmingham B31 2AP
England
121-627-8582 (work)
121-627-8623 (fax)

Home Address:
41 Serpentine Road Harborne
Birmingham B17 9RD
England
121 426 6884 (home)

Specialty/Certification: Radiology, 1983

Education:
1973–78 – Univ. of Birmingham Medical School
1980–84 –'West Midland Radiology Training Program

ISS Member 1994

ISS Committees:
Member Consulting Editorial Board
Skeletal Radiology, 1995
Rules Committee, 1997 –

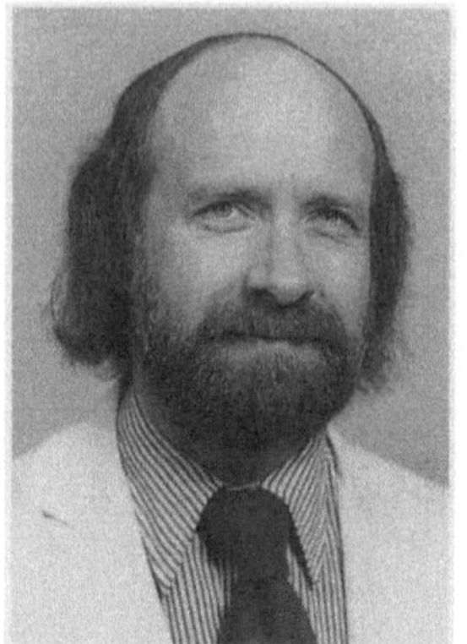

Birthdate: December 9, 1936

Academic Title: Professor of Radiology

Position at Affiliation: Attending Radiologist

Business Address:
Loyola University Chicago Medical Center
2160 South First Avenue
Maywood, IL- 60153
U.S.A.
708-216-1084 (work)
708-216-8394 (fax)
tdemos@luc.edu (email)

Home Address:
834 North Euclid Avenue
Oak Park IL 60302, U.S.A.
708-216-8625 (home)

Specialty/Certification: Radiology, 1972

Education:
1959 – Knox College,
Roosevelt University, Chicago
1963 – University of Illinois School of Medicine, Chicago
1970 – University of Wisconsin
(Radiology residency)

ISS Member 1982

Spouse: Gina

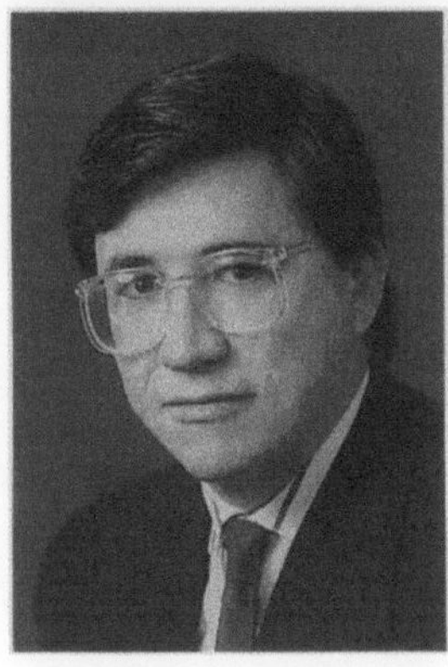

Birthdate: January 17, 1946

Position at Affiliation: Radiologist

Business Address:
Radiology Department
Memorial Hospital South West
7600 Beechnut
Houston, TX 77074
U.S.A.
713-776-4058 (work)
713-776-4043 (fax)

Home Address:
1246 Wedgewood Drive
Sugar Land, TX 77478-3338
U.S.A.
713-242-8019 (home)

Specialty/Certification: Radiology, 1976

Education:
1969 – Madrid Spain (MD)
1976 – University of Pittsburgh
(Radiology residency)

ISS Member 1978

Spouse: Gemma

Academic Title: Professor of Diagnostic
Radiology

Position at Affiliation: Section Head,
Musculoskeletal Radiology;
Vice-Chair for Program Development

Business Address:
University of Wisconsin Center for
Health Sciences
Department of Radiology, E3/311
600 Highland Avenue
Madison, WI 53792-3252
U.S.A.
608-263-9387 (work)
608-263-0876 (fax)
adesmet@facstaff.wisc.edu (e-mail)

Home Address:
25 North Yellowstone Drive
Madison, WI 53705
U.S.A.

Specialty/Certification: Radiology, 1976

Education:
University of Notre Dame, (B.S.)
University of Michigan Medical School
(M.D.)
University Hospital of San Diego County
(internship)
University of Michigan Medical Center
(house officer II – IV, Radiology)

ISS Member 1982

Spouse: Peggy

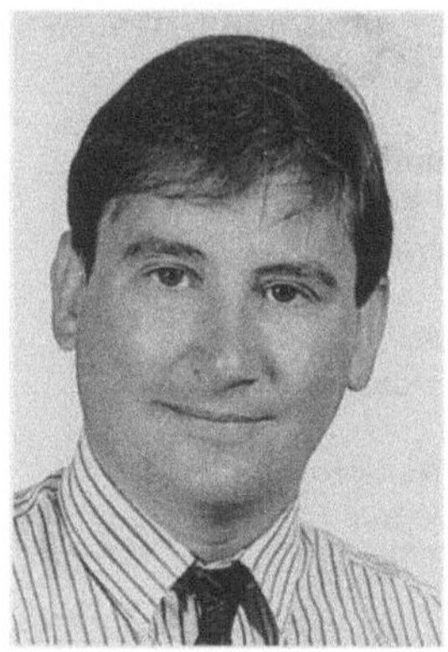

Birthdate: December 3, 1957

Academic Title: Associate Professor of Pathology

Position at Affiliation: Associate Professor of Pathology

Business Address:
University of Michigan Hospitals
Pathology, 2G332
1500 E. Medical Center Drive
Ann Arbor, MI 48109-0054
U.S.A.
313-936-6622 (work)
313-763-4095 (fax)
devaney@umich.edu (e-mail)

Home Address:
272 Harbor Way
Ann Arbor, MI 48103
U.S.A.

Specialty/Certification: Anatomic Pathology, 1987; Clinical Pathology, 1989

Education:
Tulane University, New Orleans,
Louisiana (college)
Tulane School of Medicine, New Orleans,
Louisiana (medical school)
Bethesda Naval Hospital, Bethesda,
Maryland (Pathology residency)

ISS Member 1996

Spouse: Stephanie

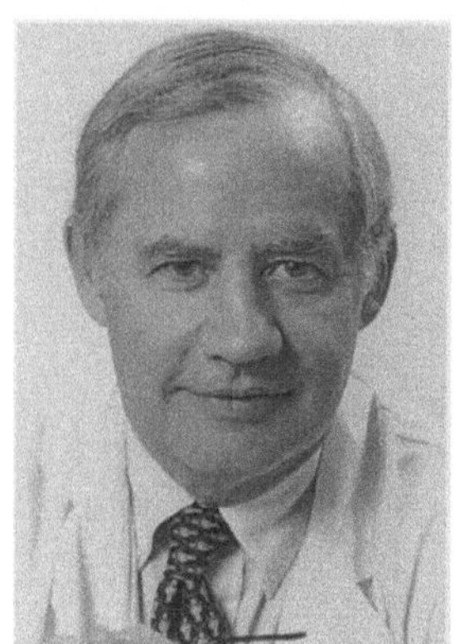

Birthdate: December 22, 1933

Academic Title: Frank E. Stinchfield Professor and Chairman

Position at Affiliation: Director of Service

Business Address:
Dept. of Orthopaedic Surgery
Columbia Presbyterian Medical Center
622 West 168th Street, PH5-Stem
New York, NY 10032
U.S.A.
212-305-3293 (work)
212-305-6193 (fax)

Home Address:
152 Ashley Place
Park Ridge, NJ 07656
U.S.A.
201-391-7785 (home)

Specialty/Certification: Orthopaedic Surgery, 1968

Education:
1952–56 – Princeton University, Princeton, NJ (A.B.)
1956–60 – New York University School of Medicine, New York, NY (M.D.)
1960–61 – The Queen's Hospital, Honolulu, Hawaii (rotating internship)
1962–66 – New York Orthopaedic Hospital, New York (resident)
1966–67 – New York Orthopaedic Hospital, New York (hand fellow)

ISS Member 1986

Spouse: Joyce Anne

DIEPPE, PAUL M.D.

Business Address:
Consultant Sr. Lecturer/Rheumatology
Department of Medicine
Bristol Royal Infirmary
Bristol BS2 8HW
England

ISS Member 1985

DIETEMANN, JEAN-LOUIS M.D.

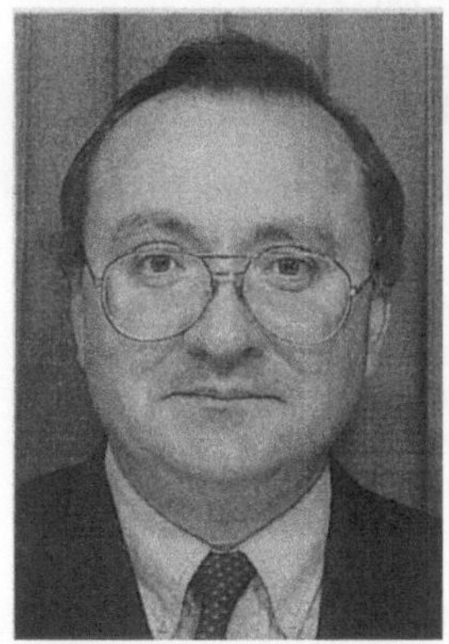

Birthdate: December 13, 1957

Academic Title: Professor

Business Address:
Chu De Hautepierre
Service De Radiologie 2
67098 Strasbourg
France
33 03 88 12 78 88 (work)
33 03 88 12 71 18 (fax)

Home Address:
7, Rue Des Tulipes
67960 Entzheim
France

Specialty/Certification: Radiology, 1982

ISS Member: 1995

DIHLMANN, WOLFGANG W.M. M.D.

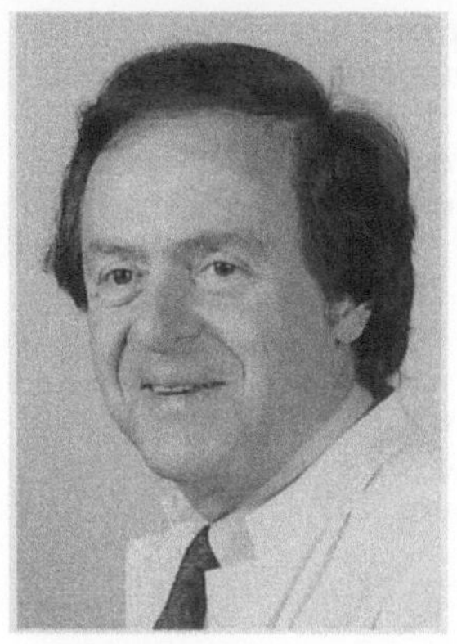

Academic Title: Professor Emeitus

Position at Affiliation: Partner

Business Address:
Radiology Associates Barmbek
D-22305 Hamburg
Hufnerstrasse 110
Germany
040-6900053 (work)
040-6900056 (fax)

Home Address:
Hollenbek 17
D-22339 Hamburg
Germany
040-538-5525 (home)

Specialty/Certification: Radiology, 1959

Education:
1952 – M.D.

ISS Member 1976

ISS Committees:
Nominating Committee

Spouse: Dr. Rosemarie Dihlmann

DIRHEIMER, YVES E.C. M.D.

Business Address:
Cabinet de Rhumatologie et de Neurologie
40, Rue du Tivoli
67000 Strasbourg
France
33 03 88 35 36 26 (work)
33 03 88 36 84 64 (fax)

Home Address:
27, Rue Goethe
67000 Strasbourg
France
33 03 88 61 88 77

Specialty: Rheumatology

ISS Member 1982

Spouse: Claudette

DORFMAN, HOWARD D. M.D.

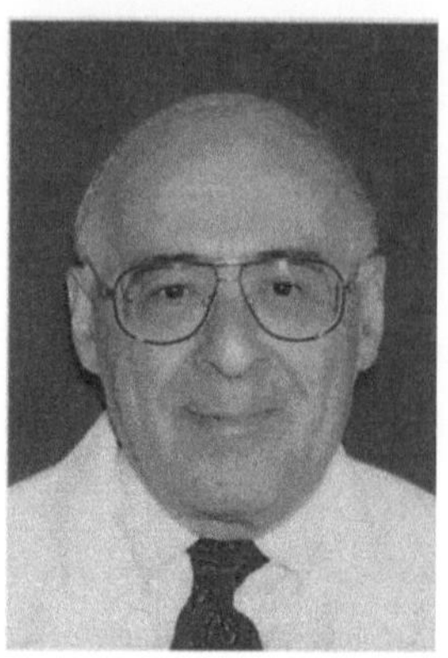

Birthdate: July 20, 1928

Academic Title: Professor of Pathology, Radiology and Orthopaedic Surgery

Position at Affiliation: Head, Division of Orthopaedic Pathology

Business Address:
Department of Orthopaedic Surgery
Albert Einstein College of Medicine
Montefiore Medical Center
111 East 210th Street
Bronx, NY 10467
U.S.A.
718-920-5622 (work)
718-231-2243 (fax)

Home Address:
530 East 72nd Street
New York, NY 10021
U.S.A.
212-535-8503 (home)

Specialty/Certification: Anatomic Pathology, 1958

Education:
1947 – New York University (B.A.)
1951 – Downstate Medical Center, Brooklyn (M.D.)

ISS Member 1973

Offices Held in ISS and Dates of Service:
President, 1986 – 88

ISS Medals and Awards:
Founders' Lecture, Toronto, 1993

ISS Committees:
Program Committee
Closed Meeting Committee-Chairman,
1975–85
Editorial Committee, 1975 – present
Executive Committee, 1986 – present
ISS Endowment Fund Trustee, 1987 –
present (chairman), 1995-97

Spouse: Esther

DOSCH, JEAN CLAUDE M.D.

Business Address:
Dept. of Radiology
Centre De Traumatologic et DF'Ortho-
pedie
Boite Postale 96,67403 Illkirch Cedex
Strasbourg
France
88.67.33.33 (work)
88.67.45.15 (fax)
88.65.12.52 (home)

Specialty: Radiology

ISS Member 1990

Spouse: Jacqueline

DUAN, CHEN-XIANG M.D.

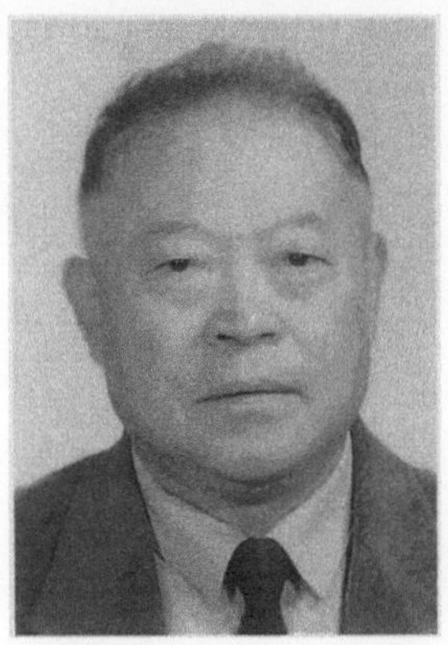

Birthdate: November 16, 1928

Academic Title: Professor

Position at Affiliation: Radiologist

Business Address:
Chinese Medical Association
Beijing
Peoples Republic of China
21-65347018 – 72519 (work)
21-58674397 (fax)

Home Address:
174 Changhai Road
Shanghai 200433
Peoples Republic of China
21 65347017-77544 (home)

Specialty: Radiology

Education:
The Second Military College

ISS Member 1987

Spouse: Shu Xin Huang

DUSSAULT, ROBERT G. M.D.

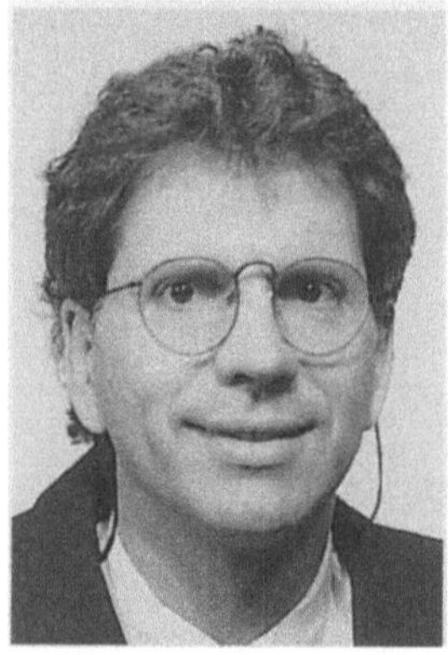

Birthdate: April 14, 1946

Academic Title: Professor of Radiology and Orthopedics

Position at Affiliation: Professor

Business Address:
University of Virginia Health Science Center
Department of Radiology
P.O. Box 170
Charlottesville, Virginia 22908
U.S.A.
804-982-3255 (work)
804-982-1618 (fax)
rgd6q@avery.med.virginia.edu (e-mail)

Home Address:
3050 Pryor's Mountain Lane
Charlottesville, VA 22903
U.S.A.
804-984-4054 (home)

Specialty/Certification: Radiology, 1976

Education:
1966 – Jean de Brébeuf College, Montreal, Quebec (B.A.)
1971 – University of Sherbrooke, Sherbrooke, Quebec (M.D.)
1971–72 – Centre Hospitalier Universitaire de Sherbrooke (internship Internal Medicine)
1972–74 – Sherbrooke University, Sherbrooke, Quebec (resident Diagnostic Radiology)
1975–76 – McGill University, Montreal, Quebec (resident Diagnostic Radiology)
1976 – Hosp. for Special Surgery, Cornell Univ., New York (visiting fellow in Bone Radiology)

ISS Member 1982

ISS Committees:
Chair, Liaison Future Planning Committee, 1995
Chair, Evaluation of Research Grants Committee, 1996–97

Spouse: Phoebe A. Kaplan, M.D.

DUURSMA, SIJMEN A. PH.D., M.D.

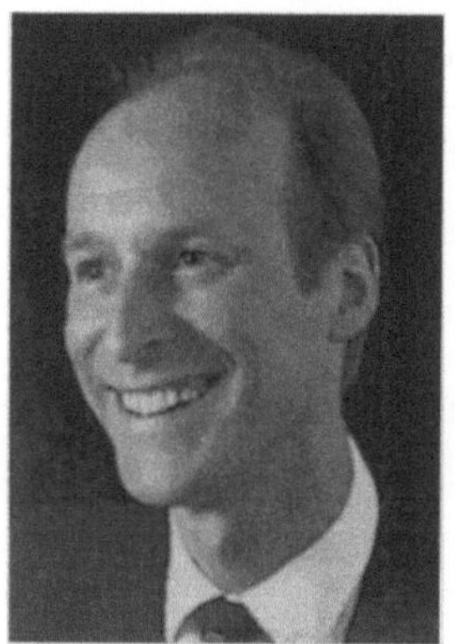

Business Address:
Department of Internal Medicine
University Hospital, University of Utrecht
P. O. Box 85500
3508 GA Utrecht
The Netherlands
30-507398 (work)
30-518328 (fax)

Home Address:
3405-63111 (home)

ISS Member 1981

Spouse: Mrs. J. A. Duursma-Nolle

EARWAKER, JOHN W.S. FRACR

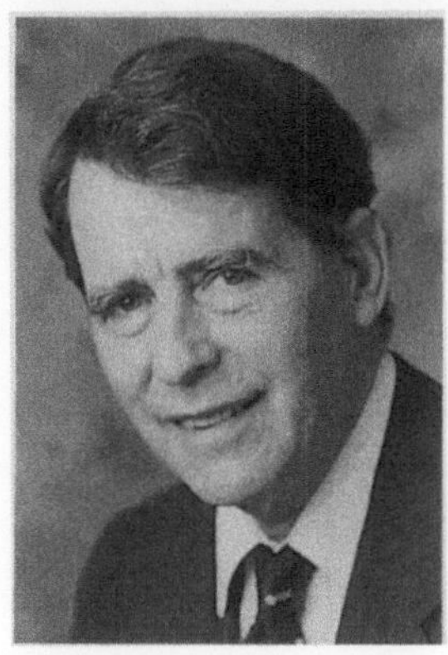

Birthdate: May 7, 1939

Academic Title: Dr.

Position at Affiliation: Consultant Radiologist

Business Address:
Holy Spirit Hospital
Department of Medical Imaging
259 Wickham Terrace
Brisbane QLD 4000
Australia
61 7 3839 5530 (work)
61 7 3831 1026 (fax)

Home Address:
101 Windsor Road
Red Hill QLD 4059
Australia
61 7 3369 5356 (home)
61 7 3217 6701 (fax)

Specialty/Certification: Radiology, 1968

Education:
1962 – University of Qld (MBBS)
1968 – FRACR
1970 – FRCR

ISS Member 1993

Spouse: Elizabeth

ECKARDT, JEFFREY J. M.D.

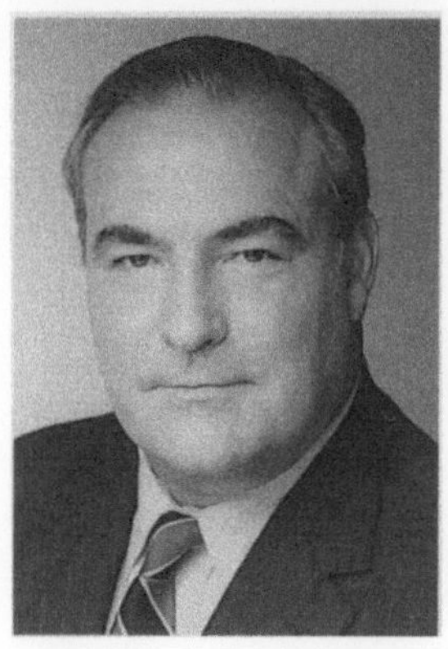

Birthdate: November 23, 1945

Academic Title: Professor of Orthopaedic Surgery

Position at Affiliation: Chief, Section of Musculoskeletal Oncology

Business Address:
U.C.L.A. Medical Center
Division of Orthopaedic Surgery
10833 Le Conte Avenue
Los Angeles, CA 90095-6902
U.S.A.
310-206-6503 (work)
310-206-0063 (fax)
Jeckardt@ortho.medsch.ucla.edu
(e-mail)

Home Address:
3308 Patricia Avenue
Los Angeles, Ca 90064
U.S.A.
310-206-6503 (home)

Specialty/Certification: Orthopaedic Surgery, 1981

Education:
1967 – Williams College
1971 – Cornell University Medical College (M.D.)
1975–79 – UCLA (residency)
1979–81 – Mayo Clinic (Orthopaedic Oncoloy fellowship)

ISS Member 1984

Spouse: Mary

Edeiken, Jack M.D.

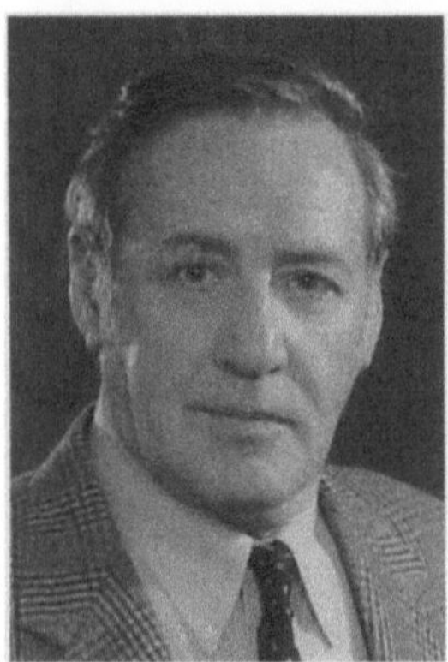

Birthdate: May 25, 1923

Academic Title: Professor

Home Address:
7 Wellington Lane
Sugar Land, TX 77478
U.S.A.
281-491-9356 (home)

Specialty/Certification: Radiology, 1951

Education:
Villanova
University of Pennsylvania Medical
School (Radiology)

ISS Member Founding member

Offices Held in ISS and Dates of Service:
Secretary Treasurer 1974-80
President Elect 1980-82
President 1982-84

ISS Committees:
Executive Committee
Editorial Committee
Endowment Committee
Future Planning Committee

ISS Medals and Awards:
Founders' Lecture, San Diego, 1991

Spouse: Toni

Edeiken-Monroe, Beth S. M.D., FACR

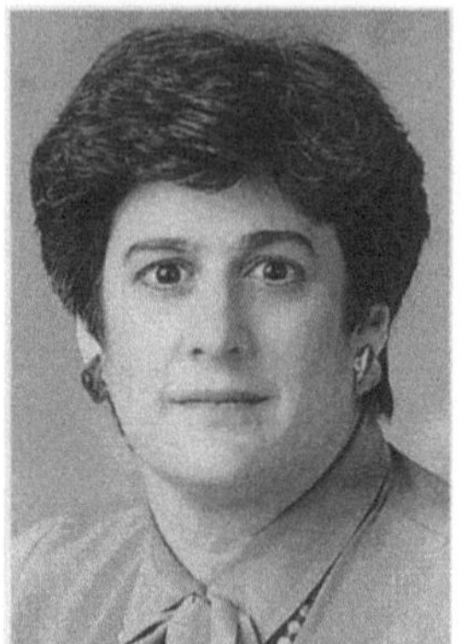

Birthdate: January 27, 1948

Academic Title: Associate Professor

Position at Affiliation: Radiologist

Business Address:
Department of Diagnostic Radiology –
Box 57
The University of Texas M.D. Anderson
Cancer Center
1515 Holcombe Boulevard
Houston, TX 77030
U.S.A.
713-792-7784 (work)
713-745-1399 (fax)
bethedeiken@diagimaging.mda.uth.tmc.
edu (e-mail)

Home Address:
12 Shadder Way
Houston, TX 77019
U.S.A.
713-524-0029 (home)
713-524-2369 (fax)

Specialty/Certification: Radiology, 1979

Education:
Temple University, Philadelphia, PA (B.S.)
Jefferson Medical College, Philadelphia,
PA (M.D.)
Jefferson Medical College, Philadelphia,
PA (residency)
University of Texas, Houston, TX
(residency)

ISS Member 1986

Spouse: Matthew T. Monroe, M.D.

EDHOLM, PAUL M.D.

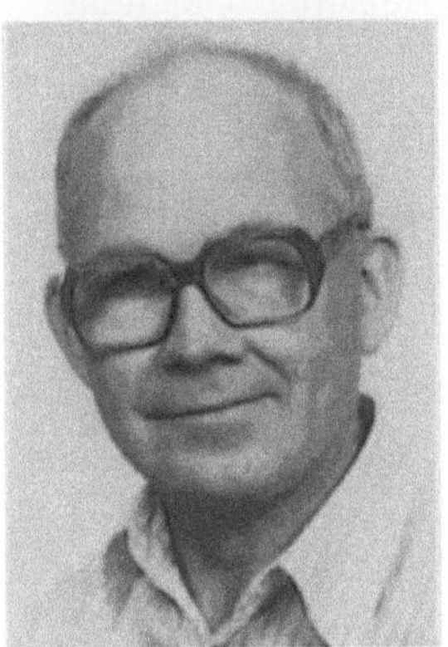

Business Address:
University of Linkoping
Regionsjukhuset
S-581 85 Linkoping
Sweden
013-192710 (work)
013-103132 (home)

ISS Member 1980

Spouse: Else

EGUND, NIELS M.D., PH.D.

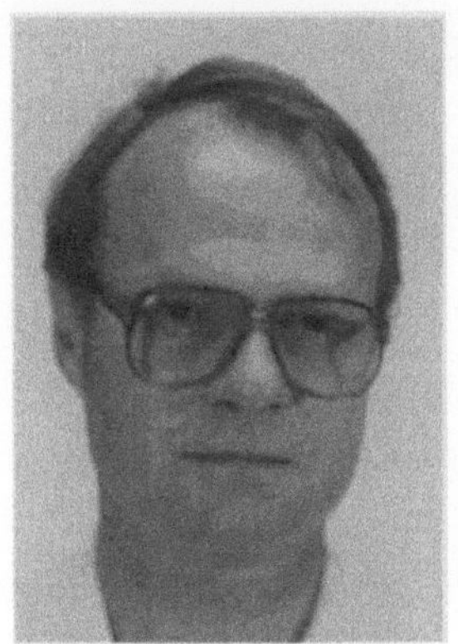

Birthdate: July 15, 1939

Academic Title: Professor

Position at Affiliation: Professor,
Chief of Division, Orthopaedic
Radiology

Business Address:
Department of Radiology R
Aarhus University Hospital
Århus Kommune Hospital
DK-8000 Århus C
Denmark
45 89 49 23 94 (work)
45 89 49 24 10 (fax)

Specialty: Radiology

Education:
1968 – University of Copenhagen (M.D.)
1968–74 University Hospital, Lund,
Sweden (Radiology residency)

ISS Member 1987

EHARA, SHIGERU M.D., D.M.Sc

ISS Member 1990

ISS Committees:
Committee for Promotion of Refresher
Course, 1994

Spouse: Keiko

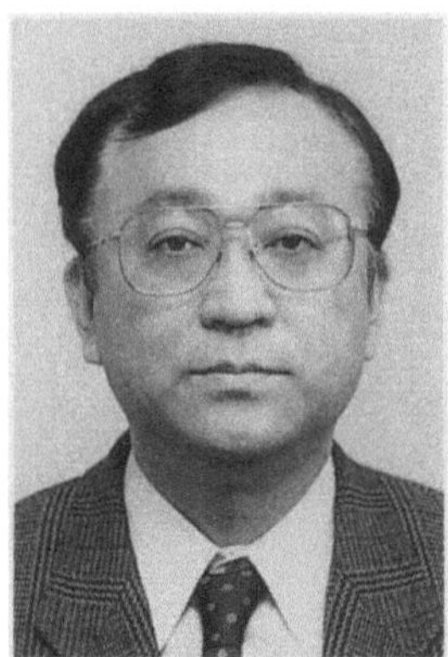

Birthdate: April 19, 1953

Academic Title: Associate Professor
of Radiology

Position at Affiliation: Associate
Director, Department of Radiology

Business Address:
Department of Radiology
Iwate Medical University School
of Medicine
19-1 Uchimaru
Morioka 020
Japan
81-196-51-5111 ext. 3689 (work)
81-196-51-7071 (fax)
ehara@iwate-med.ac.jp (e-mail)

Home Address:
2-2-12 Ueda, #102
Morioka 020
Japan
81-196-23-8394 (home)
81-196-23-8394 (fax)

Specialty/Certification: Radiology, 1986,
1990

Education:
1979 – Tohoku University School
of Medicine (M.D.)
1982–86 – St. Luke's Roosevelt Hospital
Center (residency)
1986–87 – Univ. of Iowa (fellowship
Skeletal Radiology)

EKELUND, LEIF A. M.D., PH.D.

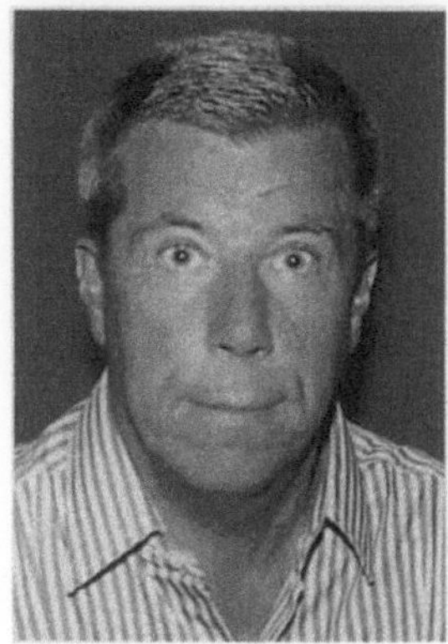

Birthdate: March 18, 1941

Academic Title: Professor of Diagnostic Radiology

Position at Affiliation: Professor and Chairman

Business Address:
Department of Radiology
FMHS
United Arab Emirates University
Al Ain
United Arab Emirates
971-3-679200 (work)
971-3-671278 (fax)
radio@medic.uaeu.ac.ae (e-mail)

Home Address:
P.O. Box 17666
Al Ain
United Arab Emirates

Specialty: Radiology, 1971

Education:
University of Lund, Sweden (specialty training)

ISS Member 1984

Spouse: Karen

EL-KHOURY, GEORGE Y. M.D., B.SC.

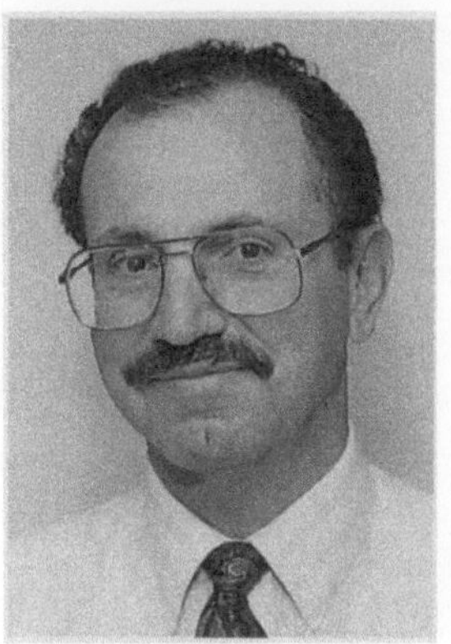

Academic Title: Professor of Radiology and Orthopaedics

Position at Affiliation: Director of Diagnosis

Business Address:
Department of Radiology
University of Iowa Hospitals and Clinics
Iowa City, IA 52242
U.S.A.
319-356-3654 (work)
319-356-2220 (fax)
george-el-khoury@uiowa.edu (e-mail)

Home Address:
44 Hunters Place
Iowa City, IA
U.S.A.
319-351-5161 (home)

Specialty/Certification: Radiology, 1973

Education:
1965–69 – American University of Beirut (B.S.)
1969 – American University of Beirut Hospital (M.D.)
1971 – American University of Beirut (Diagnostic Radiology residency)
1973 – University of Iowa (Diagnostic Radiology residency)

ISS Member 1984

ISS Committees:
Editorial Board of Skeletal Radiology
Multiple Committees

Spouse: Salam

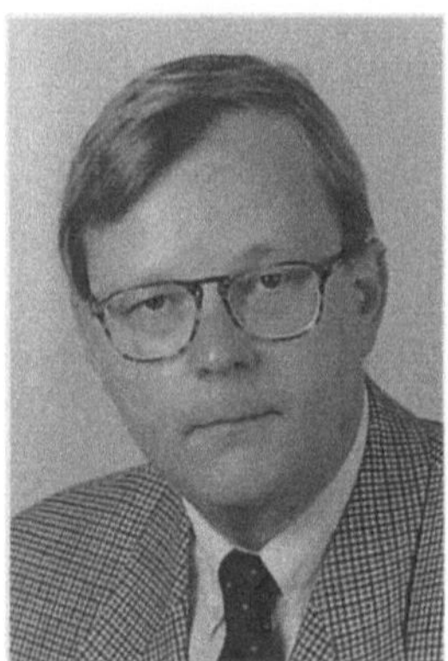

Birthdate: September 17, 1955

Academic Title: Professor of Radiology

Position at Affiliation: Chefarzt (Head of Department)

Business Address:
Institut fuer Radiologie
St. Johannes Hospital
An der Abtei 7–11
47166 Duisburg
Germany
0203-546-2660 (work)
0203-546-2659 (fax)

Home Address:
Raiffeisenstr. 26 A
46535 Dinslaken
Germany
02064-58313 (home)

Specialty/Certification: Radiology, 1987

Education:
Le University of Mulster
1982–87 – Clemens Hospital and
Dept. of Radiology
Le Univ. of Mulster, Germany (resident)

ISS Member 1992

Spouse: Rita

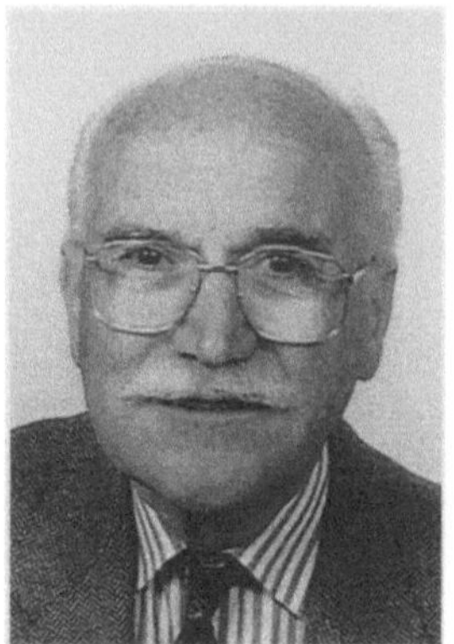

Birthdate: September 10, 1920

Academic Title: Professor (retired)

Business Address:
Hôpital d'Enfants Armand-Trousseau
26 avenue du Dr Arnold-Netter
75012 Paris
France
33-1-44736124 (work)
33-1-44736511 (fax)

Home Address:
74 rue Escudier
92100 Boulogne
France
33-1-48252351 (home)

Specialty: Radiology

Education:
1946 – Resident in Radiology

ISS Member 1977

ISS Medals and Awards:
Founders' Lecture, Cannes, 1987

Spouse: Micheline

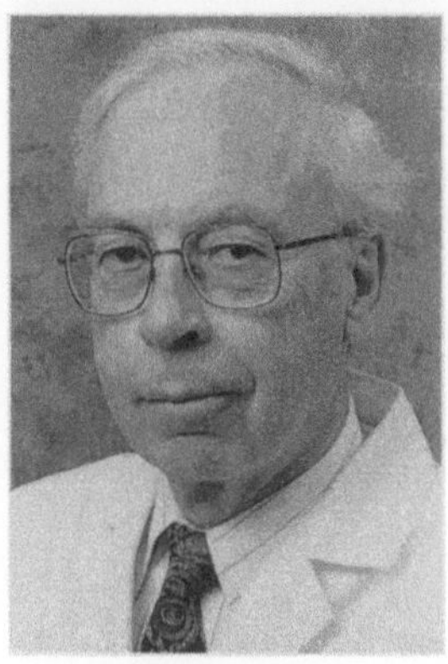

Birthdate: February 17, 1936

Academic Title: Professor of Pathology

Position at Affiliation: Director of Anatomic Pathology

Business Address:
University of Virginia Medical Center
Department of Pathology
Charlottesville, VA 22908
U.S.A.
804-982-4403 (work)
894-924-0217 (fax)
ref@virginia.edu (e-mail)

Home Address:
217 E. Jefferson Street
Charlottesville, VA 22908
U.S.A.

Specialty/Certification: Pathology, 1966

Education:
1960 – Washington University School
of Medicine (M.D.)
1960–64 – Barnes Hospital, (Pathology
residency)

ISS Member 1982

ISS Committees:
Editorial Board – Skeletal Radiology,
1984–96

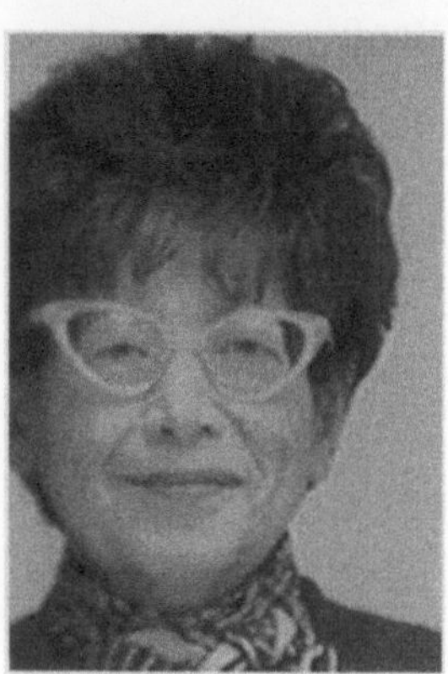

Academic Title: Professor of Radiology
and Orthopedics

Position at Affiliate: Attending Radiologist

Business Address:
Department of Radiology
Columbia-Presybterian Medical Center
622 West 168th Street
New York, NY 10032
U.S.A.
212-305-9869 or 212-305-2986 (work)
212-305-3028 (fax)

Home Address:
417 West 246th Street
Bronx, NY 10032
U.S.A.

Specialty: Radiology

Education:
New York University – Bellevue School
of Medicine
Beth Israel, Bellevue, Columbia
Presbyterian Medical (residency in
Radiology)

ISS Member: Founding Member

ISS Committees:
Refresher Course Committee
Education & Instruction Committee
Liaison Future Planning Committee

Ad Hoc Committee for Fellowship
Accreditation of Musculoskeletal
Radiology
Chairman, Ad Hoc Proceedings
Committee
Chairman, Corinne Farrel Prize
Committee
Nomenclature Committee

Spouse: Prof. Rubem Pochaczevsky,
M.D., FACR

Business Address: Radiology Department
New York University Medical Center
Tisch Hospital
560 First Avenue
New York, NY 10016
U.S.A.

Specialty: Radiology

ISS Member 1978

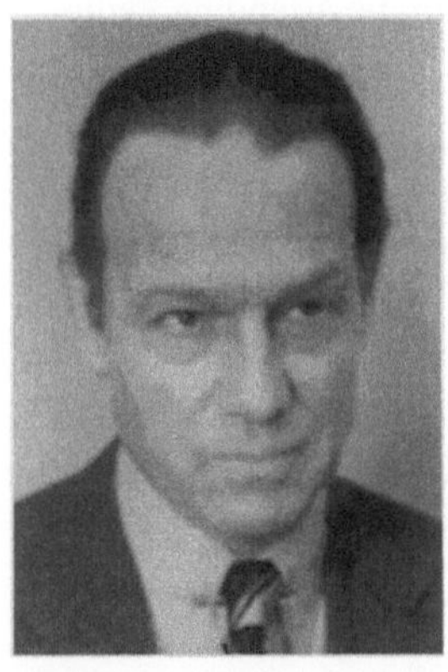

Business Address:
105 East 65th Street
New York, NY 10021
U.S.A.
212-877-3544 (home)

Specialty: Orthopaedic Surgery

ISS Member 1987

Spouse: Doris

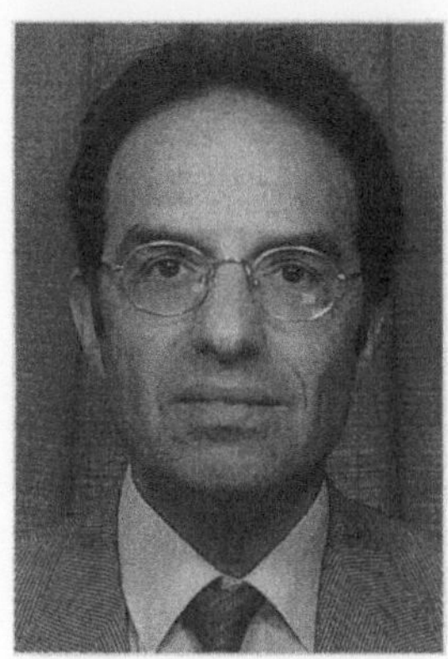

Birthdate: September 4, 1948

Academic Title: Professor

Position at Affiliation: Consultant Physician in Nuclear Medicine

Business Address:
Guy's Hospital
Department of Nuclear Medicine
St. Thomas Street
London, SE 1 9 RT
England
171-955-4593 (work)
171-955-4657 (fax)
i.fogelman@umds.ac.uk (e-mail)

Home Address:
16 Canons Drive
Edgware
Middlesex HA8 7QS
England
181-952-2966 (home)
181-381-1368 (fax)

Specialty/Certification: Internal Medicine/Endocrinology/Nuclear Medicine, 1982

Education:
University of Glasgow, Scotland (M.D.)
Royal Infirmary, Glasgow, Scotland (specialty training)

ISS Member 1988

Spouse: Coral

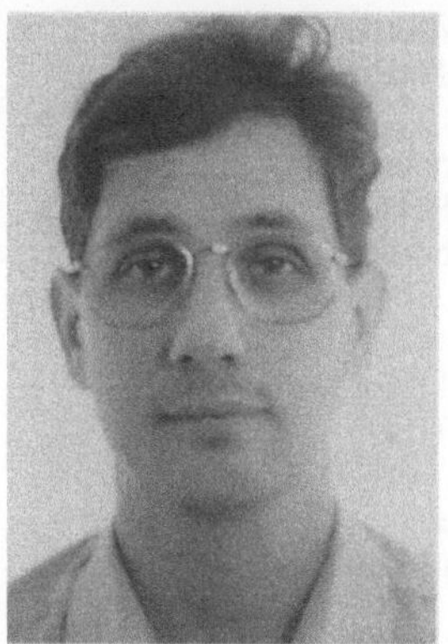

Birthdate: February 5, 1958

Position at Affiliation: Research fellow

Business Address:
Brigham and Women's Hospital
Radiology Department
75 Francis Street
Boston, MA 02115
U.S.A.
617-732-6295 (work)
617-278-6976 (fax)
karoly@bwh.harvard.edu (e-mail)

Home Address:
70 St. Paul Street #3
Brookline, MA 02146
U.S.A.
617-738-2959 (home)

Specialty/Certification: Radiology, 1988; Rheumatology, 1992

Education:
Semmelweis (M.D.)

ISS Member 1996

Spouse: Andrea

Position at Affiliation: Chairman, Department of Pathology

Business Address:
CHU Cochin-Port Royal
27 rue du Faubourg St. Jacques
75014, Paris
France
33-1-42341450 (work)
33-1-44412519 (fax)

Home Address:
153 avenue du Maine
75014 Paris
France
33-1-45393789 (home)

Specialty: Pathology

ISS Member: 1992

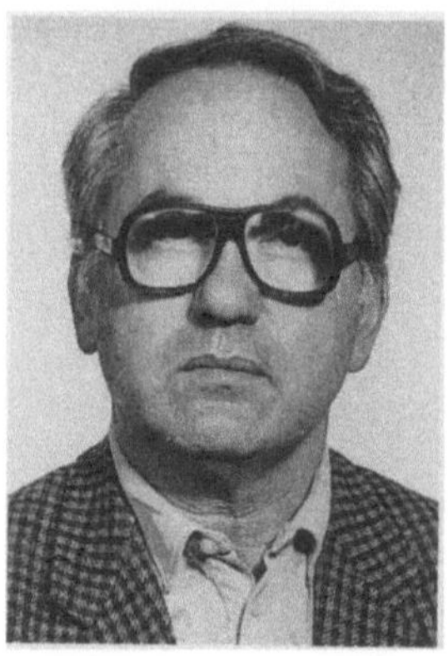

Academic Title: Professor of Radiology

Position at Affiliation: Head, Department of Radiology

Business Address:
Uzsoki Hospital
Department of Diagnostic Radiology
1145 Budapest, Uzsoki u.29.
Hungary
36 1 251 7333 or 36 1 220 9949 (work)

Home Address:
1075 Budapest
Karoly KRT 7.
Hungary
36 1-267 9639 (home)
36 1-3429-314 (fax)

Specialty: Radiology

Education:
Semmelweis Medical Univ., Budapest
(M.D.)
Radiological Clinic, Budapest (specialty
training)

ISS Member 1991

ISS Committees:
Committee for the Promotion of the
Refresher Course Outside of North
America

Spouse: Katalin

Fornage, Bruno M.D.

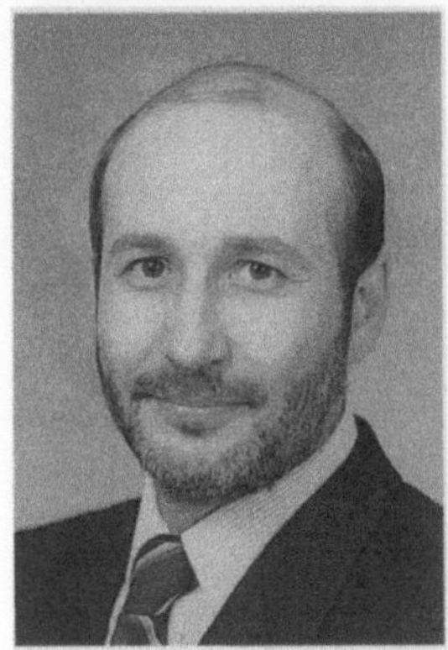

Birthdate: July 2, 1949

Academic Title: Professor of Radiology

Position at Affiliation: Chief of Ultrasound

Business Address:
The University of Texas M.D. Anderson Cancer Center
Department of Diagnostic Radiology, Box 57
1515 Holcombe Boulevard
Houston, TX 77030-4095
U.S.A.
713-794-1424 (work)
713-745-1153 (fax)
bruno_fornage@diag-imaging.mdacc.tmc.edu (e-mail)

Home Address:
4902 Palmetto
Bellaire, Texas 77401
U.S.A.
713-432-7776 (home)
713-432-1213 (fax)

Specialty: Radiology

ISS Member 1991

Spouse: Brigitte

Fornasier, Victor L. M.D., FRCPC

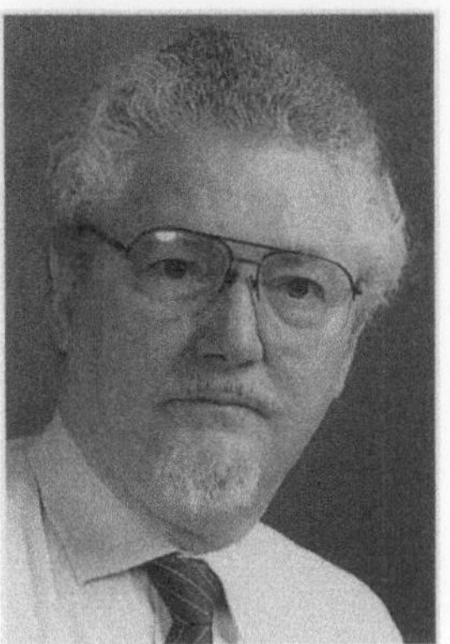

Birthdate: November 8, 1937

Academic Title: Associate Professor of Pathology & Surgery

Position at Affiliation: Pathologist-in-Chief

Business Address:
The Wellesley Central Hospital
Anatomic Pathology & Cytology
160 Wellesley Street East
Toronto, Ontario M4Y 1J3
Canada
416-926-7714 (work)
416-926-4897 (fax)
vamf@msn.com (e-mail)

Home Address:
4 Cotillion Court
Etobicoke, Ontario M9A 4S8
Canada
416-248-0870 (home)
416-248-0870 (fax)

Specialty: Pathology

Education:
University of Toronto (M.D.)
Hamilton (internship)
Toronto (FRCPC)
Royal National Institute of Orthopaedics, London, England (McLaughlin Traveling Fellow)

ISS Member 1979

ISS Committees:
Meeting Planning Committee
Local Arrangements Committee
Nomenclature Committee
Closed Program Committee

Spouse: Mary

FORRESTER, DEBORAH M. M.D.

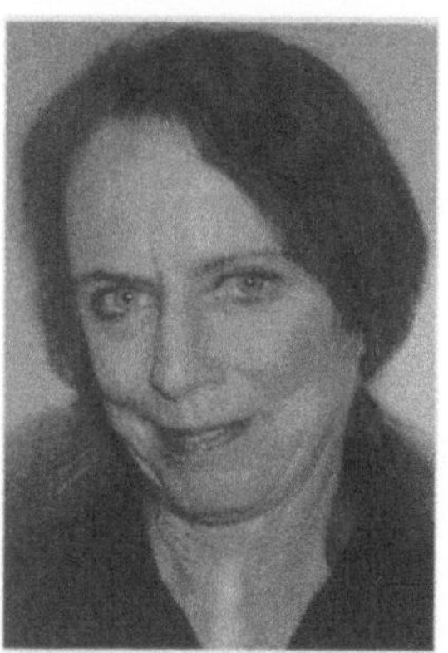

Academic Title: Associate Professor

Position at Affiliation: Chief, Musculo-skeletal Section

Business Address:
Department of Radiology
LA County USC Medical Center
1200 N. State St.
Los Angeles
CA 90033
U.S.A.
213-226-7242 (work)
213-226-2280 (fax)
forreste@usc.usc.edu

Home Address:
5900 Filare Hts. Avenue
Malibu, CA 90265
U.S.A.
310-457-2964 (home)
310-589-5939 (fax)

Specialty/Certification: Radiology, 1964

Education:
Swarthmore College (B.A.)
UCSF (MA, Physiology)
1969 – University of Pennsylvania (M.D.)

ISS Member 1987

Spouse: John C. Brown, M.D.

FOTTER, RICHARD M.D.

Birthdate: August 21, 1946

Academic Title: Professor

Position at Affiliation: Chairman

Business Address:
Department of Radiology, Division of
Pediatric Radiology
University Hospital Graz
A-8036 Graz
Austria
43 316 385 4203 (work)
43 316 385 4299 (fax)

Home Address:
Amschlgassezz
A-8010 Graz
Austria
43 316 685163 (home)

Specialty/Certification: Radiology, 1980;
Pediatric Radiology, 1982

ISS Member 1991

Spouse: Karin

FRASSICA, FRANK J. M.D.

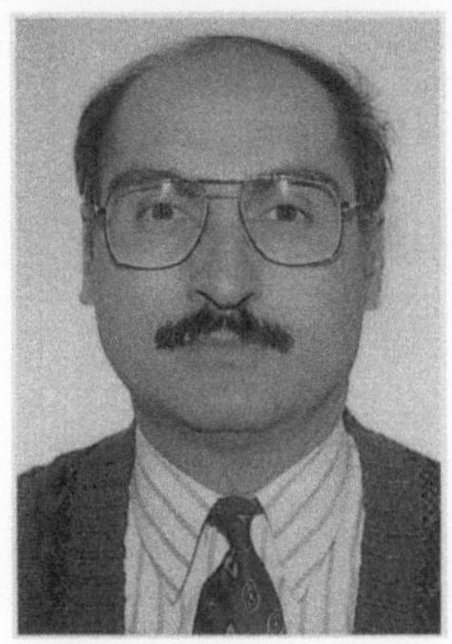

Academic Title: Associate Professor

Position at Affiliation: Chief of Adult
Orthopaedics and
Reconstructive Surgery

Business Address:
Johns Hopkins University
JHOC 5223
601 North Caroline Street
Baltimore, MD 21287-0882
U.S.A.
410-955-9414 (work)
410-955-1719 (fax)

Home Address:
46688 Willowgrove Drive
Elliott City, MD 21042
U.S.A.
410-715-1431 (home)

Specialty/Certification: Orthopaedic
Surgery, 1990

Education:
1975 – U.S. Naval Academy (B.S.)
1982 – Medical University of South
Carolina (M.D.)
Mayo Clinic – Ortho and Oncology

ISS Member 1996

Spouse: Deborah Anne

Business Address:
2208 Arden Road
Baltimore, MD 21209
U.S.A.

ISS Member 1974

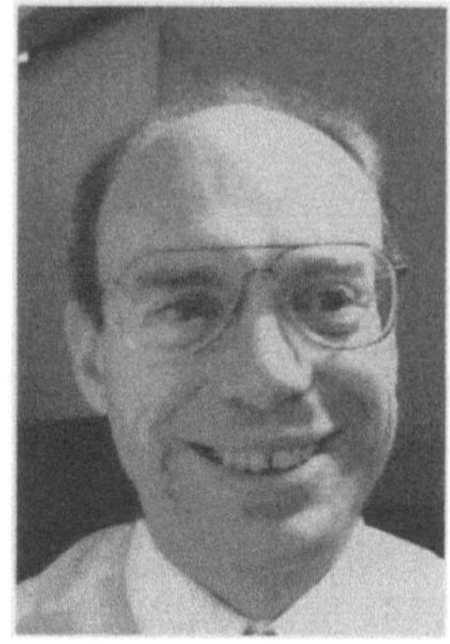

Birthdate: March 24, 1953

Academic Title: Professor

Position at Affiliation: Professor of
Osteoarticular Pathology

Business Address:
University of Manchester
Stopford Building, Oxford Road
Manchester, M139PT
England
161-275-5268 (work)
161-275-5268 (fax)
tony.freemont@man.ac.uk (e-mail)

Home Address:
10, Harewood Avenue, Sale,
Cheshire, M335BY
England
161-973-1869 (home)
161-976-6879 (fax)

Specialty/Certification: Pathology, 1976

Education:
St. Thomas Hospital Medical School,
London, England

ISS Member: 1994

Spouse: Susan

FREIBERGER, ROBERT H. M.D.

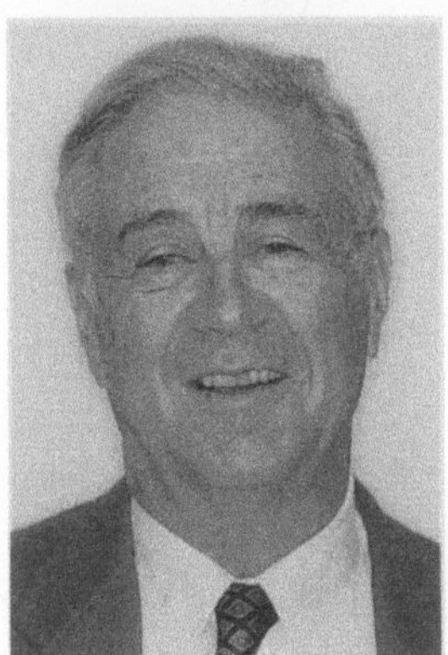

Academic Title: Professor of Radiology

Position at Affiliation: Attending Radiologist

Business Address:
Radiology Department
The Hospital for Special Surgery
535 East 70th Streets
New York, NY 10021
U.S.A.
212-606-1936 (work)
212-734-7378 (fax)

Home Address:
31 Bogart Road
Demarest, NJ 07627
U.S.A.
201-768-4013 (home)

Specialty/Certification: Radiology, 1953

Education:
1949 – Tufts University (MD)

ISS Member Founding member

ISS Medals and Awards:
Founders' Lecture, New Orleans, 1995

Spouse: Eva J.

FREYSCHMIDT, JÜRGEN W. M.D.,
PROF. DR. MED.

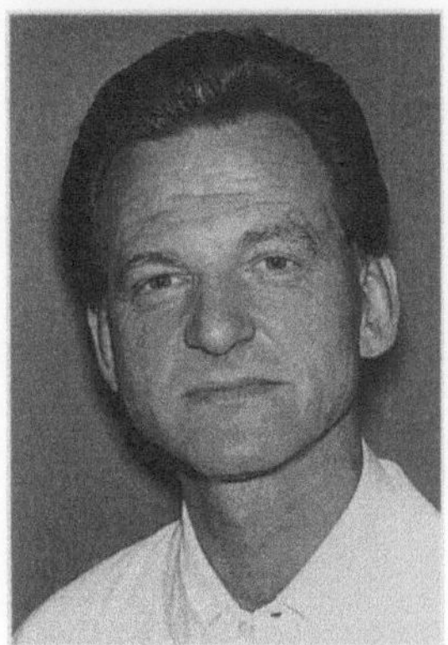

Birthdate: August 3, 1940

Academic Title: Professor Dr. med.

Position at Affiliation: Director,
Department of Radiology

Business Address:
Department of Diagnostic Radiology
Central-Kankenhaus, St.-Jürgen-Straße
28205 Bremen
Germany
0421-497-5430 (work)
0421-497-3328 (fax)

Home Address:
Oberneulanderlandstr. 58
28355 Bremen
Germany
0421-25 95 32 (home)

Specialty: Radiology

Education:
University of Goettingen
University of Hannover

ISS Member 1979

ISS Committees:
Membership Committee 1995–96

Spouse: Gisela Freyschmidt, Dr. med

Friedlaender, Gary E. M.D.

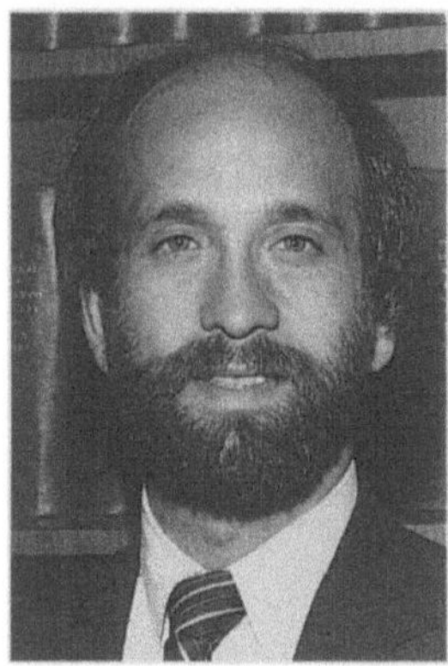

Academic Title: Professor of Orthopaedics and Rehabilitation

Position at Affiliation: Chairman, Orthopaedics and Rehabilitation

Business Address:
Yale University School of Medicine
Department of Orthopaedics
and Rehabilitation
P. O. Box 208071
New Haven, CT 06520-8071
U.S.A.
203-737-5660 (work)
203-785-7132 (fax)
gary.friedlaender@quickmail.yale.edu

Home Address:
15 Old Still Road
Woodbridge, CT 06525
U.S.A.
203-393-2873 (home)

Specialty/Certification: Orthopaedic Surgery, 1975

Education:
1967 – Kényon College/University of Michigan (B.S.)
1969 – University of Michigan (M.D.)
1971–74 – Yale New Haven Hospital (resident)
1983 – Massachusetts General Hospital (Musculoskeletal fellowship)

ISS Member 1988

Spouse: Linda

Friedman, Lawrence MBBCh, FRCPC, FACR, FFRAD,(D) SA

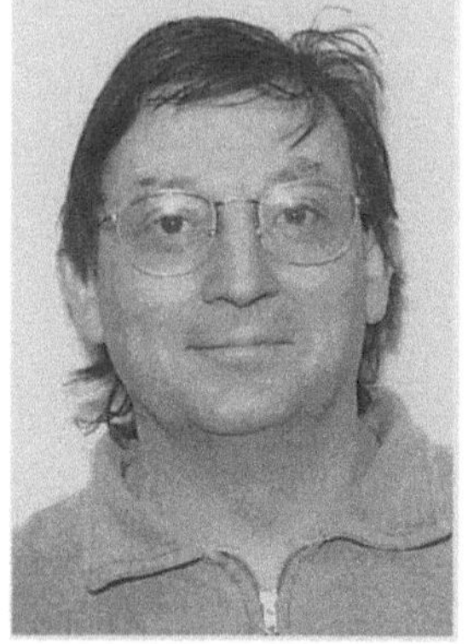

Birthdate: June 1, 1952

Academic Title: Clinical Associate Professor McMaster

Position at Affiliation: Chief of Radiology

Business Address:
Guelph General Hospital
115 Delhi Street, Guelph
Ontario N1E 4J4
Canada
519-822-5350 ext. 307 (work)
law@1com.ca (e-mail)

Home Address:
6 Parkway Place
Dundas
Ontario L9H 6K4
Canada
905-628-4591 (home)
905-627-8099 (fax)

Specialty: Radiology

Education:
1984 – FFRAD (DJSA)
1987 – FRCPC
1990 – FACR

ISS Member 1992

Spouse: Elaine

Garcia, Jean F. M.D.

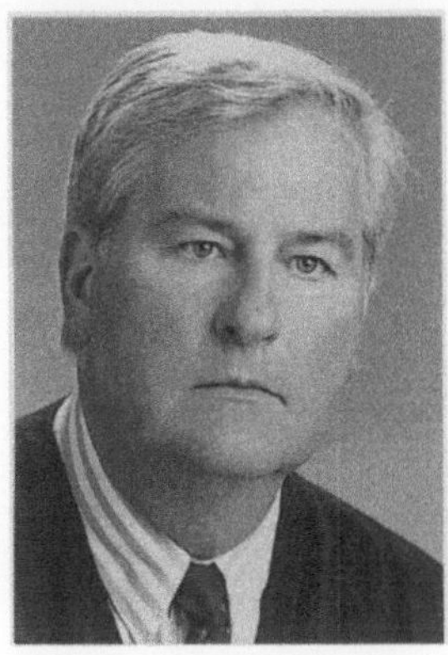

Birthdate: November 30, 1937

Academic Title: Professor of Radiology

Position at Affiliation: Vice-Chairman

Business Address:
Department of Radiologie
Hopital Cantonal Universitaire
Rue Micheli Du Crest
Geneva
Switzerland
41-22-3723311 (work)
41-22-3727072 (fax)

Home Address:
52 Route De Cara
1243 Presinge
Switzerland
41-227591382 (home)

Specialty/Certification: Radiology, 1974

Education:
University of Geneva (Medical Studies,
Radiology)
Fellowship at UCSF – Oct – Dec 1976;
RNOH in London (1977)
Special training in MRI (USA 1984),
(Belgium and USA 1987)

ISS Member 1985

Spouse: Ursula

Gebhardt, Mark C. M.D.

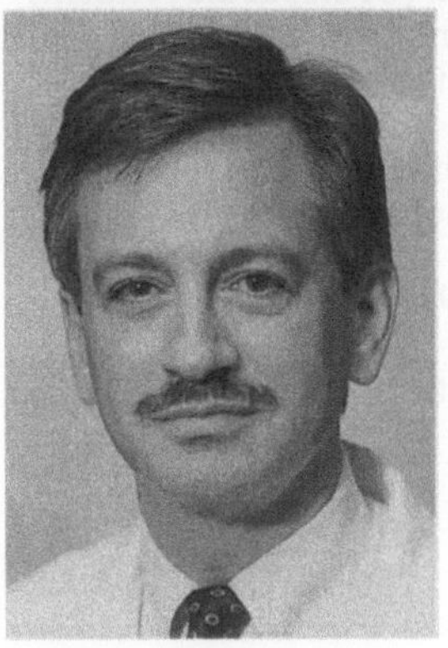

Birthdate: July 17, 1949

Academic Title: Associate Professor of
Orthopedic Surgery

Position at Affiliation: Associate Orthopaedic Surgeon, Associate Professor
of Orthopaedic Surgery

Business Address: Massachusetts
General Hospital
Orthopaedic Surgery
32 Fruit Street – Gray 606
Boston, MA 02114
U.S.A.
617-724-3700 (work)
617-726-6823 (fax)
gebhardtm@al.mgh.harvard.edu
(e-mail)

Home Address:
44 Willow Cresen
Brookline, MA 02146
U.S.A.
617-734-0048 (home)

Specialty/Certification: Orthopaedic
Surgery, 1985

Education:
1971 – Bucknell University (B.S.)
1975 – University of Cincinnati, College
of Medicine (M.D.)
1975–77 – Univ. Health Center of
Pittsburgh, Pittsburgh, PA (internship
and residency)

1977–78 – University of Pittsburgh
(surgical fellow)
1978–82 – Harvard combined orthopaedic program (Orthopaedic resident)
1982 – Children's Hospital Medical
Center (fellow in Pediatric Orthopaedic
Surgery)
1983 – Massachusetts General Hospital
(fellow in Orthopaedic Oncology)

ISS Member 1991

Spouse: Paulette

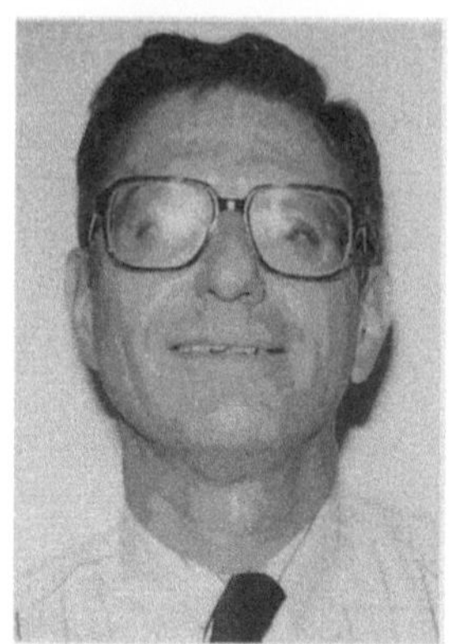

Birthdate: January 26, 1939

Position at Affiliation: Chairman,
Department of Radiology

Business Address:
Pioneer Valley Hospital
3460 South Pioneer Parkway
West Valley City, UT 84120
U.S.A.
801-964-3619 (work)
801-964-3247 (fax)
mgelman@pol.net (e-mail)

Home Address:
4504 Parkview Drive
Salt Lake City, Utah 84124
U.S.A.
801-272-2522 (home)

Specialty: Radiology

Education:
1956–60 – Temple University (B.S.)
1960–64 – Temple University Medical
School (M.D.)
1967–71 – Thomas Jefferson University
Hospital (Radiology residency)

ISS Member Founding member

Spouse: Sheila

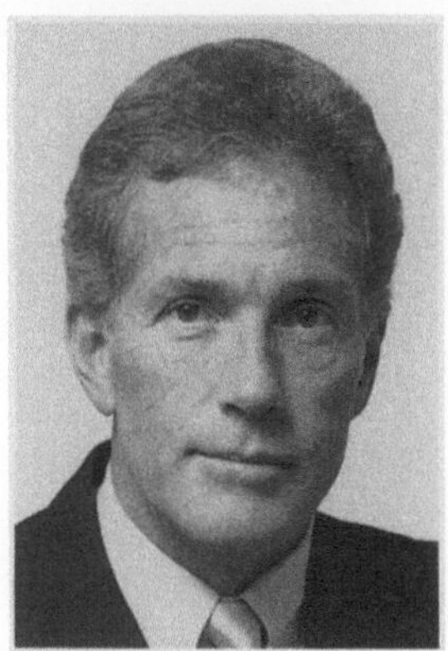

Birthdate: August 14, 1942

Academic Title: Professor

Position at Affiliation: Professor of Radiology, Medicine & Orthopaedic Surgery; Chief, Musculoskeletal Radiology; Executive Director, Osteoporosis Research Group

Business Address:
Department of Radiology
University of California San Francisco
San Francisco, CA 94143
U.S.A.
415-476-4864 (work)
415-476-8550 (fax)
harry-genant@radmac1.ucsf.edu (e-mail)

Home Address:
7 Tara Hill Road
Tiburon, CA 94920
U.S.A.
415-435-3543 (home)

Specialty/Certification: Radiology, 1973

Education:
1960 – 63 – University of Illinois, Urbana (Pre-med)
1963 – 67 – Northwestern University, Chicago, IL (B.S., M.D.)
1967 – 68 – Johns Hopkins (Osler Medical Service), Baltimore, MD (internship)
1968 – 72 – The University of Chicago, IL (resident in Radiology)

ISS Member Founding member

Offices Held in ISS and Dates of Service:
Secretary, 1996 –

ISS Committees:
Membership Committee, Chairman, 1991 – 94
Committee for Evaluation of Research Travel Grants, 1994 – 96
Executive Committee – 1993 – present

Spouse: Gail Genant, M.D.

GERSHUNI, DAVID H. M.D.

Business Address:
Department of Orthopaedic Surgery
Veterans Administration Medical Center
3350 La Jolla Village Drive
San Diego, CA 92161
U.S.A.
619-453-6933 (home)
619-552-8585 ext. 3841 (work)
619-543-2540 (fax)

Specialty: Orthopaedic Surgery

ISS Member 1989

Spouse: Nina

GIEDION, ANDRES H. PROF. DR. MED.

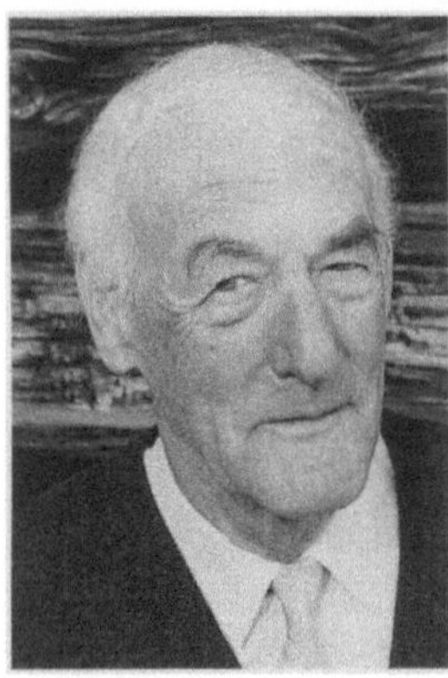

Birthdate: May 2, 1925

Academic Title: Professor of Pediatrics

Position at Affiliation: Chief Emeritus, Senior Consultant

Business Address:
Dept. of Radiology
Children's Hospital
University of Zurich
8032 Zurich
Switzerland
01-266-7111 (work)
01-266-7771 (fax)

Home Address:
Doldertal 7
8032 Zurich
Switzerland
01-251-7767 (home)

Specialty/Certification: Pediatrics, 1955

Education:
University of Zurich Medical School
University of Paris Medical School
Childrens Medical Center, Boston, MA
(Pediatrics and Pediatric Radiology)
Children's Hospital (Childrens University
Clinic), Zurich (Pediatrics)

ISS Member 1987

Spouse: Monica Risch

GILSANZ, VICENTE M.D., PH.D.

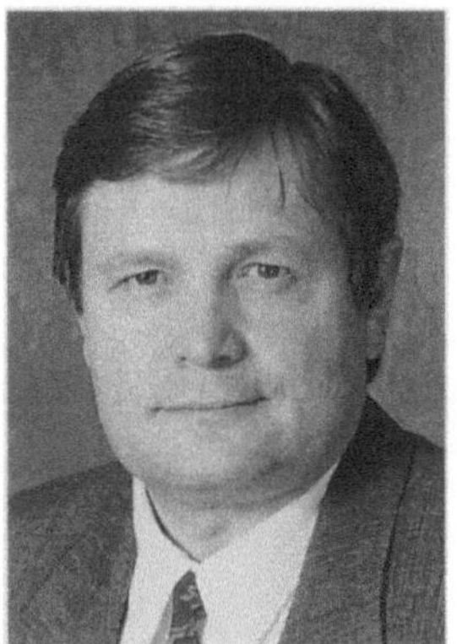

Birthdate: September 16, 1946

Academic Title: Professor of Radiology

Position at Affiliation: Radiologist

Business Address:
Childrens Hospital of Los Angeles
Radiology Department MS #81
4650 Sunset Boulevard
Los Angeles, CA 90027
U.S.A.
213-669-4571 (work)
213-666-7816 (fax)
gilsanz@hsc.usc.edu (e-mail)

Home Address:
15231 Via de las Olas
Pacific Palisades, CA 90272
U.S.A.

Specialty/Certification: Internal Medicine, 1973; Radiology 1976

Education:
1969 – Facultad de Medicina, Madrid,
Spain (M.D.)
1976 – Universidad Complutense,
Madrid, Spain (Ph.D.)
1971–73 – Mayo Medical School,
(residency internal Medicine)
1976–78 – Harvard Medical School,
Boston, MA (fellowship Pediatric
Radiology)

ISS Member 1989

Spouse: Maria Ines Boechat

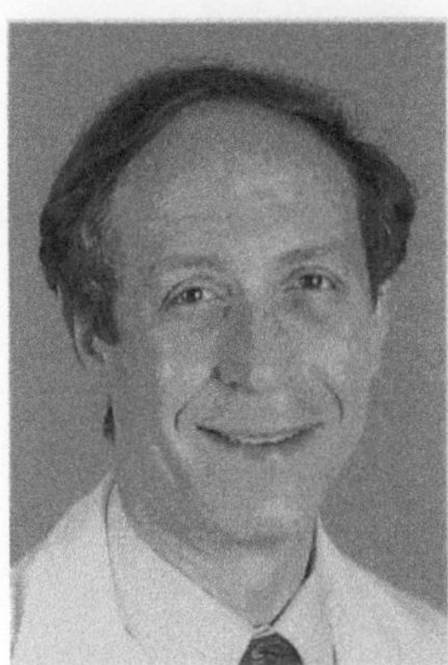

Birthdate: October 21, 1942

Academic Title: Professor of Radiology, Orthopedic Surgery and Plastic Surgery

Position at Affiliation: Director, Musculoskeletal Radiology

Business Address:
The Edward Mallinckrodt Institute of Radiology
Washington University
510 South Kingshighway Boulevard
St. Louis, MO 63110
U.S.A.
314-362-2911 (work)
314-362-4660 (fax)
gilula@mirlink.wustl.edu (e-mail)

Home Address:
250 Dielman Road
St. Louis, MO 63124
U.S.A.
314-997-4487 (home)

Specialty/Certification: Radiology, 1973

Education:
University of Illinois School of Medicine, Chicago, IL (M.D.)
San Francisco General Hospital, San Francisco, CA (internship)
Max C. Starkloff Memorial, St. Louis City Hospital, St. Louis, MO (residency)

ISS Member 1978

ISS Awards and Medals:
Medal of the ISS (Silver), Dublin, 1998

ISS Committees:
1983–85 – Member, Executive Committee
1983–89 – ISS Refresher Course Program Committee
1985–87 – Chairman, Ad Hoc Committee on Refresher Course Planning
1985–88 – Co-Chairman, Ad Hoc Convention Planning Committee
1986 – Co-Chairman, Refresher Course Committee, Vancouver
1986 – Member, Ad hoc Liaison & Future Planning Committee
1988–94 – Member, Awards Committee
1989 – present – Chairman, Convention Planning Committee

Spouse: Deborah

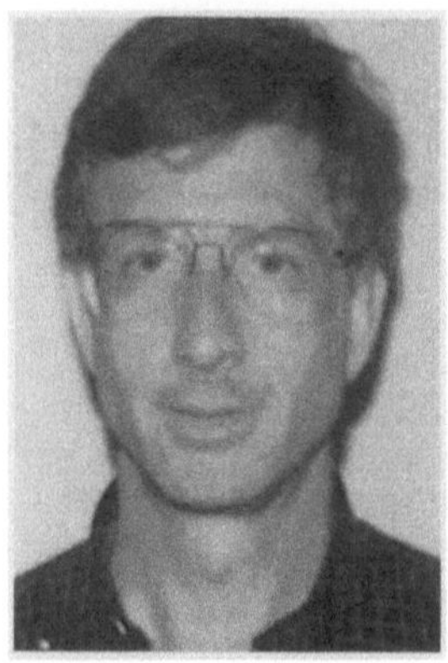

Birthdate: May 28, 1942

Academic Title: Associate Professor

Business Address:
Department of Radiology
Palomar Medical Center
555 East Valley Parkway
Escondido, CA 92025
U.S.A.
619-739-5400 (work)
619-739-3232 (fax)
tgoergen@aol.com (e-mail)

Home Address:
P.O. Box 8037
Rancho Santa Fe, CA 92067-8037
U.S.A.
619-756-3696 (home)

Specialty/Certification: Radiology, 1974;
Nuclear Medicine, 1975

Education:
University of Michigan (B.S.)
Wayne State University Medical School
(M.D.)
San Francisco General Hospital
(internship)
University of California, San Diego
(residency)

ISS Member 1985

Spouse: Carol

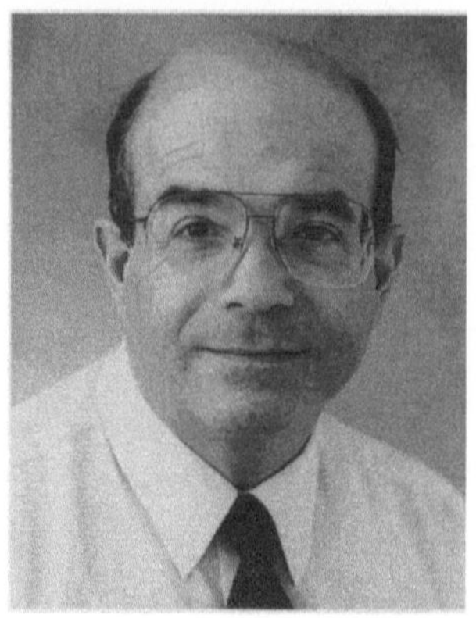

Birthdate: November 20, 1935

Academic Title: Professor

Position at Affiliation: Executive Vice
Chair Academic Programs

Business Address:
Department of Radiology
U.C.L.A. Medical Center
Los Angeles, CA 90095-1721
U.S.A.
310-825-7532 (work)
310-794-6613 (fax)
rgold@mail.rad.ucla.edu (e-mail)

Home Address:
929 Hilts Avenue
Los Angeles, CA 90024
U.S.A.
310-475-0429 (home)

Specialty/Certification: Radiology, 1969

Education:
1953–56 – New York University (B.A.)
1956–60 – University of Louisville (M.D.)
1963–66 – Yale-New Haven Hospital
(residency)
1967–68 – University of California,
San Francisco (fellowship)

ISS Member Founding member

ISS Committees:
Auditing Committee, 1992 – present,
(chair 1997 –)
Convention Planning, 1988–92
Rules Committee, 1982–84

Spouse: Gittelle

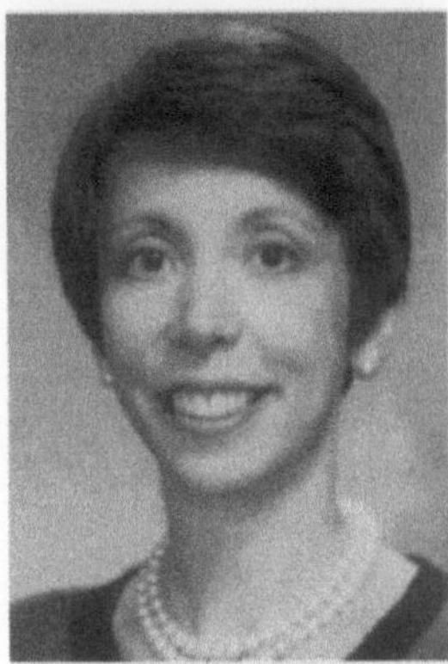

Birthdate: September 30, 1944

Academic Title: Professor of Radiology

Position at Affiliation: Attending Radiologist

Business Address:
Radiology Department
The Hospital for Special Surgery
535 East 70th Street
New York, NY 10021
U.S.A.
212 606-1130 (work)

Home Address:
333 E. 79th Street
New York, NY 10021
U.S.A.
212 734-1713 (home)

Specialty/Certification: Radiology, 1974

Education:
New York University, College
New York University, Medical School

ISS Member 1975

ISS Committees:
Chairman, Membership Committee
Chairman, Nomination Committee
Chairman, Corinne Farrell Awards
Committee
Co-Chairman, Future Planning
Committee

Spouse: David S. Goldman, M.D.

Business Address:
The Children's Hospital
Department of Radiology
2300 Children's Plaza
Chicago, IL 60614
U.S.A.

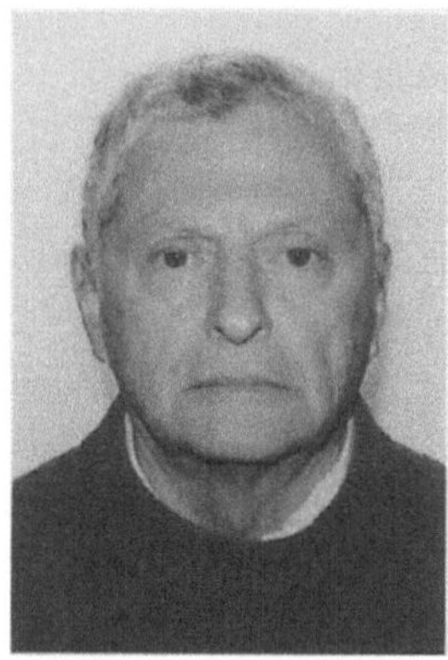

Birthdate: May 4, 1928

Academic Title: Professor

Position at Affiliation: Professor of Radiology

Business Address:
University of South Florida
College of Medicine
Tampa, FL 33612
U.S.A.
813-972-8425 (work)

Home Address:
12438 First Street West
Treasure Island, FL 33706, U.S.A.
813-360-8021 (home)

Specialty/Certification: Radiology, 1961; Nuclear Medicine, 1972

Education:
New York University (A.B.)
State University of Utrecht, Holland (Med. Drs.)
Bridgeport Hospital, CT (internship)
St. Luke's Hospital, Chicago (residency in Radiology)

ISS Member Founding member

ISS Committees:
Program Committee
Nomenclature Committee
Editorial Selection Committee
Awards Committee – current

Spouse: Barbara

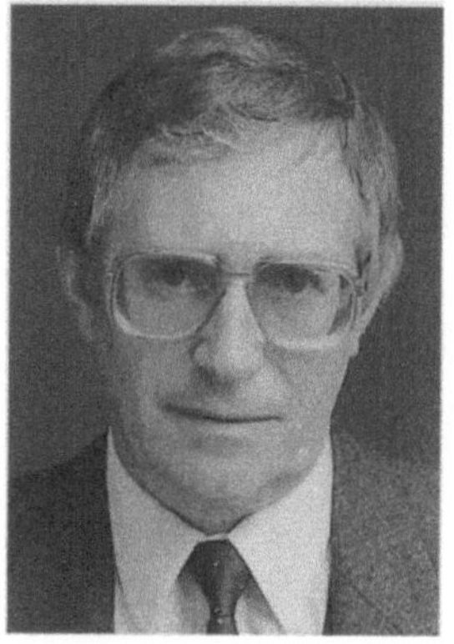

Birthdate: May 28, 1935

Academic Title: Professor

Position at Affiliation: Chief, Musculo-skeletal Radiology

Business Address:
University of California, Davis
School of Medicine
2516 Stockton Blvd, Ticon II
Sacramento, CA 95817
U.S.A.
916-734-3608 (work)
916-734-8490 (fax)

Home Address:
1036 Wilhaggin Park Lane
Sacramento, CA 95864
U.S.A.
916-973-1553 (home)

Specialty/Certification: Radiology, 1975

Education:
Medical Academy of Wroclaw, Poland

ISS Member 1983

ISS Medals and Awards:
Corinne Farell Prize, 1995

Spouse: Barbara

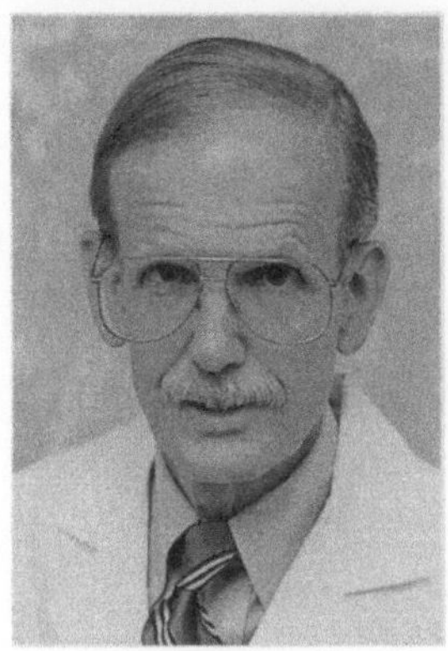

Birthdate: January 3, 1943

Academic Title: Associate Clinical Professor

Position at Affiliation: Attending Radiologist

Business Address:
Department of Radiology
Baylor University Medical Center
3500 Gaston Avenue
Dallas, TX 75246
U.S.A.
972-820-3219 (work)
972-820-7437 (fax)

Home Address:
17006 Preston Bend Drive
Dallas, TX 75248-1349
U.S.A.
972-931-0218 (home)

Specialty/Certification: Radiology, 1976

Education:
1961–65 – University of Michigan,
Ann Arbor (B.S.)
1966–70 – University of Michigan
Medical School, Ann Arbor (M.D.)
1970–71 – University Hospital,
Ann Arbor (internship)
1971–72; 74–76 – University Hospital,
Ann Arbor (residency)
1976–77 – University of California
San Diego, San Diego, CA
(Musculoskeletal Radiology fellowship)

ISS Member 1984

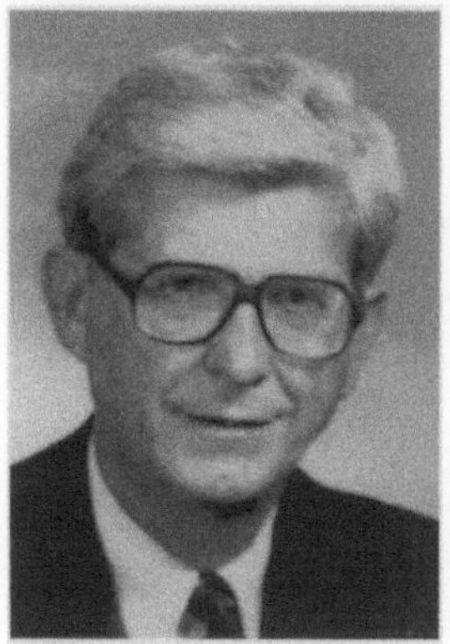

Academic Title: Professor Orthopaedic Surgery

Position at Affiliation: Professor Orthopaedic Surgery

Business Address:
Medical University of South Carolina
171 Ashley Avenue
708 C.S.P.
Charleston, South Carolina 29645
U.S.A.
803-792-9435 (work)
803-792-3674 (fax)

Home Address:
4 Hidden Green Lane
Isle of Palms, SC 29451
U.S.A.
803-886-4672 (home)

Specialty/Certification: Orthopaedic Surgery, 1962

Education:
Wake Forest University (B.S.)
Bowman Gray School of Medicine (M.D.)

ISS Member 1983

Spouse: Margaret

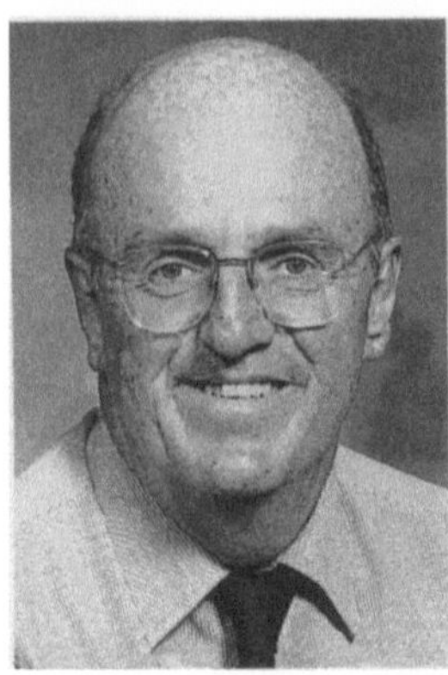

Academic Title: Professor

Position at Affiliation: Staff physician

Business Address:
Department of Radiology
University of Missouri Hospital
One Hospital Drive
Columbia, MO 65212
U.S.A.
573-882-1026 (work)
573-884-4729 (fax)
105550.712@compuserve.com (e-mail)

Home Address:
3225 Holmes Avenue South
Minneapolis, MN 55408
U.S.A.
612-822-4167 (home)

Specialty/Certification: Radiology, 1971

Education:
1957 – Epsom College, Surrey, England
('O&'A' Levels)
1963 – Guy's Hospital Medical Center,
London, England (MRCS,
LRCP, MbBs)
1967 – Hammersmith Hospital, London,
England (DMRD)

ISS Member 1975

ISS Committees:
Membership Committee, 1985–88
Program Committee, 1992–93

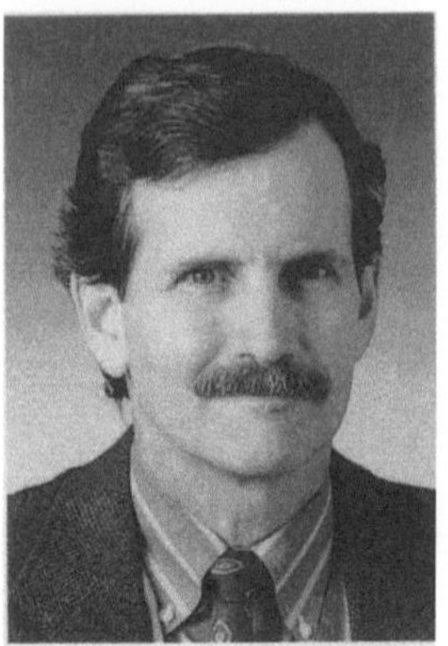

Birthdate: December 2, 1946

Position at Affiliation: Musculoskeletal
Radiologist

Business Address:
Charlotte Radiology
3030 Latrobe Drive
P.O. Box 36937
Charlotte, NC 28236
U.S.A.
704-355-3140 (work)
704-362-7081 (fax)
bguil@aol.com (e-mail)

Home Address:
1371 Perth Road
Troutman, NC 28166
U.S.A.

Specialty/Certification: Radiology, 1977

Education:
UNC, Chapel Hill, NC
(residency Radiology)
Tufts NEMCH; Royal National Ortho-
paedic Hospital
(Skeletal Radiology fellowships)

ISS Member 1986

Spouse: Diane

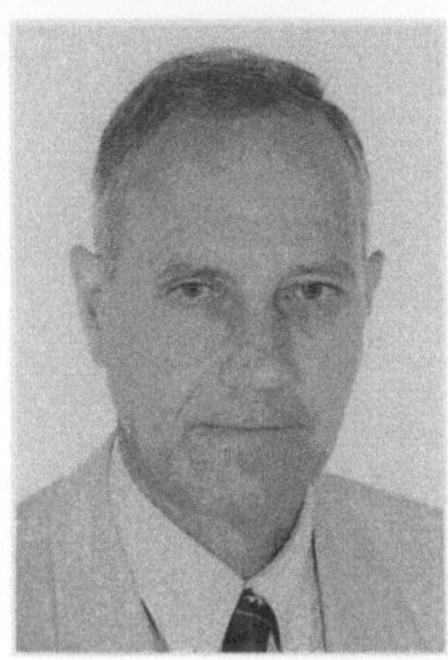

Birthdate: July 10, 1938

Academic Title: Associate Professor

Position at Affiliation: Director, Orthopaedic Oncology

Business Address:
Department of Orthopaedics
Sahlgren University Hospital
41345 Gothenburg
Sweden
46-31-601971 (work)
46-31-416701 (fax)

Home Address:
Torgilsgatan 40
43136 Molndal
Sweden
46-31-278414 (home)

Specialty/Certification: Orthopaedic Surgery, 1973

ISS Member 1991

Spouse: Christina

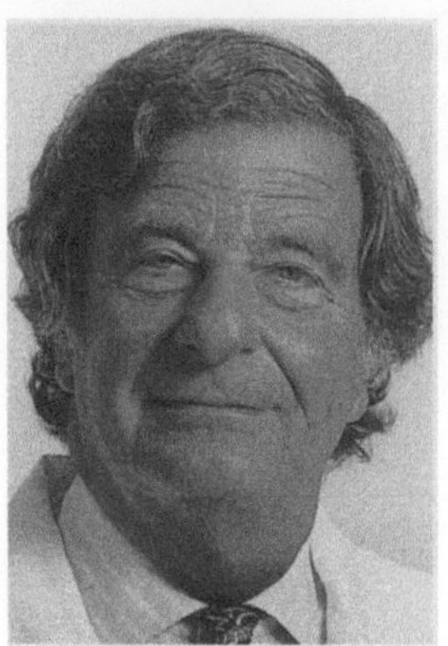

Birthdate: May 7, 1933

Academic Title: Professor & Chairman Department of Orthopaedic Surgery

Position at Affiliation: Chairman, Department of Orthopaedic Surgery

Business Address:
Albert Einstein College of Medicine and Montefiore Medical Center
Department of Orthopaedic Surgery
111 East 210th Street
Bronx, NY 10467
U.S.A.
718-920-4961 or 4962 (work)
718-231-2243 (fax)

Home Address:
335 Whippoorwill Road
Chappaqua, NY 10514
U.S.A.
914-238-5530 (home)
914-238-5917 (fax)

Specialty/Certification: Orthopaedic Surgery, 1968, 1985, 1995

Education:
1955 – Johns Hopkin University (A. B.)
1959 – State University of New York at Syracuse (M. D.)
1959–60 – University of California Medical Center San Francisco (internship)
1962–66 – Hospital for Joint Disease (Orthopaedic residency)
1967 – Wrightington Hospital, England (fellowship)

ISS Member 1977

Spouse: Susan

Business Address:
6727 Edmonton Avenue
San Diego, CA 92122
U.S.A.

ISS Member 1989

HALL, CHRISTINE MARGARET M.D.

Business Address:
Apex Lodge Fitzroy Park
Highgate Village
London N6 6JA
England

ISS Member 1987

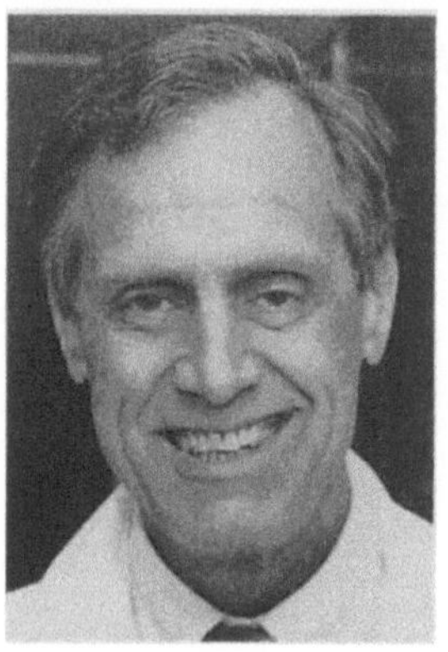

Birthdate: January 19, 1936

Academic Title: Professor

Position at Affiliation: Radiologist

Business Address:
Radiology Department
Beth Israel Deaconess Medical Center
330 Brookline Avenue
Boston, MA 02215
U.S.A.
617-667-3532 (work)
617-667-8212 (fax)

Home Address:
14 Amory Street
Brookline, MA 02146
U.S.A.
617-232-3047 (home)

Specialty/Certification: Internal
Medicine, 1968; Radiology, 1971

Education:
1957 – Swarthmore College
1961 – University Pennsylvania Medical
School (M.D.)
1965 – Philadelphia General Hospital
(Internal Medicine residency)
1971 – Peter Bent Brigham Hospital
(Radiology residency)

ISS Member 1979

Spouse: Nancy

Haller, Jorg M.D.

Business Address:
I. Medizinische Universitatsklinik
A-1090 Wien, Lazarcttgasse 14
University Clinic of Vienna-Austria
Vienna
Austria

ISS Member 1990

Harcke, Jr., H. Theodore M.D., FACR

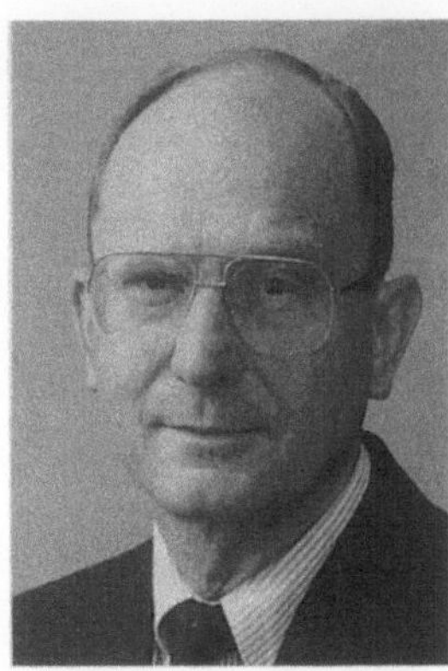

Birthdate: May 12, 1938

Academic Title: Professor of Radiology
and Pediatrics

Position at Affiliation: Chief of Imaging
Research

Business Address:
Alfred I. Dupont Institute
Department of Medical Imaging
1600 Rockland Road
P. O. Box 269
Wilmington, DE 19899
U.S.A.
302-651-4640 (work)
302-651-4626 (fax)
tharcke@aidi.nemours.org

Home Address:
3205 Coachman Road
Wilmington, DE 19803
U.S.A.
302-478-4729 (home)

Specialty/Certification: Radiology, 1975;
Pediatric Radiology, 1995

Education:
1956–60 – United States Military
Academy, West Point, NY (B.S.)
1965–66 – Pennsylvania State University, University Park, PA (M.Ed)
1967–71 – Penna. State Univ. College of
Medicine, Hershey, PA (M.D.)
1971–72 – Childrens Hospital of
Philadelphia, Philadelphia, PA
(internship in Pediatrics)
1972–74 – Temple University Medical
Center, Philadelphia, PA (resident in
Diagnostic Radiology)
1974–76 – St. Christopher's Hospital for
Children, Phila., PA (fellowship
in Pediatric Radiology)

ISS Member 1986

Spouse: Virginia

HARRIS, JR., JOHN H. M.D., D.Sc., FACR, FRACR (HON.)

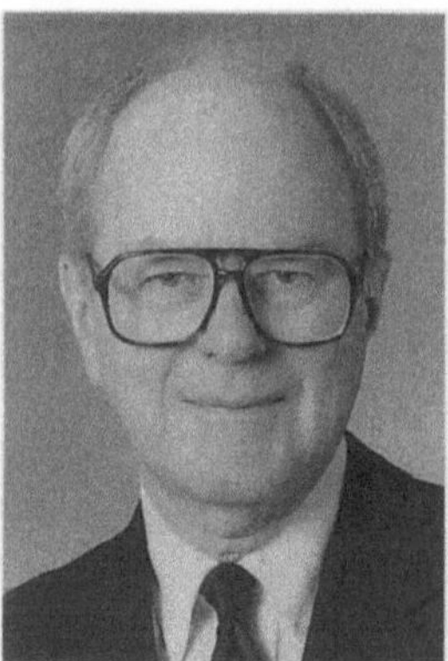

Birthdate: October 16, 1925

Academic Title: Professor

Position at Affiliation: Chief, Emergency Radiology

Business Address:
Radiology Department
The University of Texas Medical School
at Houston
6431 Fannina, 2.100
Houston, TX 77030
U.S.A.
713-704-3539 (work)
713-704-5734 (fax)
jharris@msrad3.med.uth.tmc.edu
(e-mail)

Home Address:
2351 Underwood
Houston, TX 77030
U.S.A.
713-665-7415 (home)
713-665-2326 (fax)

Specialty/Certification: Radiology, 1957

Education:
1948 – Dickinson College, Carlisle, PA
(Bsc)
1953 – Jefferson Medical College (M.D.)
1957 – Hospital University of PA
(Radiology residency)
1953 – 1957 – U of PA Graduate School of
Medicine (MSc & DSc)

ISS Member 1978

ISS Committees:
Chair, Auditing Committee, 1992 – present
Honors Committee

Spouse: Cathy

Hashimoto, Hiroshi M.D.

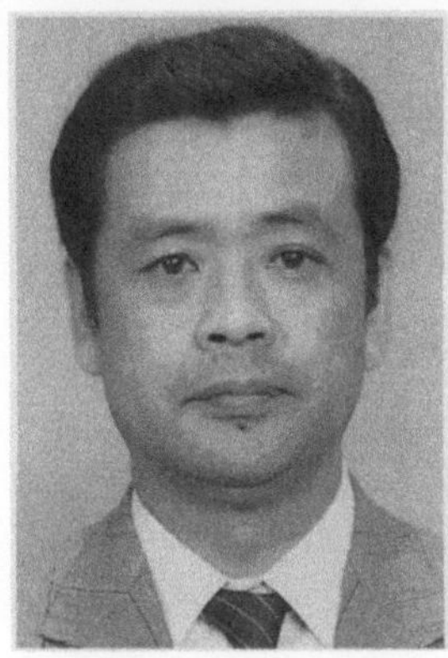

Birthdate: August 1, 1948

Academic Title: Professor

Position at Affiliation: Professor and Chairman of Pathology

Business Address:
Dept. of Pathology
School of Medicine
Univ. of Occupational and Environmental
Health
1-1 Iseigaoka, Yahatanishi-ku
Kitakyushu 807
Japan
93-691-7239 (work)
93-692-0189 (fax)
@med.uoeh-u.ac.jp

Home Address:
5-12-23 Torikai, Jonan-ku
Fukuoka 814-01
Japan
92-831-4477 (home)

Specialty: Pathology

Education:
1974 – Kyushu University Faculty of
Medicine (M.D.)
1975–79 – Graduate School of Kyushu
University
1985–86 – Research Fellow of the
Alexander von Humboldt Foundation;
Pathologie der
Universität Frankfurt am Main

ISS Member: 1995

Spouse: Mieko

Healey, John H. M.D.

Academic Title: Associate Professor
Orthopaedic Surgery

Position at Affiliation: Chief, Orthopaedic Surgery

Business Address:
Memorial Sloan Kettering Cancer Center
1275 York Avenue
New York, NY 10021
U.S.A.
212-639-7610 (work)
212-794-4015 (fax)

Home Address:
333 E. 68th Street
New York, NY 10021
U.S.A.

Specialty/Certification: Orthopaedics
Surgery, 1986

Education:
1974 – Yale University (BS)
1978 – University of Vermont (MD)
1983 – Hospital for Special Surgery
(residency Orthopaedic Surgery)

ISS Member 1992

Spouse: Paula Olsiewski

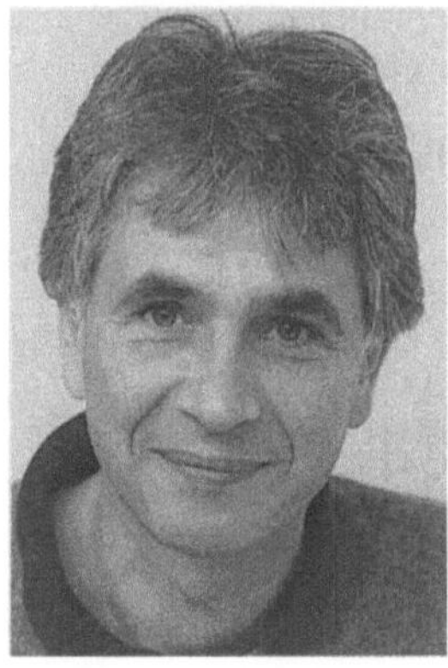

Birthdate: November 29, 1946

Academic Title: Professor Dr.

Position at Affiliation: Chairman and Director

Business Address:
Klinik für Radiologische Diagnostik
Christian-Akbrechts-Universität zu Kiel
Arnold-Heller-Str.9
D-24105 Kiel
Germany
49 431 597-3153 (work)
49 431 597-3151 (fax)

Home Address:
Dörpfeldstr. 39
D-22609 Hamburg
Germany
49 40 8078000 (home)
49 40 8078001 (fax)

Specialty/ Certification: Radiology, 1980

Education:
1966 – Altsprachliches Gymnasium Worms
1974 – Universität Mainz; Medizinische Hochschule Lübeck;
Universität Wien (Austria); Universität Heidelburg
Universitäts-Strahlenklink Heidelberg; Radiologische Klinik
Universitätskrankenhaus Hamburg-Eppendorf
Department of Radiology, University of California San Francisco

Membership: 1992

Spouse: Michèle Richartz-Heller, M.D.

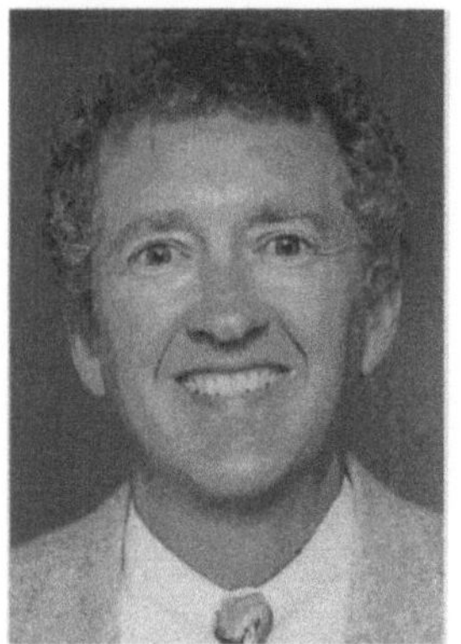

Birthdate: April 12, 1946

Academic Title: Professor

Position at Affiliation: Chief, Musculo-skeletal Section

Business Address:
Dept. of Radiology,
Duke University Medical Center
P.O. Box 3808
Durham, NC 27710
U.S.A.
919-684-7453 (work)
919-684-7138 (fax)
helms002@mc.duke.edu (e-mail)

Home Address:
16114 Morehead
Chapel Hill, NC 27514
U.S.A.
919-929-7392 (home)

Specialty/Certification: Radiology, 1977

Education:
Nicholls State College, Louisiana
University of Texas Medical Center, San Antonio, TX (M.D.)
University of California San Francisco (residency and bone fellowship)

ISS Member 1981

ISS Committees:
Chair, Liaison Future Planning Committee, 1994–97

Spouse: Nancy M. Major, M.D.

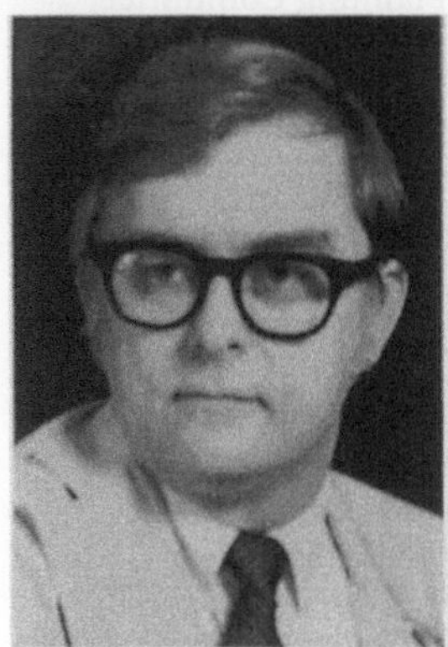

Business Address:
Section Musculoskeletal Radiology
710 North Fairbanks Ct.
Chicago, IL 60611
U.S.A.
312-908-5134 (work)
708-986-0418 (home)
Specialty: Radiology

ISS Member 1984

Spouse: Miriam

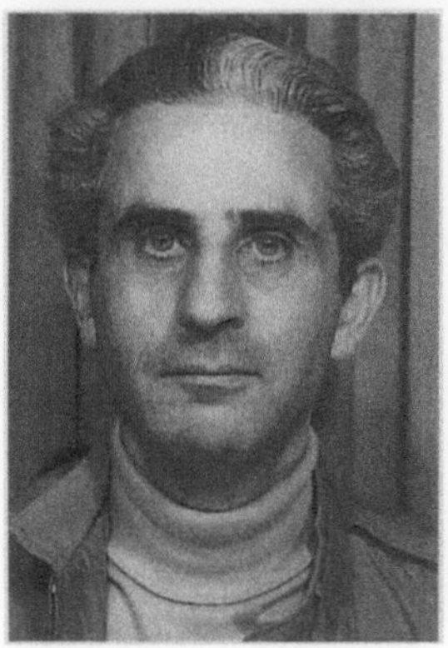

Academic Title: Professor

Position at Affiliation: Professor
of Radiology

Business Address:
Mt. Sinai Medical Center
Annenberg B-1
One Gustave L. Levy Place
5th Ave. at 100th Street
New York, NY 10029
U.S.A.
212-241-5798 or 212-241-7446 (work)
212-427-8137 (fax)

Home Address:
61-20 Grand Central Parkway
Apartment A1105
Forest Hills, NY 11375
U.S.A.
718-271-2729 (home)

Specialty/Certification: Radiology, 1976

Education:
Semmelweis Medical University,
Budapest, Hungary (M.D.)
Hadassah Medical Center of the Hebrew
University, Jerusalem, Israel
(residency, Diagnostic Radiology)
Hospital for Joint Diseases, New York,
NY (fellowship)

ISS Member 1983

ISS Committees:
Refresher Course Committee, 1996 –
present

Spouse: Eva

HERNANDEZ, RAMIRO M.D.

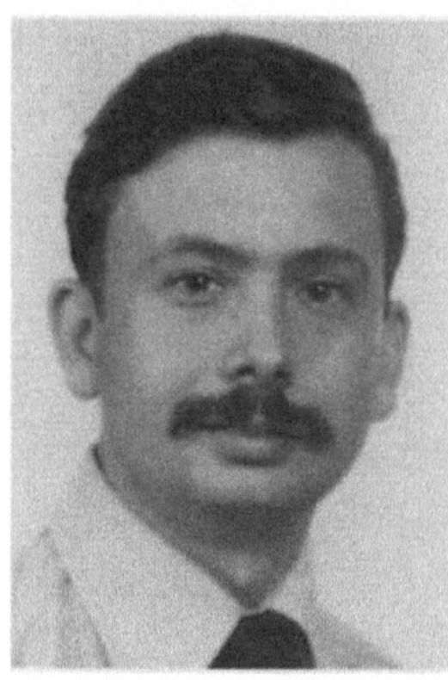

Birthdate: July 30, 1946

Academic Title: Professor

Position at Affiliation: Professor of Radiology; Director, Pediatric Radiology section

Business Address:
Section of Pediatric Radiology
C.S. Mott Children's Hospital.
C3123/0252
1500 E. Medical Center Drive
Ann Arbor, MI 48109-0252
U.S.A.
313-763-2570 (work)
313-764-9351 (fax)
Ramer-Hernandez.radiology@mailgw.
surg.med.umich.edu (e-mail)

Home Address:
2996 Devonshire
Ann Arbor, MI 48104
U.S.A.
313-971-3248

Specialty/Certification: Radiology 1975;
Pediatric Radiology 1994

Education:
1957–64 – Academia Castellano, Valencia,
Spain
1964–70 – Facultad de Medicina, Valencia,
Spain (M.D.)
1989–91 – Univ. of Michigan, Ann Arbor,
MI (M.S.)

ISS Member 1984

ISS Committees:
Liaison Future Planning Committee,
1992-96

Spouse: Mary Bozynski

HERNDON, JAMES H. M.D.

Business Address:
Orthopaedic Department
M 272 Scafe Hall
3550 Terrace Street
Pittsburgh, PA 15261
U.S.A.
412-648-2311 (work)
412-963-9443 (home)
412-687-0802 (fax)

ISS Member 1982

Spouse: Gerry

HERRLIN, KRISTIAN M.D., PH.D

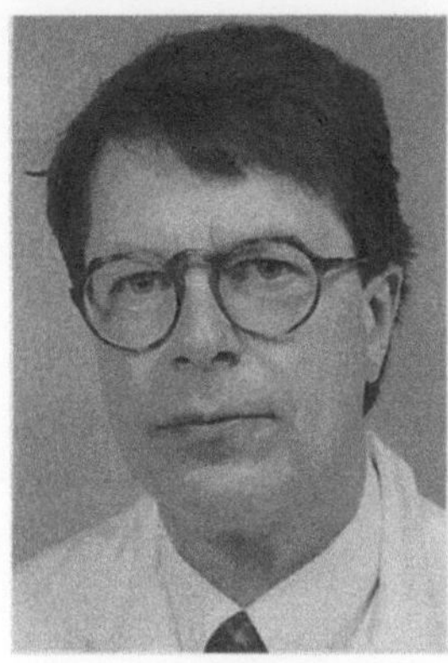

Birthdate: September 21, 1946

Academic Title: Associate Professor

Position at Affiliation: Consultant Radiologist

Business Address:
Department of Radiology
University Hospital
S-22185 Lund
Sweden
46-46171000 (work)
46-462116956 (fax)
drad.@drad.lu.se (e-mail)

Home Address:
Clemenstorget 2
22221 Lund
Sweden
46-462116057 (home)
46-462116057 (fax)

Specialty/Certification: Radiology, 1981

ISS Member: 1993

ISS Committees:
Refresher Course Committee

HEUCK, ANDREAS F. PRIV. DOZ. DR. MED.

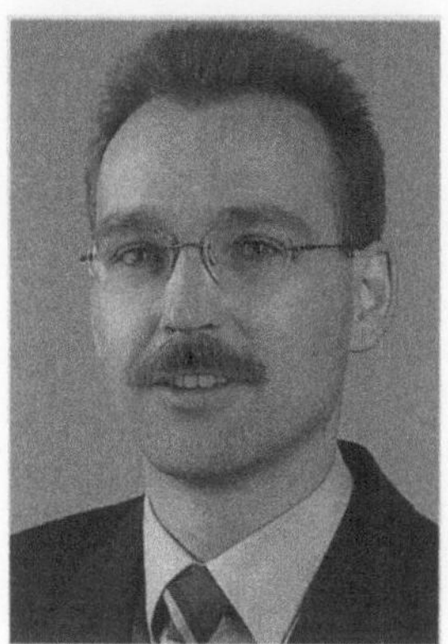

Birthdate: October 29, 1956

Position at Affiliation: Assistant Professor

Business Address:
Institut fuer Radiologische Diagnostik
Klinikum Grosshadren, Universitaet
Muenchen
Marchioninistr. 15
D-81377 Muenchen
Germany
49-89-70953250 (work)
49-89-70958822 (fax)

Home Address:
Albanistr. 2
D-81541 Muenchen
Germany
49-89-657876 (home)
49-89-656373 (fax)

Specialty/Certification: Radiology, 1989

Education:
Medical School Universities
of Regensburg, Heidelberg, Freiburg,
and Muenchen
Radiology Training at Technical University Muenchen

ISS Member: 1995

ISS Committees:
Committee for Evaluation of Research
Grants, 1996 – 98
Committee for Promotion of Refresher
Course Outside North America, 1996 – 98

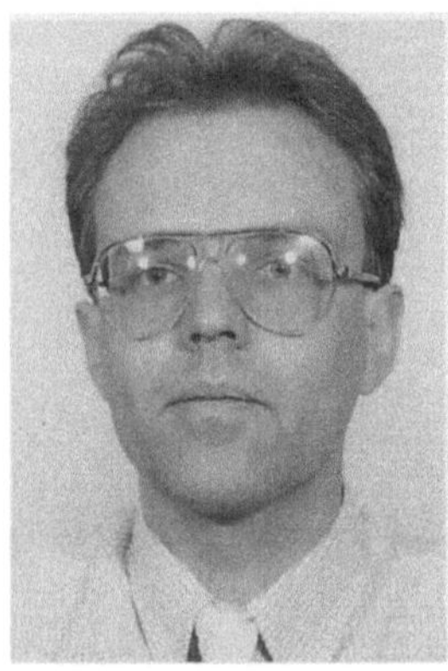

Birthdate: February 7, 1957

Position at Affiliation: Chief of Section

Business Address:
Radiology
Balgrist Clinic
University of Zurich
Forchstrasse 340
CH-8008 Zurich
Switzerland
41-1-386-3311 (work)
41-1-386-3319 (fax)
hodlerzh@bluewin.ch (e-mail)

Home Address:
In der Fadmatt 64
CH-8902 Urdorf
Switzerland
41-1-734-2725 (home)

Specialty/Certification: Radiology, 1987

Education:
College/Medical School University
of Berne'
1983–87 – University of Berne,
(residency in Radiology
1990–91 – UCSD, San Diego, (Research
Fellowship)

ISS Member: 1993

Spouse: Esther

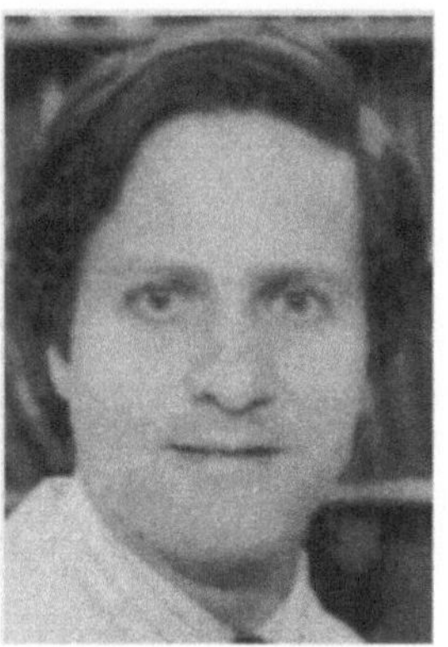

Birthdate: October 27, 1957

Academic Title: Associate Professor

Position at Affiliation: Chief of Orthopaedic Oncology

Business Address:
Allegheny University Hospitals-
Hahnemann
Department of Orthopaedic Surgery
230 N. Broad Street, Mail Stop 420
Philadelphia, PA 19102
U.S.A.
215-762-4275 (work)
215-762-1731 (fax)
HOROWITZS@allegheny.edu (e-mail)

Home Address:
17 Lucerne Court
Cherry Hill, NJ 08003
U.S.A.
609-751-8321 (home)

Specialty: Orthopaedic Surgery

Education:
1983 – New York Medical College (M.D.)
1984 – Beth Israel Medical Center
New York, NY (internship)
1988 – Johns Hopkins Hospital, (Orthopaedic Surgery residency)
1988–90 – Memorial Sloan Kettering
Cancer Center, Hospital for Special
Surgery, Cornell University School
of Medicine, (fellowship in
Musculoskeletal Oncology)

ISS Member: 1995

Spouse: Nancy

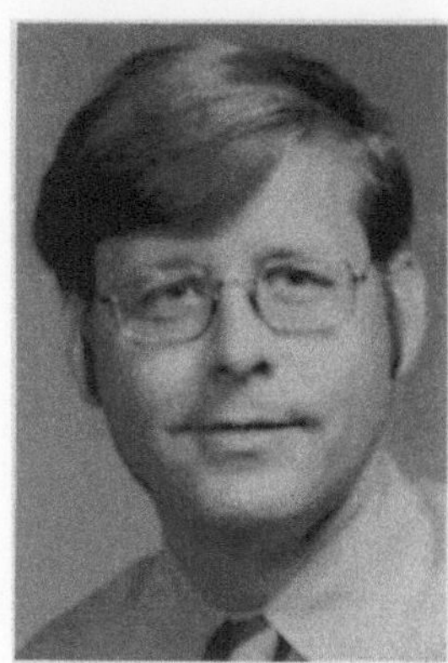

Business Address:
Radiology Section
Emory Clinic
1365 Clifton Road NE
Atlanta, GA 30322
U.S.A.
404-248-5834 (work)
404-248-5058 (fax)

Specialty: Radiology

ISS Member 1984

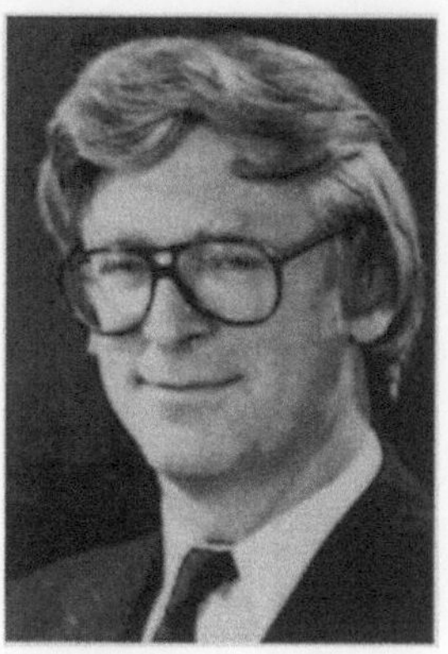

Business Address:
Royal Postgraduate Medical School
University of London
Hammersmith Hospital
81 Abbotsbury Road
London W14 8EP
England
071-603-7904 (home)
081-740-3215 (work)
081-740-3215 (fax)

ISS Member 1983

Spouse: Felicity

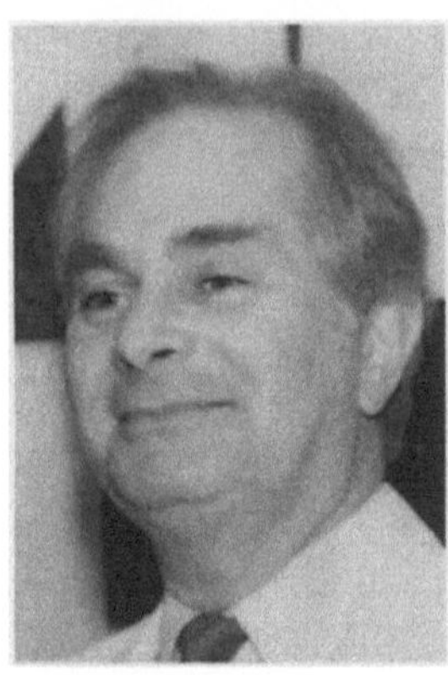

Business Address:
Department of Pathology
Memorial Sloan Kettering
Cancer Center
1275 York Avenue
New York, NY 10021
U.S.A.
212-639-5905 (work)
212-717-3203 (fax)

Specialty: Pathology

ISS Member 1980

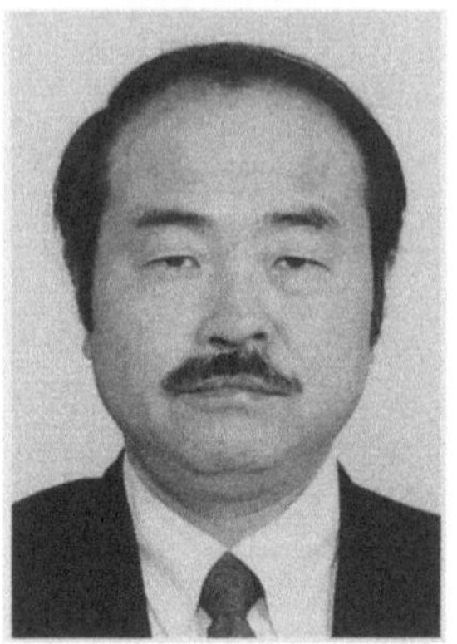

Birthdate: August 1, 1946
Academic Title: Professor of Surgical Pathology
Position at Affiliation: Director and Professor
Business Address:
Department of Surgical Pathology
Teikyo University School of Medicine
2-11-1 Kaga
Itabashi-ku
Tokyo 173
Japan
81-03-3964-1211 ext. 3686 (work)
81-03-3961-9518 (fax)
Home Address:
5-34-7 Taishido
Setagaya-ku
Tokyo 154
Japan
81-03-3795-0162 (home)
Specialty/Certification: Pathology, 1981
Education:
1971 – Kanazawa University School of Medicine (M.D.)
1971–74 – Tokyo University, Department of Pathology, Faculty of Medicine, and Department of Pathology, Cancer Institute, Tokyo (resident)
1983–85 – Department of Pathology, Sinal Hospital of Baltimore and Department of Orthopaedic Surgery, Montefiore Hospital, New York (fellow)
ISS Member 1996
Spouse: Tomoko

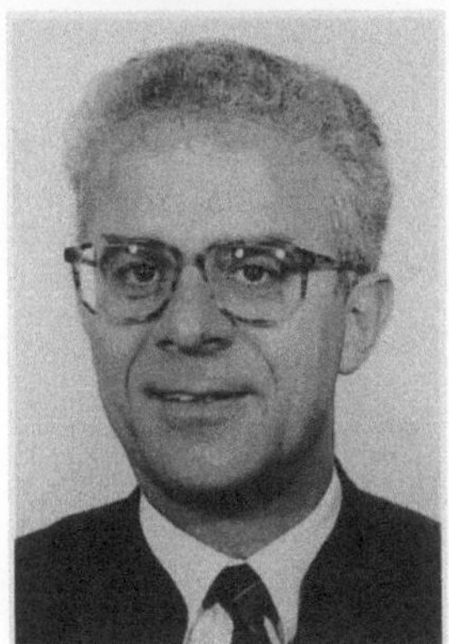

Birthdate: February 9, 1943

Academic Title: Professor

Position at Affiliation: Chief

Business Address:
Osteology 3 MRI/Univ. Klinik. f.
Radiodiagnostik
AKH-Vienna (Univ. Hospitals)
Austria
A-1090 Wahringergurtel 18-20
43-1-40400-5801 (work)
43-1-40400-3777 (fax)
mr@univie.ac.at (e-mail)

Home Address:
Delugstr. 18
A-1190 Vienna
Austria
43-1-3203961 (home)

Specialty/Certification: Radiology, 1975

Education:
1968 – University of Vienna (M.D.)
University Hospitals (residency)

ISS Member: 1992

Spouse: Dr. Ilse

Business Address:
University of Götheburg
Lilla Askimsvagen 6
S-43640 Askim
Sweden

ISS Member 1990

Ishida, Tsuyoshi M.D

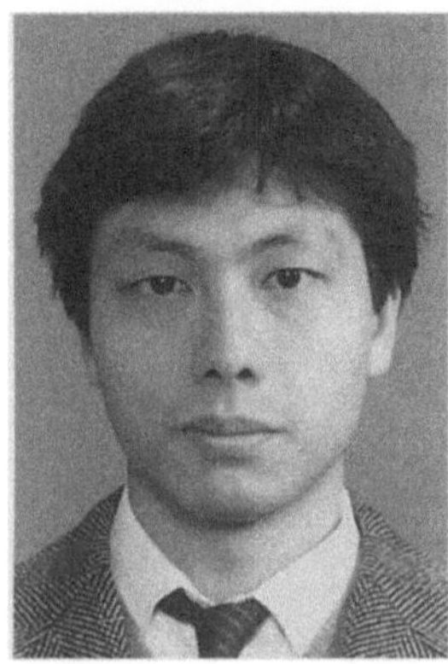

Birthdate: December 8, 1961

Academic Title: Assistant Professor

Position at Affiliation: Assistant Professor

Business Address:
Department of Pathology
University of Tokyo Hospital
7-3-1 Hongo, Bunkyo-ku
Tokyo 113
Japan
81-3-3815-5411 ex.5231 (work)
81-3-3815-8379 (fax)
ishida-pat@h.u-tokyo.ac.jp (e-mail)

Home Address:
1-2-3-103 Higashisugano, Ichikawa
Chiba 272
Japan
81-47-322-6074 (home)

Specialty/Certification: Pathology, 1991

Education:
1980–86 – Teikyo University, School of
Medicine (M.D.)
1986–90 – Tokyo University (residency)

ISS Member 1996

Spouse: Noriko

Jacobson, Harold G. M.D.

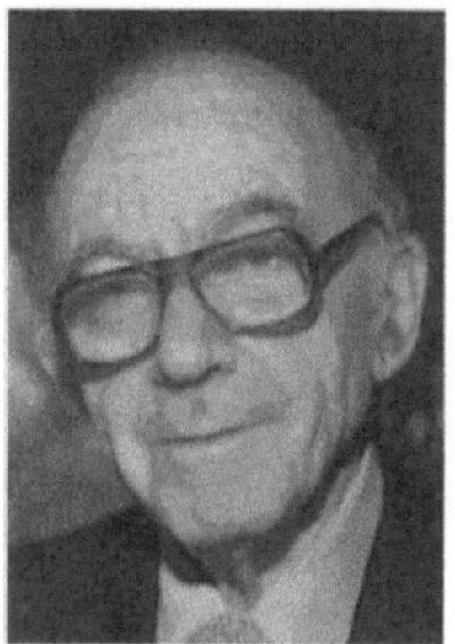

Birthdate: October 12, 1912

Academic Title: Emeritus Professor
Chairman

Position at Affiliation: Emeritus
Professor Chairman

Business Address:
Montefiore Medical Center
111 East 210th Street
Bronx, NY 10467
U.S.A.
718-547-4121 (work)
718-798-7983 (fax)

Home Address:
3240 Henry Hudson Pkwy.
Apartment 7D
Bronx, NY 10463, U.S.A.
718-543-5951 (home)

Specialty/Certification: Radiology, 1941

Education:
1934 – University of Cincinnati (B.S.)
1936 – University of Cincinnati College
of Medicine (B.M.)
1937 – University of Cincinnati College
of Medicine (M.D.)
1936–38 – Los Angeles County General
Hospital (internship)
1939–41 – Mount Sinai Hospital
(Radiology residency)

ISS Member: Founding member

Offices Held in ISS and Dates of Service:
President 1974-76

ISS Committees:

ISS Medals and Awards:
Founders' Lecture, New York, 1989

Jensen, Pamela S. M.D.

Business Address:
Radiology Service
HCR 60 - Box 3170
Camden, MA 04843
U.S.A.
207-236-4825 (home)
207-623-5735 (work)
Specialty: Radiology

ISS Member 1975

Spouse: Stephen A. Ross, M.D.

Jevtic, Vladimir V. M.D., Ph.D.

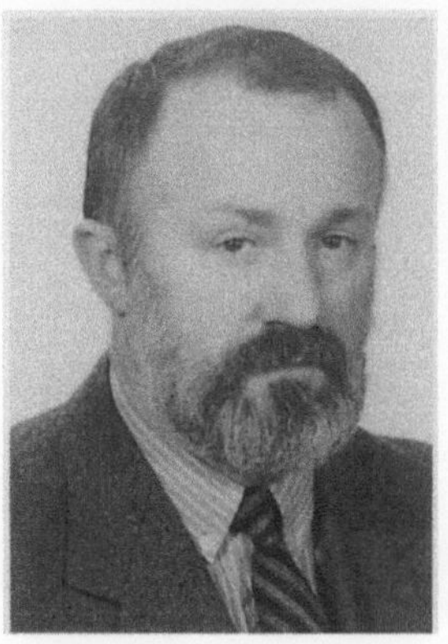

Birthdate: September 2, 1944

Academic Title: Professor, Diagnostic
Radiology

Position at Affiliation: Head

Business Address:
Clinical Radiology Institute, University
Medical Centre
Zaloska 7,
SI 0 1525 Ljubljana
Slovenia, Europa
386 61-325-570 (work)
386 61-13 31-044 (business fax)

Home Address:
Stirnova 8
SI-1000 Ljubljana
Slovenia, Europa
386 61-579-464 (home)

Specialty/Certification: Radiology, 1979

Education:
Faculty of Medicine, University of
Zagreb, Croatia
1975 – 79 Faculty of Medicine, Univ. of
Ljubljana, Slovenia (speciality training)

ISS Member 1992

ISS Committees:
Committee for the Promotion
of the Refresher Course outside
of North America

Spouse: Wanda

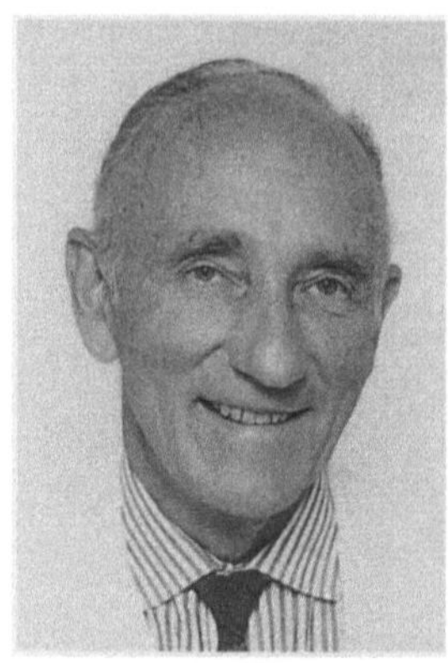

Birthdate: January 24, 1931

Academic Title: Professor of Clinical Orthopedics

Position at Affiliation: Professor of Orthopedic Oncology

Business Address:
Department of Orthopaedic Surgery
University of California San Francisco,
Rm. MU320W
500 Parnassus Avenue
San Francisco, CA 94143-0728
U.S.A.
415-476-2495 (work)
415-323-7751 (fax)
mbeec5@aol.com (e-mail)

Home Address:
30 Toro Ct.
Portola Valley, CA 94028
U.S.A.
415-851-1153 (home)
415- 851-1109 (fax)

Specialty/Certification: Orthopaedic Surgery, 1964

Education:
1951 – Albion College (B.S.)
1951 – 55 – University of Michigan Medical School (M.D.)
1956 – 60 – University of Michigan Medical School (residency in Orthopedics)

ISS Member 1989

Spouse: Mary Bee

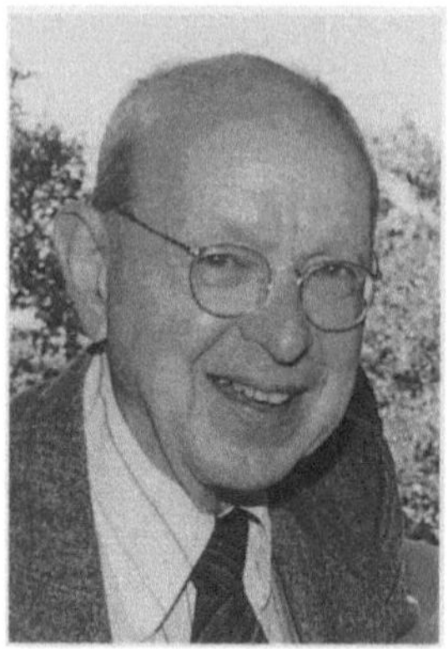

Birthdate: June 9, 1917

Academic Title: Professor of Radiology, Emeritus, Active

Position at Affiliation: Professor of Radiology, Emeritus, Active

Business Address:
Department of Radiology
Stanford University School of Medicine
Palo Alto, CA 94305
U.S.A.
415-72 5-4937 (work)

Home Address:
723 Mayfield Avenue
Stanford, CA 94305
U.S.A.
415-858-1574 (home)

Specialty/Certification: Radiology, 1951

Education:
1939 – Haverford College (B.A.)
1943 – Yale University School of Medicine (M.D.)
1944 – Metropolitan Hospital, New York (internship)
1944 – 46 – Yale (Radiology residency)

ISS Member 1980

Spouse: Margaret

Jonsson, Kjell F. J. M.D., Ph.D.

Birthdate: July 18, 1939

Academic Title: Professor

Position at Affiliation: Professor

Business Address:
Department of Radiology
University Hospital
S-221 85, Lund
Sweden
46-46 173090 (work)
46 46211 69 56 (fax)

Home Address:
Holmgangen 11
S-224 75 Lund
Sweden
46-46 12 01 27 (home)

Specialty/Certification: Radiology, 1972

Education:
Medical School, Lund, Sweden
University Hospital, Lund, Sweden

ISS Member 1990

ISS Committees:
Program Committee, 1992

Spouse: Ann-Christine

Jurik, Anne Grethe M.D., DMSc

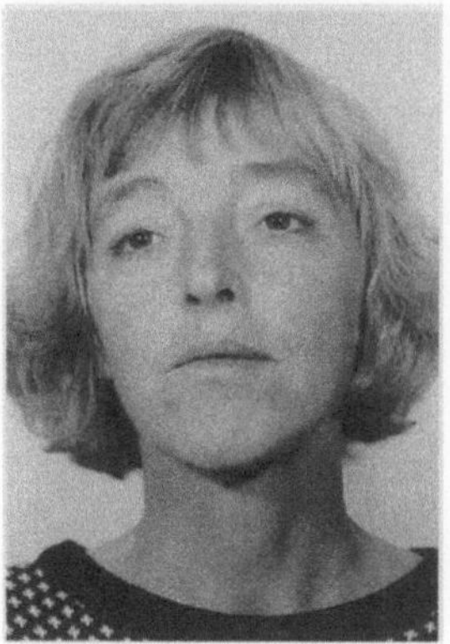

Birthdate: March 29, 1948

Academic Title: Associate Professor

Position at Affiliation: Head of
Department

Business Address:
Department of Radiology
Municipal Hospital
University of Aarhus, Noerrebrogade 44
DK-8000 Aarhus C
Denmark
45 89 49 23 92 (work)
45 89 49 24 10 (fax)

Home Address:
Bredkaer Parkvej 8
DK-8250 Egaa
Denmark
45 86 22 32 01 (home)

Specialty/Certification: Radiology, 1987

ISS Member 1993

Kahn, Leonard B. MB,BCh, M. Med., FRC (Path)

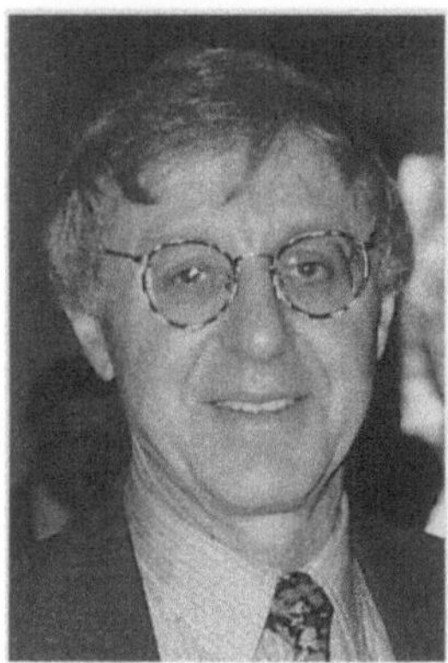

Birthdate: July 20, 1937

Academic Title: Professor, Albert Einstein College Medicine

Position at Affiliation: Chairman, Department of Pathology

Business Address:
Department of Pathology
Long Island Jewish Medical Center
270-05 76th Avenue
New Hyde Park, NY 11040
U.S.A.
718-470-7491 (work)
718-347-9171 (fax)

Home Address:
18 Oak Drive
Great Neck, NY 11021
U.S.A.
516-482-1837 (home)

Specialty/Certification: Anatomic Pathology, 1980

Education:
1960 – University of Witwatersrand (M.B.B.Ch.)
1964 – University of Cape Town (Pathology)
1967–69 – Washington University School of Medicine (Pathology)

ISS Member 1982

ISS Committees:
Program Committee, 1990
Chairman, Program Committee, 1996 –

Spouse: Louise Jean

Kaitila, Ilkka Ilmari M.D., Sc.D.

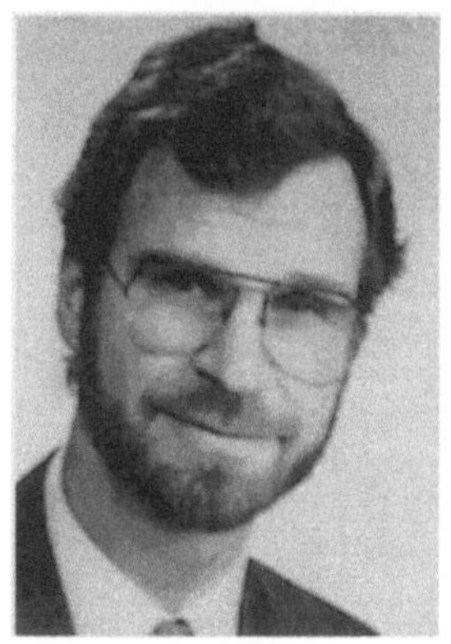

Business Address:
Department of Clinical Genetics
Helsinki University Hospital
Tukholmankatu 8 F
SF-00290 Helsinki
Finland
358-0-4712186 (work)
358-0-4715500 (fax)

ISS Member 1987

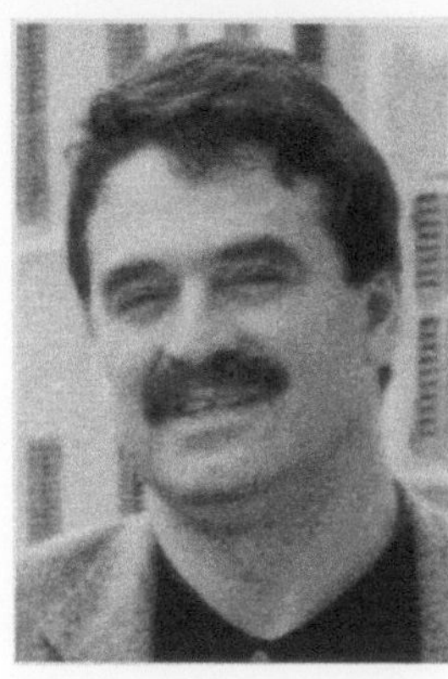

Birthdate: June 20, 1946

Academic Title: Professor

Position at Affiliation: Chairman

Business Address:
Department of Radiology
Hopital Saint-Vincent, De Paul
82 avenue Denfert, Rochereau
75014 Paris
France
33-1-4048-8188 (work)
33-1-4048-8346 (fax)

Home Address:
27 Rue Cecile Vallet
92340 Bourg La Reine
France

Specialty: Radiology

Education:
University of Paris (medical school)
UCSF (fellow in research)

ISS Member 1994

Spouse: Chantal

Birthdate: May 20, 1953

Academic Title: Associate Professor

Position at Affiliation: Staff Pathologist

Business Address:
Department of Pathology & Laboratory
Medicine
Mount Sinai Hospital
600 University Avenue
Toronto, Ontario M5G 1X5
Canada
416-586-8516 (work)
416-586-8628 (fax)

Home Address:
430 Heath Street E.
Toronto, Ontario M4G 1B5
Canada
416-421-6535 (home)

Specialty/Certifcation: Pathology, 1983

Education:
1978 – M.D.
1983 – FRCP (C)

ISS Member: 1997

Spouse: Gabor Kandel

Kang, Heung Sik M.D.Ph.D.

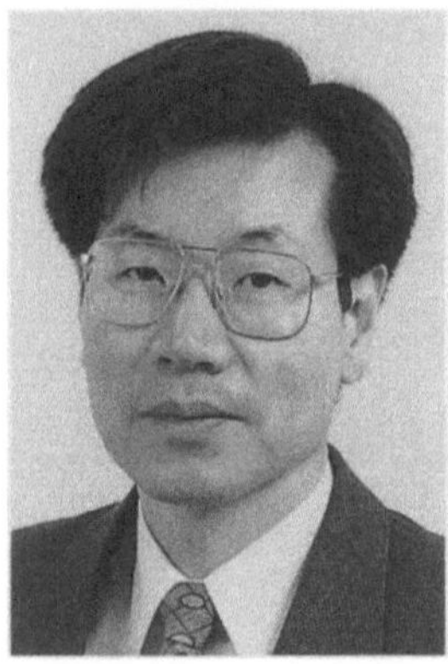

Birthdate: October 15, 1952

Academic Title: Professor

Position at Affiliation: Chief, Musculo-skeletal Section

Business Address:
Department of Radiology
Seoul National University Hospital
28 Yongon-Dong, Chongno-Gu
Seoul 110-744
Korea
82 2-760-3217 (work)
82 2-743-6385 (fax)
kanghs@snu.ac.kr (e-mail)

Home Address:
310-1404 Gangchon-Maeul, Madu-Dong
Goyang-Shi, Gyunggi-Do 411-350
Korea
82-344-903-5760 (home)

Specialty/Certification: Radiology, 1982

Education:
Seoul National University College of
Medicine
Seoul National University Hospital
University of California, San Diego

ISS Member 1991

Spouse: Young Sun

Kaplan, Phoebe A. M.D.

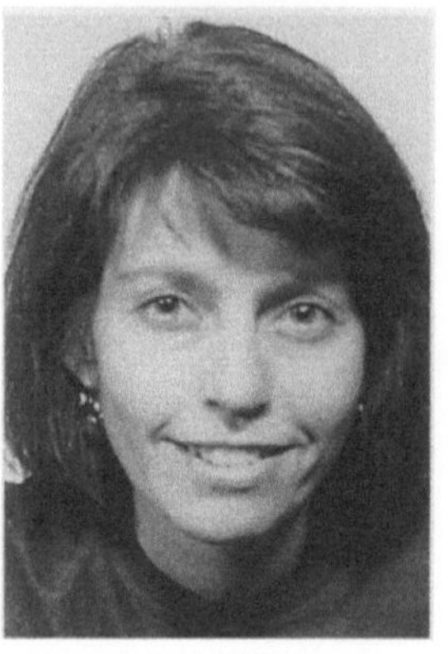

Academic Title: Professor

Position at Affiliation: Professor of
Radiology and Orthopedics

Business Address:
Radiology Department
University of Virginia Health Sciences
Center
P.O. Box 170
Charlottesville, Virginia 22908
U.S.A.
804-982-3255 (work)
804-982-1618 (fax)

Home Address:
3050 Pryor's Mountain Lane
Charlottesville, Va 22903
U.S.A.
804-984-4054 (home)

Specialty/Certification: Radiology, 1983

Education:
University of Nebraska Medical Center

ISS Member 1988

ISS Medals and Awards:
President's Medal, Toronto, 1993

ISS Committees:
Membership Committee, 1995

Spouse: Robert Dussault, M.D.

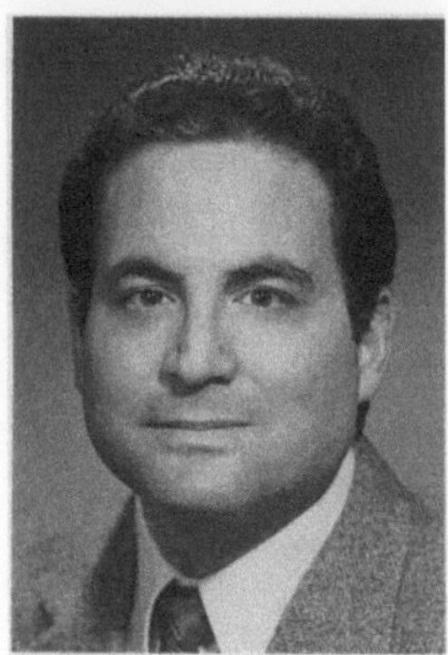

Birthdate: December 21, 1948

Academic Title: Professor of Radiology

Position at Affiliation: Chief, Musculo-skeletal Section

Business Address:
Department of Radiology
Thomas Jefferson Univ. Hospital and
Jefferson Medical College
111 South 11th Street
Philadelphia, PA 19107
U.S.A.
215-955-8167 (work)
215-923-1562 (fax)

Home Address:
1410 Colton Road
Gladwyne, PA
U.S.A.
610-527-9380 (home)

Specialty/Certification: Radiology, 1978

Education:
Temple University (undergraduate)
Jefferson Medical College (M.D.)
Thomas Jefferson University Hospital
(Radiology residency)

ISS Member 1984

ISS Committees:
Liaison Future Planning Committee,
1995–96

Spouse: Madelyn

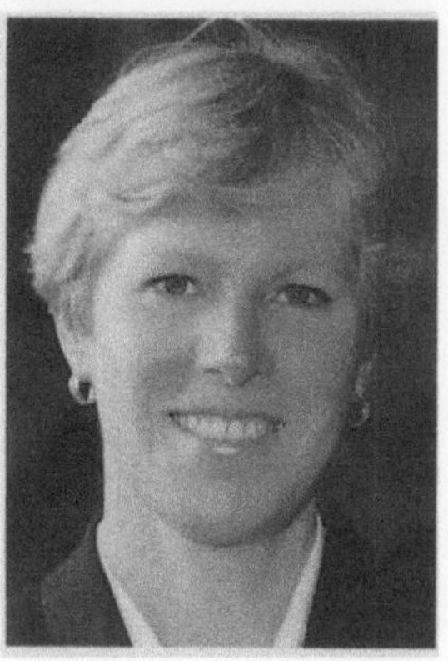

Academic Title: Associate Professor

Position at Affiliation: Section Chief,
Musculoskeletal Radiology

Business Address:
Department of Radiology
University of Iowa Hospitals and Clinics
200 Hawkins Drive
Iowa City, IA 52242
U.S.A.
(319) 356-3655 (work)
(319) 356-2220 (fax)
mary-kathol@uiowa.edu (e-mail)

Home Address:
321 Lexington Avenue
Iowa City, IA 52246
U.S.A.
319-337-5639 (home)
319-337-8660 (fax)

Specialty/Certification: Radiology, 1979

Education:
University of Kansas (B. A., Mathematics)
University of Kansas School of Medicine
(M.D.)
University of Iowa Hospitals and Clinics
(Diagnostic Radiology)

ISS Member: 1994

Spouse: Roger

KATTAN, KENNETH R. M.D.

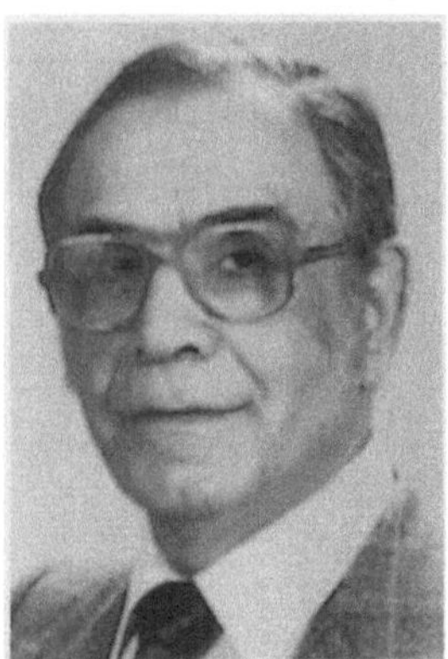

Business Address:
Radiology Service (114)
VA Medical Center
3200 Vine Street
Cincinnati, OH 45220
U.S.A.

ISS Member 1980

KATTAPURAM, SUSAN V. M.D.

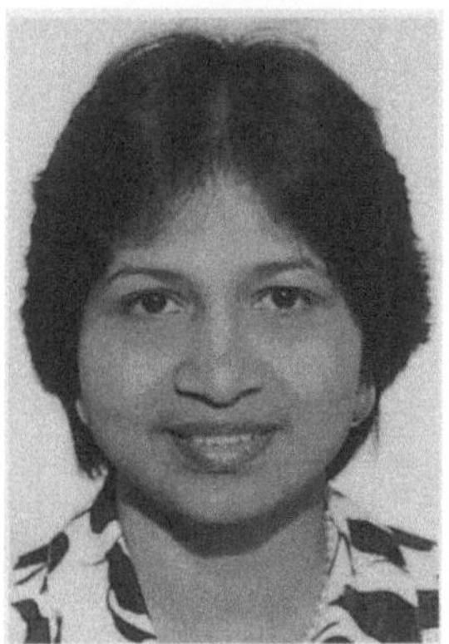

Birthdate: October 3, 1948

Academic Title: Associate Professor

Position at Affiliation: Staff Radiologist

Business Address:
Department of Radiology
Massachusetts General Hospital
15 Parkman Street
Boston, MA 02114
U.S.A.
617-726-8305 (work)
617-726-5282 (fax)
kattapuram@sisu.mgh.harvard.edu

Home Address:
19 Gavin Circle
Andover, MA 01810
U.S.A.
508-475-5765 (home)

Specialty: Radiology

Education:
1964 – Institute of Medical Sciences BHU.
India (MBBS)
Boston City and University Hospital
(Radiology residency)

ISS Member 1986

Spouse: George

KAUFMANN, HERBERT J. M.D.

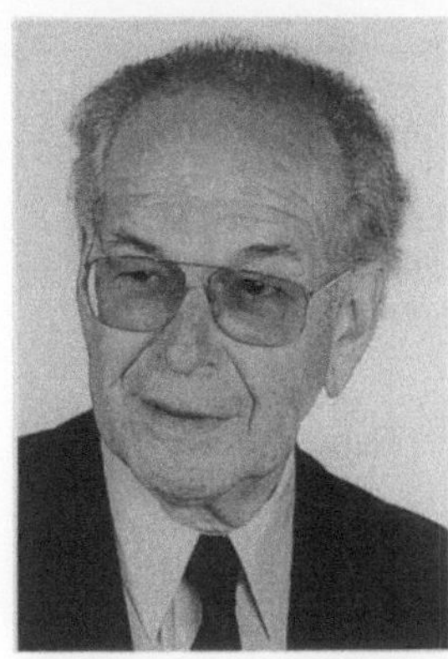

Birthdate: June 10, 1924

Academic Title: Professor of Radiology

Position at Affiliation: Chief, Pediatric Radiology (retired)

Business Address:
Free Univ. Berlin (retired)

Home Address:
Haupstrasse 56
D-01762 Ammelsdorf
Germany
49-35052-64252 (home)
49-35052-64252 (fax)

Specialty/Certification: Radiology, 1977

Education:
Medical School University of Basel,
Genreva (M.D.)
Pediatrics and Pediatric Radiology,
Boston
BCH and Childrens Medical Center
(BU & Harvard)
1953–59 and 1960–61

ISS Member Founding member

ISS Committees:
1972–74 – Steering Committee, Program
Committee,
Membership Committee
Organizer ISS Meeting Berlin, 1994

Spouse: Anita

KAYAYAMA, HITOSHI M.D.

Business Address:
Radiology
Juntendo Univ. School of Medicine
Takagi-cho, 2-10-19 Kokubunji-city
Tokyo 185
Japan
3-5802-1096 (work)
3-3812-6035 (fax)
0425-76-2039 (home)

Specialty: Radiology

ISS Member 1993

Spouse: Yasuku

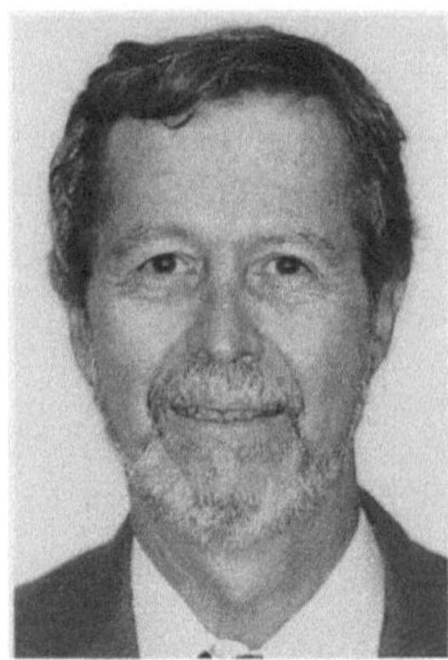

Academic Title: Professor of Radiology

Position at Affiliation: Chairman, Department Radiology

Business Address:
St. Vincents Hospital and Medical Center
153 West 11th Street
New York, NY 10011
U.S.A.
212-604-8717 (work)
212-604-2929 (fax)

Home Address:
1175 York Avenue, PH B-8
New York, NY 10021
U.S.A.
212-751-2634 (home)

Specialty/Certification: Radiology, 1970

Education:
1961 – University of Notre Dame (BS)
1965 – Cornell University Medical College (MD)
1966–69 –The New York Hospital – Cornell Medical Center (Radiology residency)

ISS Member 1975

Offices Held in ISS and Dates of Service:
Assistant Secretary – 1995–

ISS Committees:
Executive Committee – Member at Large
1991–93; 1996–97
Program Committee – 1993 – present;
Co-Chairman 1993–1996
Membership Committee – Chairman
1994–1996
Refresher Course Committee –
Chairman 1996–97
Convention Planning Committee –
1996–
Committee for Evaluation of Research
Grants – 1994–96
Board of Trustees of the Endowment
Fund 1996

Spouse: Margaret Bernadette

KEATS, THEODORE E. M.D.

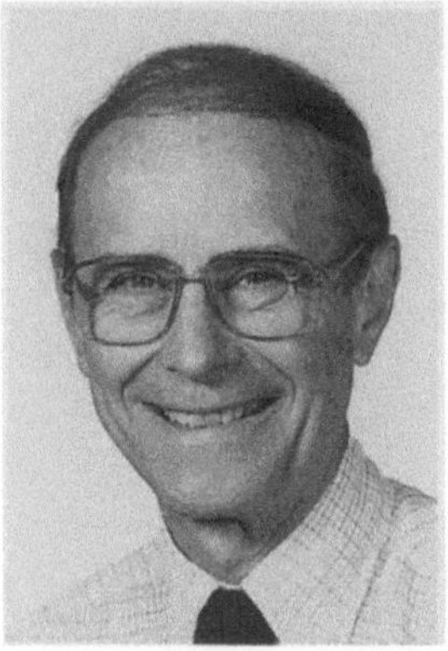

Birthdate: June 26, 1924

Academic Title: Professor of Radiology and Orthopedics

Position at Affiliation: Professor of Radiology

Business Address:
Department of Radiology
University of Virginia Health Sciences
Center
Charlottesville, VA 22908
U.S.A.
804-924-9377 (work)
804-982-1618 (fax)
tek@virginia.edu (e-mail)

Home Address:
421 Key West Drive
Charlottesville, VA
U.S.A.
804-296-2361 (home)

Specialty/Certification: Radiology, 1951

Education:
1945 – Rutgers University (B.S.)
1947 – University of Pennsylvania
School of Medicine (M.D.)
1947–48 – University of Pennsylvania
School of Medicine (internship)
1948–51 – University of Michigan
Hospital (Radiology residency)

ISS Committees:
North American Editor of Skeletal
Radiology
Editorial Committee, chairman

ISS Member Founding member

ISS Medals and Awards:
Medal of the ISS (Silver), New Orleans,
1995

Spouse: Patricia

KENAN, SAMUEL M.D.

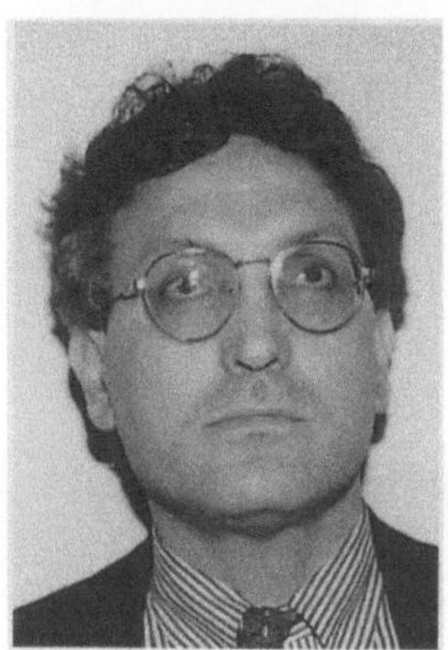

Academic Title: Associate Professor of
Orthopaedic Surgery

Position at Affiliation: Chief,
Orthopaedic Oncology

Business Address:
Hospital for Joint Diseases
Orthopaedic Oncology
301 E. 17th Street
New York, NY 10003
U.S.A.
212-598-6350 (work)
212-598-6276 (fax)

Home Address:
16 Old Seringtown Rd.
Albertson, NY 11507
U.S.A.
516-248-7756 (home)

Specialty/Certification: Orthopaedic
Surgery, 1984

Education:
Hadassah Medical Center, Jerusalem
(Medical School)
1978–84 – Hadassah Medical Center,
Jerusalem (residency)

ISS Member 1988

Spouse: Hedva

KERR, ROGER M. M.D.

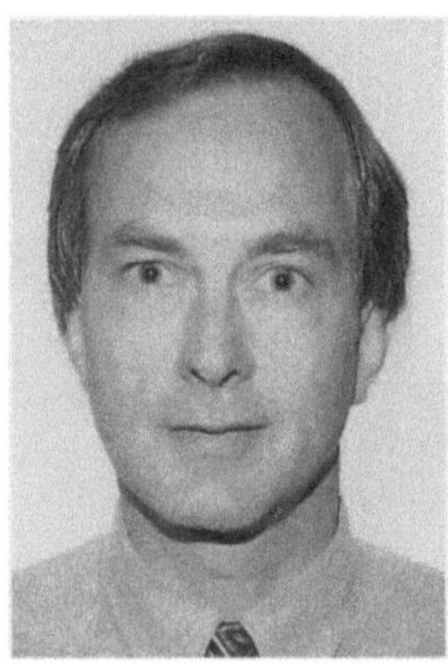

Birthdate: April 6, 1951

Academic Title: Clinical Professor of Radiology

Position at Affiliation: Director, Department of Radiology

Business Address:
Orthopaedic Hospital
Department of Radiology
2400 South Flower Street
Los Angeles, CA 90007
U.S.A.
213-742-1186 (work)
213-742-1473 (fax)

Home Address:
2612 34th Street
Santa Monica, CA 90405
U.S.A.
310-396-6175 (home)

Specialty/Certification: Radiology, 1984

Education:
SUNY at Stony Brook (B.S.)
Princeton University (Graduate Student
UMDNJ Rutgers Medical School (M.D.)
Hahnemann University Hospital
(Radiology residency)
University of Calif., San Diego
(fellowship in Osteoradiology)

ISS Member 1991

Spouse: Heidi Solz, M.D.

KILCOYNE, RAY F. M.D.

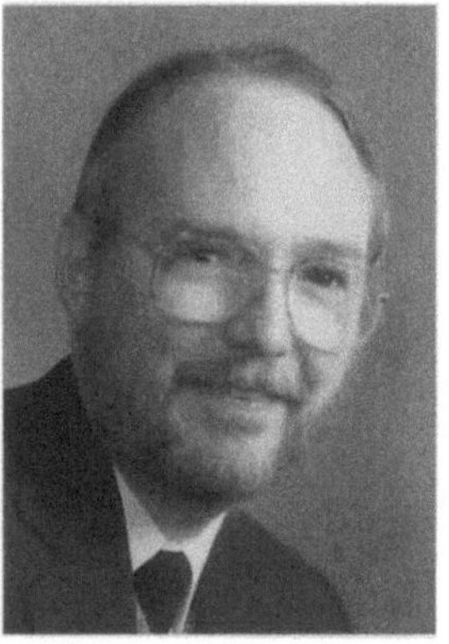

Birthdate: May 14, 1937

Academic Title: Professor

Position at Affiliation: Vice Chairman

Business Address:
Univ. Colorado Health Sciences Center
Department of Radiology
4200 East Ninth Avenue, Box A030
Denver Colorado 80262
U.S.A.
303-372-6136 (work)
303-372-6275 (fax)
Ray.Kilcoyne@UCHSC.edu (e-mail)

Home Address:
96 South Lupine
Golden, CO 80401
U.S.A.
303-278-4084 (home)
303-986-3951 (fax)

Specialty/Certification: Radiology, 1971

Education:
Marquette University School of
Medicine (M.D.)
Medical College of Wisconsin
(Radiology residency)

ISS Member 1984

Spouse: Claire

Business Address:
Department of Pathology II
Sahlgrenska University Hospital
University of Gothenburg
41345 Gothenburg
Sweden
46-31-601928 (work)
46-31-827194 (fax)

Home Address:
Engelbrektsgatan 6
41127 Gothenburg
Sweden
46-31-138584 (home)
46-31-138584 (fax)
Specialty: Anatomic Pathology

Education:
1971 – Gothenburg University (M.D.)
1975 – Gothenburg University (Ph.D)

ISS Member 1991

Spouse: Jeanne M. Meis-Kindblom M.D.

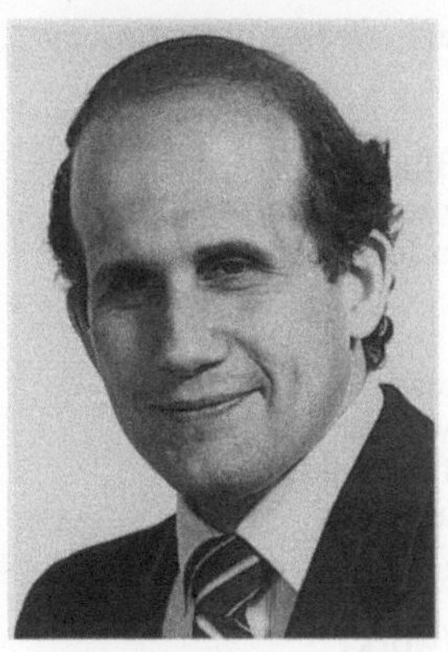

Birthdate: July 28, 1947

Academic Title: Professor of Pathology and Orthopaedics

Position at Affiliation: Attending Pathologist

Business Address:
Department of Pathology – Box 1194
Mount Sinai School of Medicine
One Gustave Levy Place
New York, NY 10029, U.S.A.
212-241-9129 (work)
212-534-7491 (fax)

Home Address:
1435 Lexington Avenue
New York, NY 10128, U.S.A.
212-289-8251 (home)

Specialty/Certification: Pathology, 1978

Education:
1969 – Rutgers University (AB)
1973 – Temple University (M.D.)
1973–77 – New York University School of Medicine (residency)
1977–78 – College of Physicians & Surgeons of Columbia University (fellowship in Orthopaedic Pathology)

ISS Member 1986

ISS Medals and Awards:
Corinne Farrell Award (1995)

ISS Committees:
Closed Program Committee, 1995–96

Spouse: Sheila

Academic Title: Professor of Radiology and Pediatrics

Position at Affiliation: Director, Pediatric Radiology; Director, Imaging Center for Child Abuse and Neglect

Business Address:
University of Massachusetts
Department of Radiology
55 Lake Avenue North
Worcester, MA 01655
U.S.A.
508-856-3124 (work)
508-856-4669 (fax)
paul.kleinman@banyan.ummed.edu
(e-mail)

Home Address:
Box 73
105 Angelica Avenue
Mattapoisett, MA 02739
U.S.A.
508-758-2274 (home)

Specialty/Certification: Radiology and Pediatrics, 1976

Education:
1967 – Boston University, Boston, MA
1971 – Downstate Medical Center, New York, NY (M.D.)
1971–72 – New York Hospital, New York, NY (internship in Pediatrics)
1972–73 – New York Hospital, New York, NY (residency/fellowship in Pediatrics)

ISS Member 1990

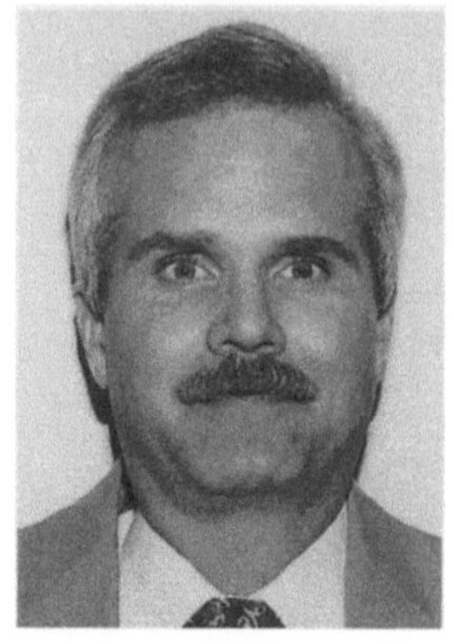

Birthdate: April 23, 1952

Academic Title: Associate Professor

Position at Affiliation: Radiologist

Business Address:
Department of Radiology
University of Pennsylvania Medical Center
3400 Spruce Street
Philadelphia, PA. 19104, U.S.A.
215-662-3037 (work)
215-662-7011 (fax)
kneeland@oasis.rad.upenn.rad (e-mail)

Home Address:
180 Berwind Circle
Radnor, PA. 19087, U.S.A.
610-971-0792 (home)

Specialty/Certification: Radiology, 1982

Education:
1970–1974 – Stanford University (B.S.)
1974–1978 – Jefferson Medical College (M.D.)
1978–1979 – University of Southern California Medical Center (internship)
1979–1982 – New York Hospital/Cornell Medical Center (resident in Radiology)
1982–1983 – Cornell Medical Center (fellow in CT and Ultrasound)

ISS Member 1992

ISS Medals and Awards:
President's Medal, Berlin, 1994

Spouse: Nancy

Kolár, Jaromir M.D., Sc.D., Prof.

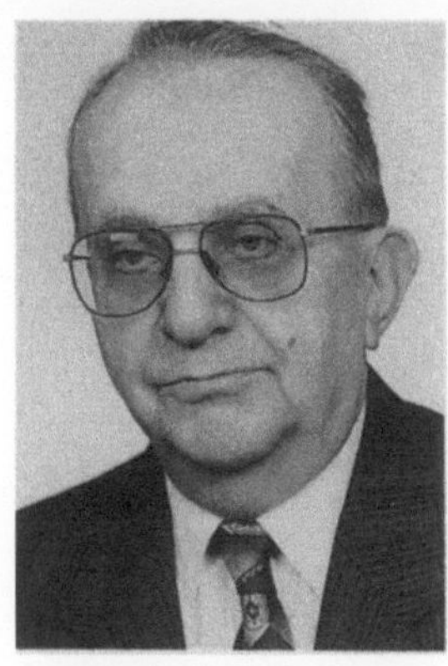

Birthdate: July 30, 1926

Academic Title: Professor

Position at Affiliation: Lecturer

Business Address:
Postgraduate Medical School
Clinic for Diagnostic Radiology
Budínova 2
Praha 8 Bulovka 180 81
Czech Republik
4 20 82-24-31 (work)
4 20 82 24 31 (fax)

Home Address:
Preslickova 5
Praha 10 10600
Czech Republik
4 20 75-51-022 (home)

Specialty/Certification: Radiology, 1954

Education:
1945–50 – Medical Faculty, Charles
University, Prague (student)
1950–M.D.

ISS Member 1979

Spouse: Olga Kolárová

Kozlowski, Kazimierz S. M.D.

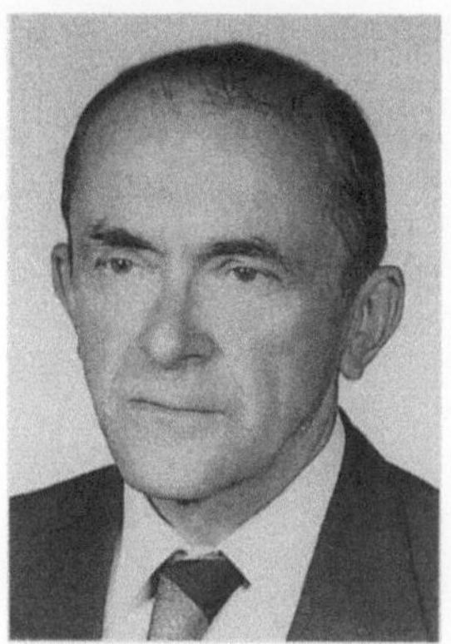

Birthdate: June 6, 1928

Academic Title: Doc. Dr. med.;
Hon. Dr. Univ. of Sydney

Position at Affiliation: Honorary
Radiologist

Business Address:
New Children's Hospital
P.O. Box 3515 – Parramatta
NSW 2124
Australia
(02) 9845-0000 (work)
(02) 845-3489 (fax)

Home Address:
8 Wilona Av
Wolstonecraft 2065 NSW
Australia
(02) 9438-2562 (home)

Specialty/Certification: Radiology, 1958

Education:
Poznan, Poland (Medical School)
Rockefeller Fellowship, Babies Hospital,
NY

ISS Member 1986

Spouse: Daniela

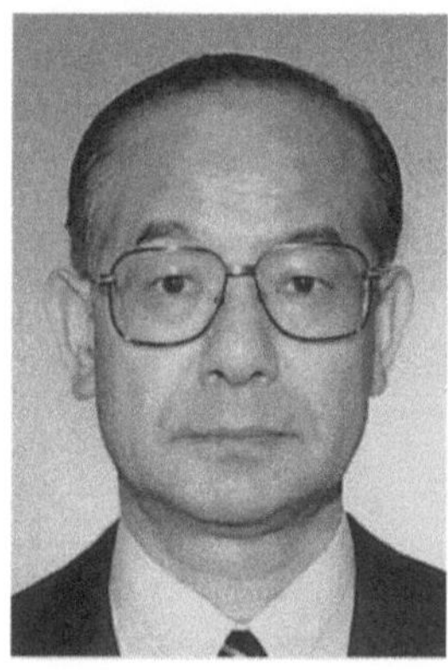

Birthdate: August 26, 1935

Academic Title: Professor

Position at Affiliation: Professor

Business Address:
Akita University School of Medicine
Hondo 1-1-1
010 Akita
Japan
81 188 34-1111 ext. 3331 (work)
81 188 36-2617 (fax)

Home Address:
Yanagida
Aza-Nukazuka 42
4-103
Akita 010
Japan
81-188-33-8788 (home)

Specialty/Certification: Orthopaedic
Surgery, 1983

Education:
Tohoku University, Sendai

ISS Member 1979

Spouse: Mitsue

Business Address:
Department of Radiologic Pathology
Armed Forces Institute
Washington, D.C. 20307
U.S.A.
202-576-2889/2973 (work)
301-924-0231 (home)
202-576-2164 (fax)

ISS Member 1991

Spouse: Judith

KRICUN, MORRIE E. M.D.

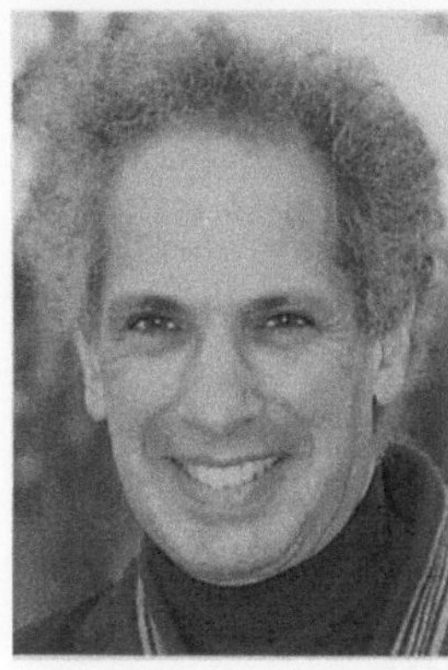

Birthdate: February 23, 1938

Academic Title: Professor

Position at Affiliation: Radiologist, Musculoskeletal Section

Business Address:
University of Pennsylvania Medical Center
Department of Radiology
1 Silverstein
3400 Spruce Street
Philadelphia, PA 19104
U.S.A.
215-662-3572 (work)
215-662-7011 (fax)
kricun@rad.upenn.edu (e-mail)

Home Address:
750 E. Weadley Road
Radnor, PA 19087
U.S.A.
610-687-3337 (home)

Specialty: Radiology, 1970

Education:
1955 – 59 – Muhlenberg College (B.S.)
1959 – 63 – Jefferson Medical College
(M.D.)
1963 – 64 – Albert Einstein Med. Ctr.,
Philadelphia, PA (internship)
1966 – 69 – Albert Einstein Med. Ctr.,
Philadelphia, PA (Radiology residency)

ISS Member Founding member

ISS Committees:
ISS Historian 1995 –
Auditing Committee, chairman
Membership Committee, co-chairman,
1986 – 90
Ad Hoc Liaison Committee for Future
Planning, 1987 – 96;
co-chairman, 1987 – 89, 1992 – 94;
chairman 1990 – 92
Ad Hoc Committee on Recruitment
of Skeletal Radiologists,
Co-Chair1989 – 92
Ad Hoc Proceedings Committee,
1992 – 93
Refresher Course Committee, 1983 – 84
Editor ISS Book of Members, 1995 –
Nomenclature Committee, 1996 –
Closed Program Committee, 1983 – 85;
1988 – 93

Spouse: Virginia (Ginny)

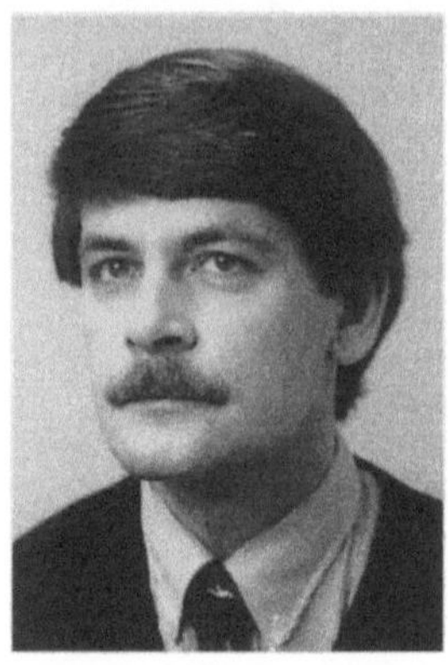

Birthdate: July 28, 1954

Position at Affiliation: Head of the Department of Skeletal Radiology

Business Address:
University Hospital Leiden
Albinusdreef 2
2333 ZA Leiden
The Netherlands
31-71-5262993 / 31-71-5262042 (work)
31-71-5248256 / 31-71-5248245 (fax)

Home Address:
Krefeldlaan 1
2314 EC Leiden
The Netherlands
31-71-5415859 (home)

Specialty/Certification: Radiology, 1983

Education:
1966–71 – College
1971–78 – Leiden University
(Graduate School)
1979–83 – University Hospital Leiden
(specialty training)

ISS Member 1996

Spouse: Ernestine Mensinga Wieringa

Birthdate: April 17, 1944

Academic Title: Professor

Position at Affiliation: Faculty
(Professor)

Business Address:
University of Texas Medical Branch
Department of Radiology
301 University Blvd, Room 2.120 OCH
Galveston, TX 77555-0709
U.S.A.
409-772-1873 (work)
409-747-2825 (fax)
raj.kumar@utmb.edu (e-mail)

Home Address:
16211 Brookvilla
Houston, TX 77059
U.S.A.
713-280-8153 (home)

Specialty/Certification: Radiology, 1975;
Nuclear Medicine, 1976

Education:
All India Institute of Medical Sciences,
New Delhi, India (M.D.)

ISS Member 1988

Spouse: Kusum

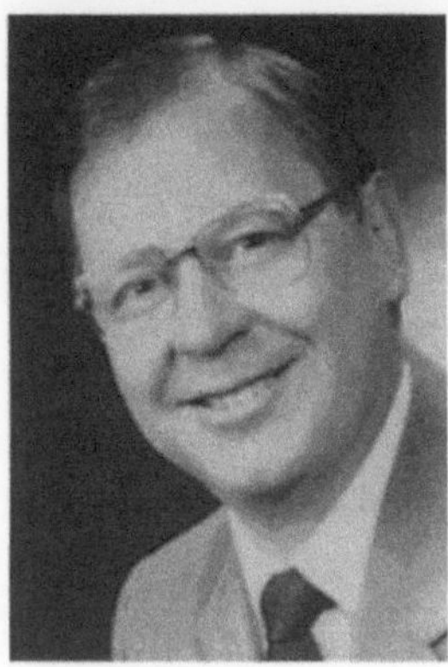

Business Address:
Radiology
Central Military Hospital
PL 5
00281 Helsinki
Finland

Specialty: Radiology

ISS Member 1983

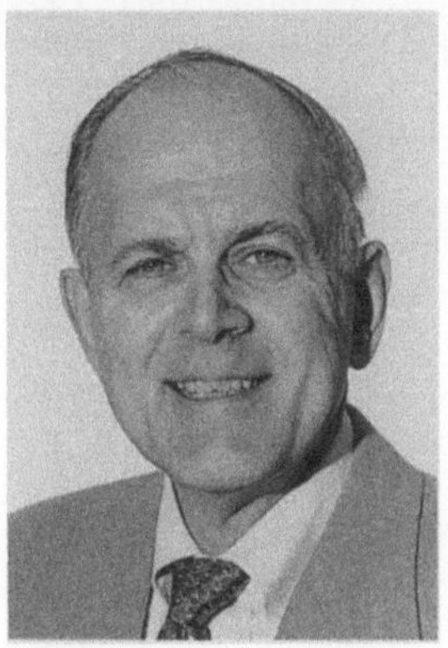

Birthdate: January 18, 1938

Academic Title: Professor of Surgical
Pathology

Position at Affiliation: Senior Surgical
Pathologist

Business Address:
Department of Pathology
Washington University School of
Medicine
Box 8118
St. Louis, MO 63110
U.S.A.
314-362-0119 (work)
314-362-8950 (fax)

Home Address:
217 Huntleigh Drive
Kirkwood, MO 63122
U.S.A.
314-822-4619 (home)

Specialty/Certification: Anatomic
Pathology, 1968

Education:
1958 – City College of New York (B.S.)
1962 – Albert Einstein College of
Medicine (M.D.)
1962–64 – Washington Univ./Barnes
Hosp. (internship/resident, pathology)
1964–66 – NIH (Research Associate)
1966–67 – Washington Univ./Barnes
Hosp. (Fellow, Surgical Pathology)

ISS Member 1981

ISS Committees:
Liaison Planning Committee 1992–1995
Closed Program Committee 1995–1996
Membership Committee 1997–
Editorial Board, Skeletal Radiology
1997–

Spouse: Jamie

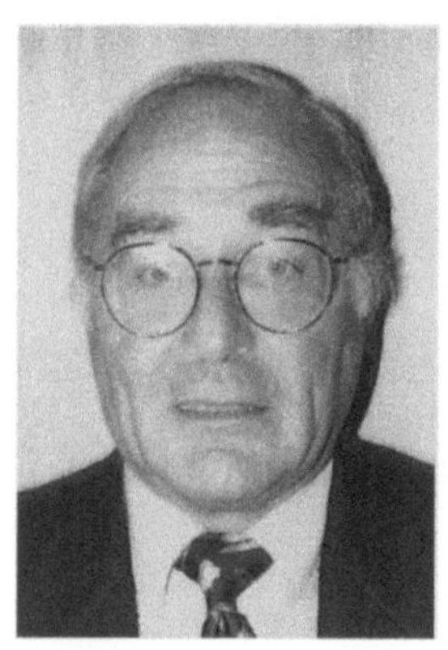

Birthdate: May 12, 1935

Academic Title: Professor of Radiology
and Pediatrics

Position at Affiliation: Pediatric
Radiologist; Co Investigator

Business Address:
International Skeletal Dysplasia Registry
and Harbor UCLA Medical Center
444 S. San Vincente Blvd. Rm. 1001
Los Angeles, CA 90048, U.S.A.
310-222-2806 (work)
213-651-5381 or 310-618-9500 (fax)

Home Address:
1636 Dalton Road
Palos Verdes Estate
Palos Verdes, CA 90274, U.S.A.
310-378-8037 (home)

Specialty/Certification: Pediatrics 1968;
Radiology 1970; Pediatric Radiology 1995

Education:
Temple University
Meharry Medical College (M.D.)
1962–64 Mt. Sinai Hospital, New York,
NY (Pediatric residency)
1966–68 Children's Hospital Medical
Center, Boston, MA (Pediatric
Radiology residency)

ISS Member 1978

ISS Committees:
Editorial Board Skeletal Radiology,
1989–95

Spouse: Rose

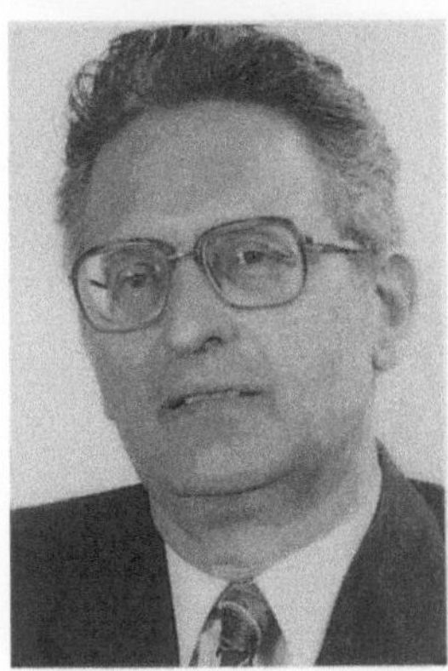

Birthdate: July 18, 1925

Academic Title: Professor Emeritus

Position at Affiliation: Pensioned

Business Address:
Department of Pathology
Genèva School of Medicine
CMU 1, rue Michel-Servet
CH-1211, Genève 4
Switzerland
4122 372 4929 (work)
4122 3724 920 (fax)

Home Address:
118 Rue de Genève
F74240 Gaillard
France

Specialty/Certification: Rheumatology, 1959

Education:
Graduate of Lyon School of Medicine
(Lyon, France)

ISS Member 1983

ISS Committees:
Future Planning Committee, 1988–89

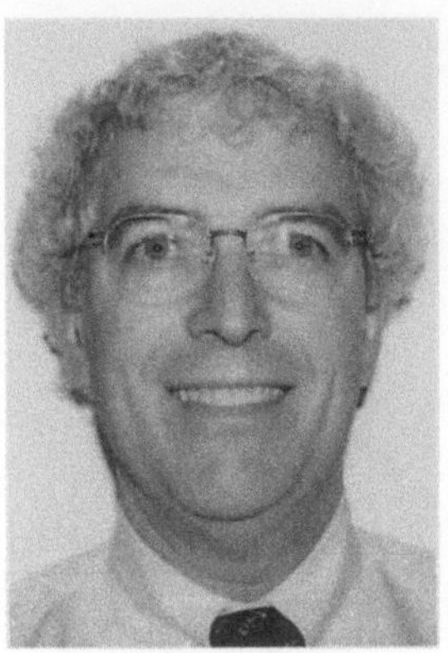

Birthdate: September 17, 1941

Academic Title: Associate Professor of
Radiology

Business Address:
SMBD Jewish General Hospital
3755 Côte St. Catherine Road
Montreal, Quebec, H3T 1E2
Canada
514-340-8233 (work)
514-340-7907 (fax)
pilander@object.people.on.ca (e-mail)

Home Address:
5637 Eldridge Avenue
Montreal, Quebec H4W 2C9
Canada
514-487-4078 (home)

Specialty/Certification: Radiology, 1971

Education:
McGill University, Montreal, Quebec,
Canada

ISS Member 1991

Spouse: Freema

LANE, JOSEPH M. M.D.

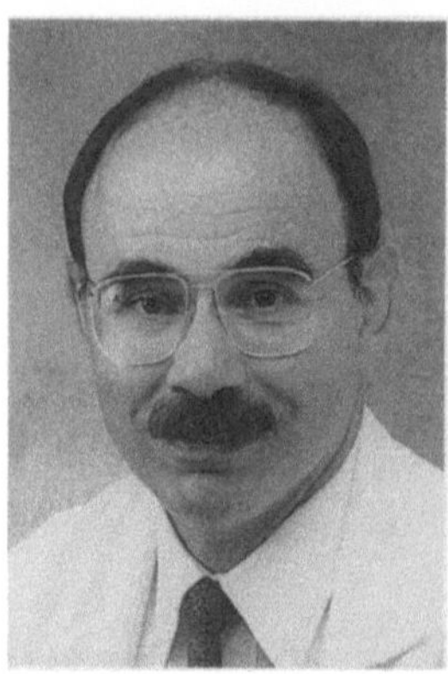

Birthdate: October 27, 1939

Academic Title: Professor Orthopedic Surgery

Position at Affiliation: Chief, Metabolic Bone Disease

Business Address:
Hospital for Special Surgery
535 East 70th Street
New York, NY 10021
U.S.A.
212-606-1172 (work)
212-772-1061 (fax)
lanej@hss.edu (e-mail)

Home Address:
38 Saw Mill Hill Road
Ridgefield, CT 06877
U.S.A.
203-894-8338 (home)
203-894-8339 (fax)

Specialty/Certification: Orthopedic Surgery, 1974

Education:
1961 – Columbia College (A.B.)
1965 – Harvard Medical School (M.D.)
1969–73 – Hospital University of Pennsylvania (Orthopedic residency)

ISS Member 1985

Spouse: Barbara

LANGER, JR., LEONARD O. M.D.

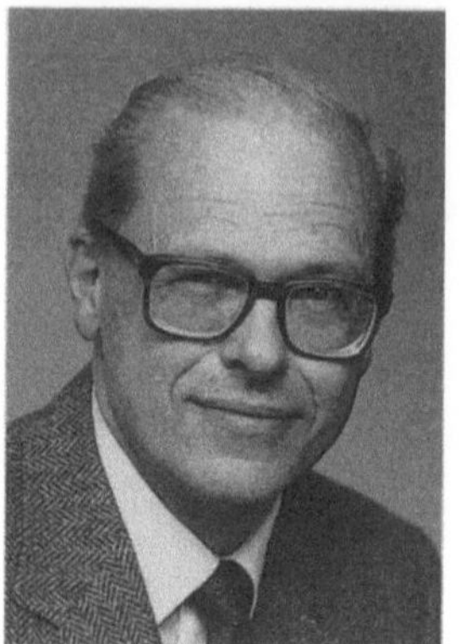

Birthdate: October 16, 1928

Academic Title: Clinical Professor

Position at Affiliation: Consultant-Pediatric Radiology

Business Address:
University of Minnesota Hospital
Box 292
Minneapolis, MN 55455
U.S.A.
612-338-6850 (work)
612-626-1951 (fax)

Home Address:
1235 Yale Place, 710
Minneapolis, MN 55403
U.S.A.
612-338-6850 (home)
612-338-3172 (fax)

Specialty/Certification: Radiology, 1960

Education:
University of Minnesota (B.A.)
University of Minnesota Medical School (B.S., M.D.)
University of Michigan (Radiology residency)

ISS Member 1974

Spouse: Rollie

LAREDO, JEAN-DENIS M.D.

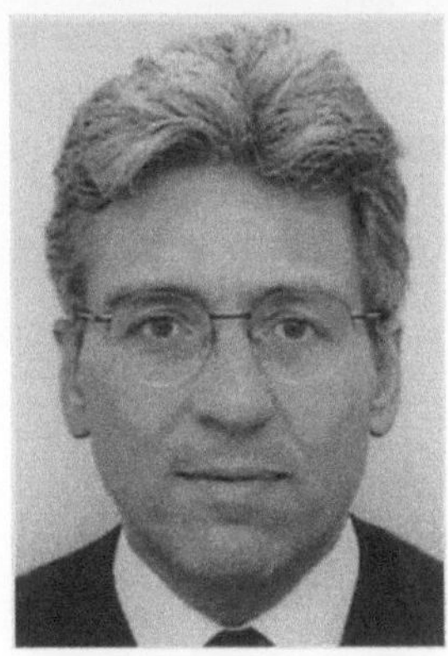

Birthdate: August 7, 1951

Academic Title: Professor of Radiology

Position at Affiliation: Chief

Business Address:
Radiologie Ostéo-Articulaire
Hôpital Lariboisière
2, rue Ambroise-Paré
Paris 75010
France
33-1-49-95-61-78 (work)
33-1-49-95-86-99 (fax)
jean-denis.laredo@prb.ap-hp-paris.fr
(e-mail)

Home Address:
1 rue D'Alencon
Paris 75015
France
33-1-45-49-19-12 (home)

Specialty/Certification: Rhumatology
1982; Radiology, 1983

Education:
Chu Broussais – Hotel Dieu, Paris VI
Chu Lariboisiere – Saint Louis, Paris VII

ISS Member 1987

ISS Medals and Awards:
President's Medal, Salzburg, 1990

ISS Committees:
Promotion of Overseas Meetings
Committee, 1995

Spouse: Lynda

LAVAL-JEANTET, M. M.D.

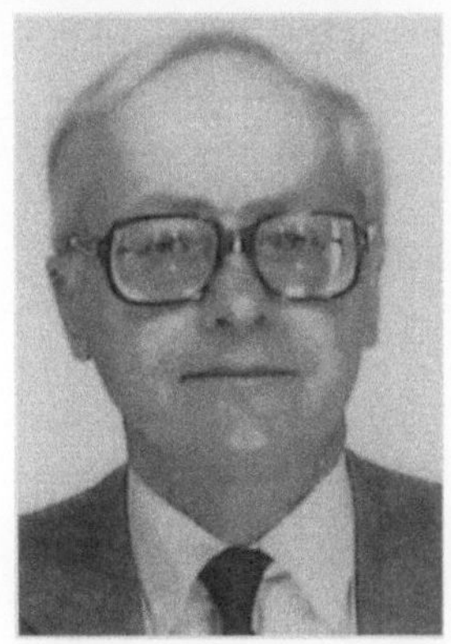

Business Address:
Department of Radiology
Hopital Saint-Louis
38, Rue Bichat
75010 Paris
France

Specialty: Radiology

ISS Member 1978

LAWSON, JACK P. MB, CHB, FRCR

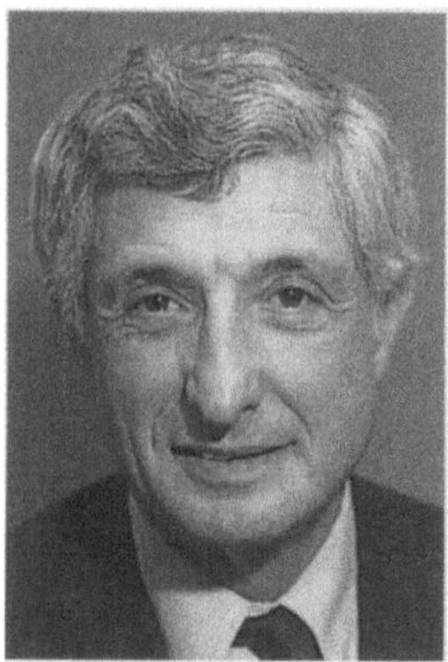

Birthdate: October 22, 1930

Academic Title: Professor of Radiology and Orthopedic Surgery

Business Address:
Department of Radiology
Yale University School of Medicine
333 Cedar Street
New Haven, CT 06520
U.S.A.
203-785-2384 (work)
203-785-7015 (fax)
jack.lawson@yale.edu (e-mail)

Home Address:
30 Brierwood Drive
Woodbridge , CT 06525
U.S.A.
203-387-5310 (home)

Specialty/Certification: Radiology
(U.K.), 1961, 1964;
Radiology (U.S.), 1968

Education:
University of Manchester School
of Medicine
Radiology residency University of
Liverpool
fellowship in Neuroradiology, University
of Newcastle upon Tyne
fellowship in Pediatric Radiology,
Children Hospital, Cincinnati

ISS Member 1982

ISS Committees:
Co-Chairman, Closed Program
Committee 1986–93
(Chairman 1988–93)
Archives Committee 1988–91
Corinne Farrell Awards Committee 1991
Consulting editor, Skeletal Radiology
1986–96

Spouse: Elaine

LEE, RUI-ZONG M.D.

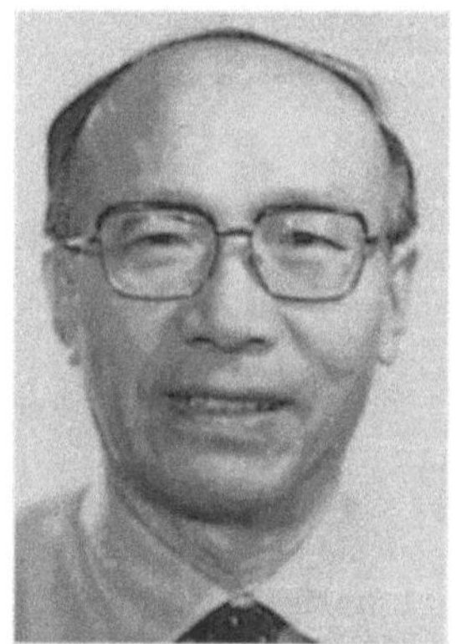

Business Address:
Department of Pathology
Orthopaedic Research Institute
Tianjin Hospital
Jie Fang Nan Lu
He Xi-District
Tianjin
Peoples Republic of China
282917-18 (work)
3454-3 (home)

ISS Member 1987

Spouse: Lee Ku Jung

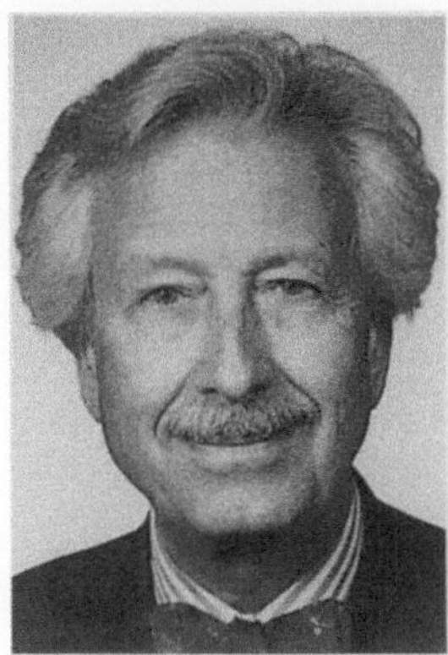

Birthdate: December 20, 1924

Academic Title: Professor

Position at Affiliation: Consultant

Business Address:
33 rue Guilleminot
75014 Paris
France
33-1-43-35-23-33 (work)
33-1-43-22-66-46 (fax)

Home Address:
33 rue Guilleminot
75014 Paris
France
33-1-43-35-23-33 (home)
33-1-43-22-66-46 (fax)

Specialty/Certification: Rheumatology, 1961

ISS Member 1976

Spouse: Natacha

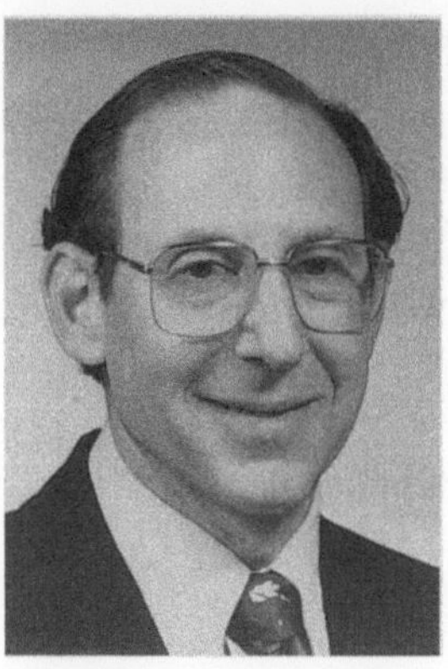

Birthdate: July 24, 1941

Academic Title: Clinical Professor

Position at Affiliation: Chief, Musculo-skeletal Radiology

Business Address:
Crouse Hospital & SUNY Health Science Center
736 Irving Avenue
Syracuse, NY 13210
U.S.A.
315-470-7551 (work)
315-470-5757 (fax)

Home Address:
5105 Muirfield Drive
Fayetteville, NY 13066
U.S.A.
315-637-8799 (home)

Specialty/Certification: Radiology, 1975

Education:
University of Washington, Seattle (BA)
University of Washington, Seattle (MD)
Baltimore City Hospital, Baltimore, MD
(Internal Medicine resident)
University of Vermont Hospitals,
Burlington, VT (Radiology resident)

ISS Member 1984

Spouse: Jeannette

Levy, Walter M. M.D.

Business Address:
Department of Pathology
Cooper Hospital Univ. Med. Center
One Cooper Plaza
Camden, NJ 08103
U.S.A.
609-342-2514 (work)

Specialty: Pathology

ISS Member Founding member

Lewis, Michael M.D.

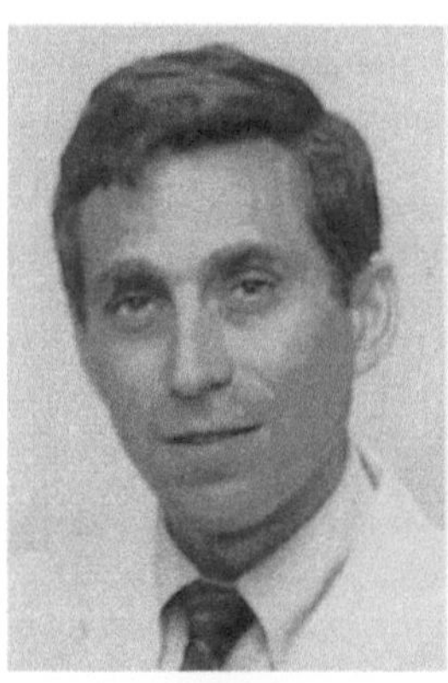

Business Address:
Dept. of Orthopaedics
Mt. Sinai Hospital
One Gustave L. Levy Place
Box 1188
New York, NY 10029
U.S.A.

Specialty: Orthopaedic Surgery

ISS Member 1985

Lingg, Gerwin M. M.D.

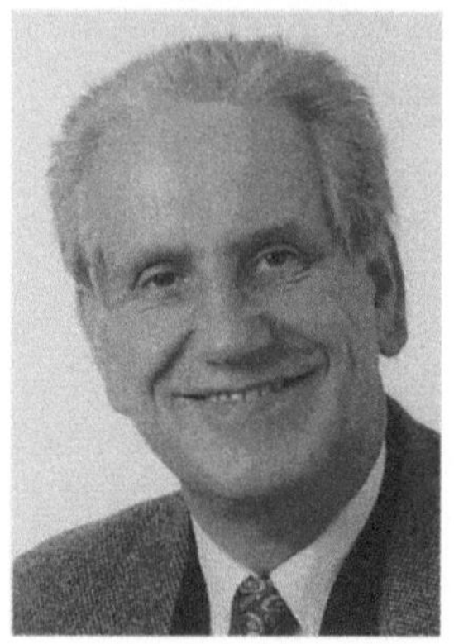

Position at Affiliation: Chief of Department

Business Address:
Zentrales Röntgeninstitut in
Rheuma-zentrum Bad Kreznach
Dr. Alfons-Gamp-Str. 1-5
D-55543 Bad Kreuznach
Germany
0671-931260 (work)
0671-932992 (fax)

Home Address:
Nelli-Schmithals-Str. 52
D-55543 Bad Kreuznach
Germany
0671-73239 (home)

Specialty/Certification: Radiology, 1981

Education:
1972–74 – St. Georg Hamburg (Radiation Therapie AK)
1976–81 – AK Barmbek (Diagnostic Radiology)

ISS Member 1985

Spouse: Eva-Maria

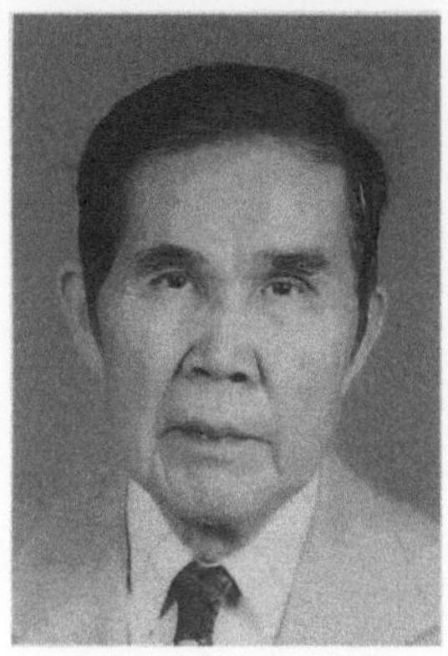

Birthdate: December 1, 1925

Academic Title: Professor

Position at Affiliation: Sr. Pathologist and Chairman

Business Address:
Department of Pathology
Animal Medical Center
510 East 62nd Street
New York, NY 10021
U.S.A.
212-838-8100 (work)
212-832-9288, 832-9630 (fax)

Home Address:
182-49 80th Road
Jamaica Estates
New York, NY 11432
U.S.A.
718-380-4787 (home)
718-380-4787 (fax)

Specialty: Pathology

Education:
Veterinary College of the Chinese Army, DVM
University of California, PhD
1964–67 – Bronx General Veteran Hospital (Pathology fellow)

ISS Member 1985

Spouse: Sing-ping Chueh, M.D.

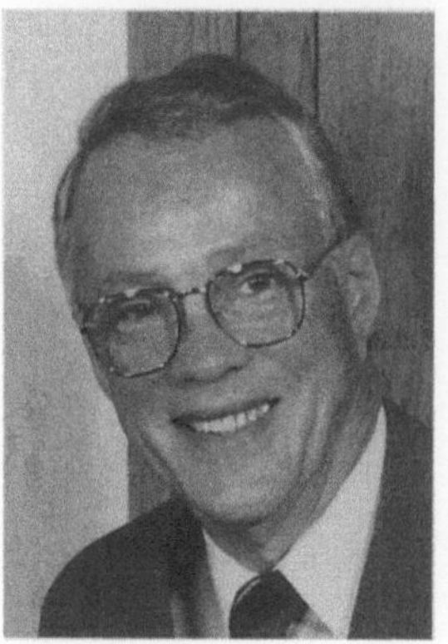

Birthdate: August 30, 1917

Academic Title: Professor Emeritus

Position at Affiliation: Honorary Radiologist

Business Address:
Massachusetts General Hospital
Boston, MA 02114
U.S.A.
lodwick@worldnet.att.nct (e-mail)

Home Address:
3900 Gulf Ocean Mile, Drive #307
Ft. Lauderdale, FL 33308
U.S.A.
954-565-1824 (home)
954-565-1804 (fax)

Specialty/Certification: Radiology, 1950

Education:
1943 – University of Iowa (B.A., M.D.)
After service in World War II,
University of Iowa (residency in Pathology and Radiology)
1951 – Armed Forces Institute of Pathology (fellowship)

ISS Member Founding member

ISS Medals and Awards:
Founders' Gold Medal, Salzburg, 1990

Spouse: Maria Antonia

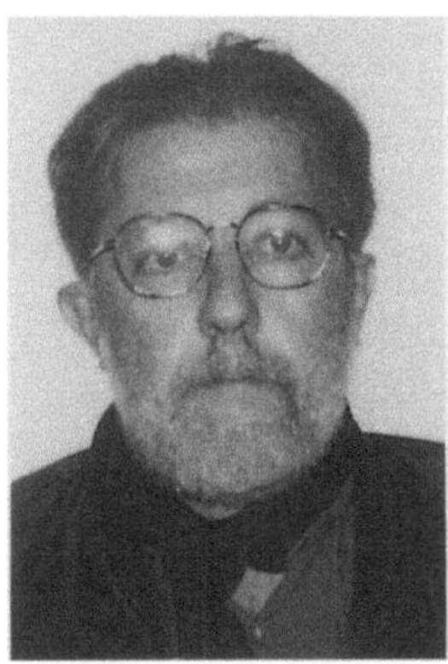

Birthdate: September 4, 1943

Academic Title: Associate Professor of Anatomic Pathology

Position at Affiliation: Chief of Surgical Pathology

Business Address:
Hospital Universitan "Germans Trids i Pujol" Carretera del Canyet s/n
Badalona, Barcelona
Spain
43-3-418 2191 (work)
43-3-418 1095 (fax)
43-3-418 2191 (home)
jlorenzo@ns.hugtip.scs.es (e-mail)

Specialty/Certification: Anatomic Pathology, 1973

Education:
Universidad de Barcelona
Facultad de Medicina de Barcelona

ISS Member 1986

ISS Committees:
Promotion of the Refresher Course Outside North America

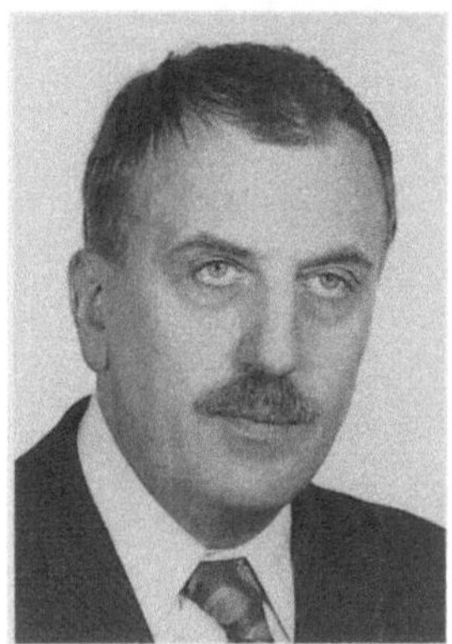

Academic Title: Dozent Dr. med. habil.

Position at Affiliation: Chefarzt

Business Address:
Semmelweiss University, Radiologic Clin.
National Institute of Rheumatology and Physiotherapy
H-1525
Budapest 114 Pf.54
Hungary
36-1212-4627 (work)
h-1052budapestpetofis.u.10.III/2 (e-mail)

Home Address:
1052 Budapest
Petofi S.u.10.III/2
Hungary
36-1-1376-168 (home)

Specialty/Certification: Radiology, 1957

Education:
Semmelweiss University, Radiologic Clinic

ISS Member 1991

Spouse: Maria Istvànffy, M.D.

MABILLE, JEAN-PIERRE M.D.

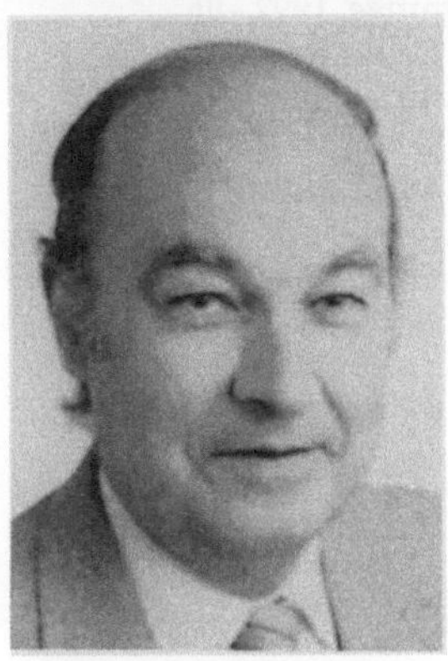

Business Address:
Hospital du Bocage
Service radiologie
10, Boulevard de Lattre-de-Tassigny
21035 Dijon
France

ISS Member 1986

MACHINAMI, RIKUO M.D., D.M.SCI.

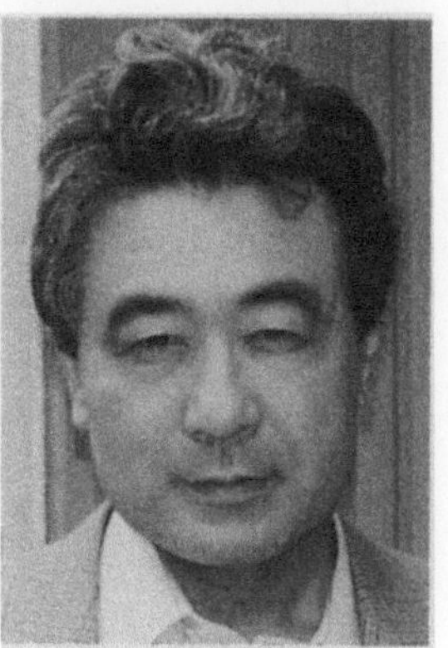

Birthdate: March 10, 1939

Academic Title: Professor of Pathology

Position at Affiliation: Professor and
Chairman

Business Address:
Department of Pathology
Graduate School and Faculty of Medicine
University of Tokyo Hospital
Hongo 7-3-1, Bunkyo-Ku
Tokyo 113
Japan
81-3-3812-9877 (work)
81-3-3815-8379(fax)

Home Address:
Gotokuji 2-16-24
Setagaya-ku
Tokyo 154
Japan
81-3-3426-1229 (home)
81-3-3426-5206 (fax)

Specialty/Certification: Pathology, 1980

Education:
1965 – Faculty of Medicine,
The University of Tokyo (MD)
1972–74 – British Council Scholar,
Chester Beatty Research Institute in
London

ISS Member 1983

Spouse: Kimiko

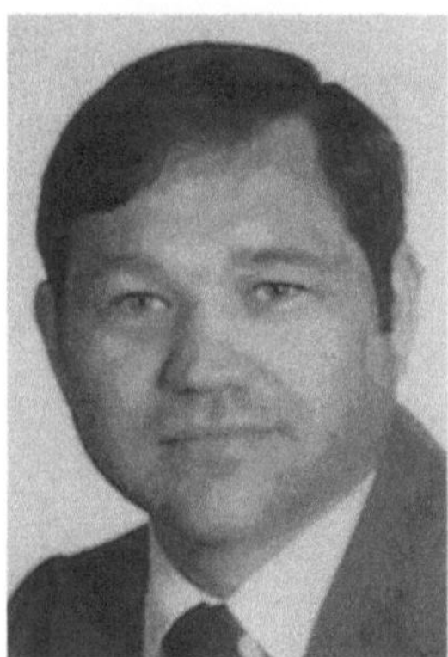

Birthdate: November 16, 1941

Academic Title: Professor and Chair, Department of Radiology

Position at Affiliation: Professor and Chair, Department of Radiology

Business Address:
Department of Radiology
The Milton S. Hershey Medical Center
Penn State University Hospital
500 University Drive
Hershey, PA 17033
U.S.A.
717-531-8044 (work)
717-531-5596 (fax)
jmadewell@xray.hmc.psu.edu (e-mail)

Home Address:
P.O. Box 895
Hershey, PA 17033
U.S.A.
717-533-6405 (home)

Specialty/Certification: Radiology, 1970

Education:
1965 – Central State College, Edmond, OK (college)
1969 – University of Oklahoma School of Medicine (M.D.)
1970 – Madigan General Hospital, Tacoma, WA (internship in medicine)
1973 – Walter Reed Army Medical Center, Washington, DC (residency Diagnostic Radiology)
1974 – Armed Forces Institute of Pathology (fellowship in radiologic pathology)

ISS Member 1975

ISS Committees:
Program Committee, 1992–96
Nomenclature Committee, 1994
Auditing Committee, 1996

Spouse: Theodora (Teddy)

Magid, Donna M.D.

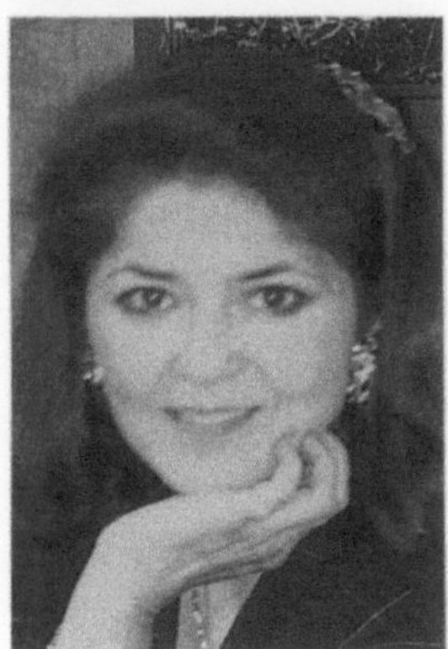

Academic Title: Associate Professor
of Radiology; Associate Professor
of Orthopaedic Surgery

Position at Affiliation: Associate
Professor of Radiology and Orthopaedic
Surgery; Deputy Editor, Radiology

Business Address:
Department of Radiology
The Johns Hopkins Medical Institutions
600 North Wolfe Street
Baltimore, MD 21205
U.S.A.
410-955-6500 (work)
410-955-5564 (fax)
dmagid@rad.jhu.edu (e-mail)

Home Address:
101 Swanhill Court
Baltimore, MD 21208
U.S.A.
410-486-8998 (home)

Specialty: Radiology

Education:
Child Psychology (Masters Med.)
Tufts University, Boston, MA (B.S.)
John Hopkins University, Baltimore, MA
(M.D.)

ISS Member 1988

Mahboubi, Saroosh M.D., FACR

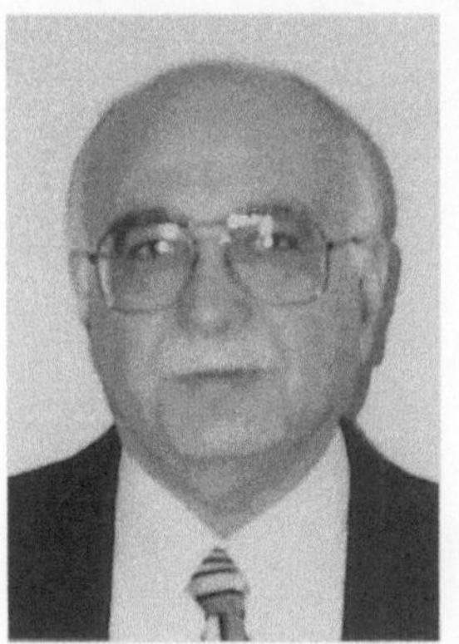

Birthdate: November 22, 1940

Academic Title: Professor of Radiology,
University of Pennsylvania

Position at Affiliation: Director,
Body CT, CHOP

Business Address:
Department of Radiology
Children's Hospital of Philadelphia
34th St. and Civic Center Blvd.
Philadelphia, PA 19104
U.S.A.
215-590-2561 (work)
215-590-4318 (fax)
mahboubi@chop.edu (e-mail)

Home Address:
104 Rock Rose Lane
Radnor, PA 19087
U.S.A.
610-688-2385 (home)

Specialty/Certification: Radiology, 1976;
Pediatric Radiology,
re-certification, 1994

Education:
Thomas Jefferson University –
Diagnostic Radiology
Children's Hospital of Philadelphia –
Pediatric Radiology

ISS Member 1994

ISS Committees:
Refresher Course, 1996 – 98

Spouse: Soheila

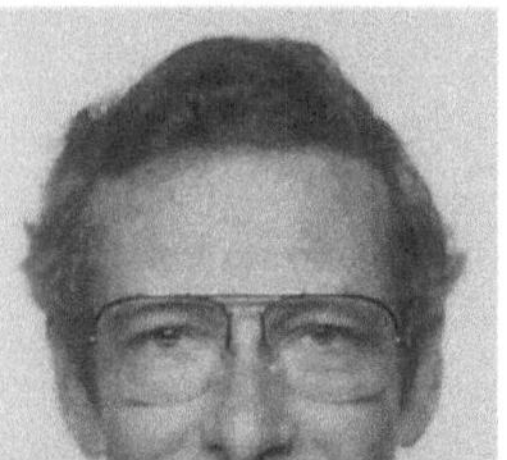

Birthdate: February 23, 1939

Academic Title: Clinical Professor, Radiology

Position at Affiliation: Chairman, Department of Radiology

Business Address:
Radiology Department
St. Francis Memorial Hospital
900 Hyde Street
San Francisco, CA 94109
U.S.A.
415-353-6390 (work)
415-441-5076 (fax)

Home Address:
254 29th Avenue
San Francisco, CA 94121
U.S.A.
415-387-4623 (home)
415-387-4623 (fax)

Specialty/Certification: Radiology, 1973

Education:
New York University (MD)
UCSF – San Francisco
(radiology residency)

ISS Member 1973

Spouse: Lonnie Zwerin

Position at Affiliation: Chairman

Business Address:
Histopathology Subgroup
MRCC/EORTC Bone Sarcoma Traials
University of Newcastle upon Tyne
Newcastle upon Tyne
England
91-232-5131 ext. 24445 (work)
91-222-8100 (fax)
91-258-6961 (home)

Specialty: Pathology

ISS Member 1991

Spouse: Patricia

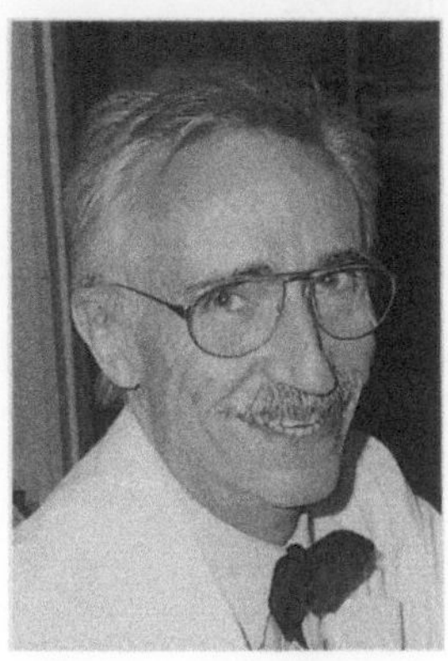

Birthdate: April 25, 1941

Academic Title: Professor of Radiology

Position at Affiliation: Professor and Chairman, Department of Radiology

Business Address:
Department of Radiology
St Luc University Hospital
B-1200 Brussels
Belgium
32-2-764-2940 (work)
32-2-764-8947 (fax)
maldague@rdgn.ucl.ac.be (e-mail)

Home Address:
Avenue des Bouvreuils
24, B-1301 Bierges
Belgium
32-10-417683 (home)
32-10-417683 (fax)

Specialty/Certification: Radiology, 1970

Education:
Catholic University of Louvain

ISS Member 1980

Spouse: Szendrei E

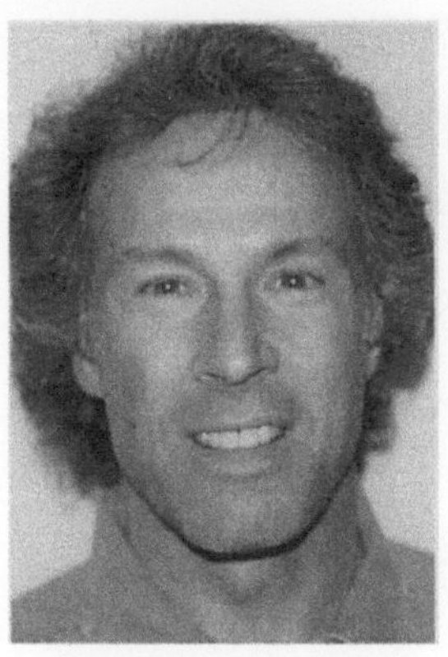

Birthdate: July 14, 1942

Academic Title: Clinical Professor of Radiology

Position at Affiliation: Vice-Chairman Department of Radiology

Business Address:
Department of Radiology
California Pacific Medical Center
3700 California Street
San Francisco, CA 94118
U.S.A.
415-750-6025 or 415-923-3232 (work)
415-750-5000 (fax)

Home Address:
43 Geldert Court
Tiburon, CA 94920
U.S.A.
415-435-2374 (home)
415-435-2375 (fax)

Specialty/Certification: Radiology, 1972

Education:
University of Illinois (undergraduate)
Northwestern University (MD)
University of Chicago (residency in Radiology)

ISS Member 1977

Spouse: Susan

MANASTER, B.J. M.D., PH.D.

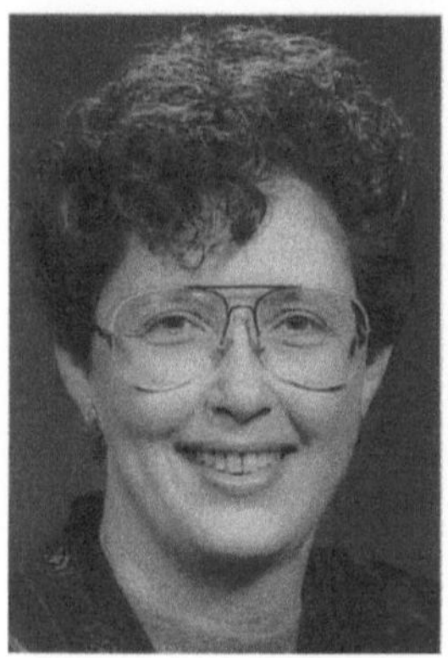

ISS Member 1985

ISS Committees:
Liaison Committee, 1992

Spouse: Steve Manaster, Ph.D.

Birthdate: July 14, 1949

Academic Title: Professor of Radiology

Position at Affiliation: Professor and
Vice Chair of Radiology

Business Address:
Department of Radiology
University of Utah School of Medicine
1A71 Health Sciences Center
50 North Medical Drive
Salt Lake City, UT 84132
U.S.A.
801-581-7553 (work)
801-581-2414 (fax)
bj.manaster@hsc.utah.edu

Home Address:
1416 Wasatch Drive
Salt Lake City, UT 84108
U.S.A.
801-583-4465 (home)

Specialty/Certification: Radiology, 1982

Education:
1970 – Oberlin College, Oberlin, OH
(BA Biology)
1975 – University of Chicago, Chicago, IL
(Ph.D. Anatomy)
1978 – University of Florida, Gainesville,
FL (M.D.)
1982 – University of Chicago, Chicago, IL
(Diagnostic Radiology residency)
1983 – Hospital for Joint Disease, Orthopedic Institute, New York, NY
(Musculoskeletal Radiology fellowship)

Mandell, Gerald A. M.D., FACR, FAAP

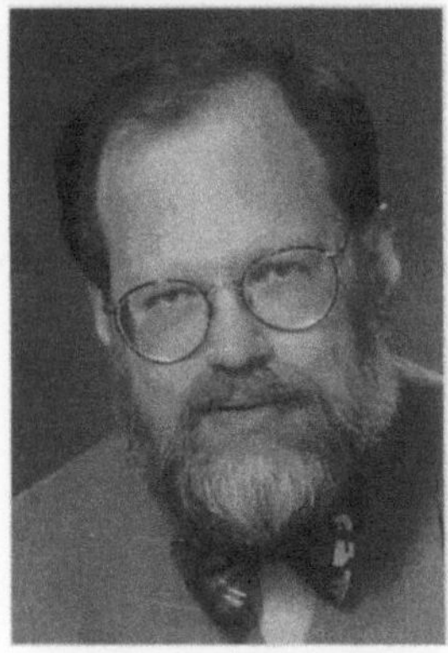

Academic Title: Professor of Radiology and Nuclear Medicine

Position at Affiliation: Chief of Nuclear Medicine

Business Address:
Department of Medical Imaging
Alfred I. Dupont Institute
P.O. Box 269
Wilmington, DE 19899
U.S.A.
302-651-4644 (work)
302-651-4626 (fax)
gmandell@nemours.aidi.org (e-mail)

Home Address:
383 Jenissa Drive
West Chester, PA 19382
U.S.A.
610-430-6630(home)
610-430-6632 (fax)

Specialty/Certification: Radiology, 1974;
Nuclear Medicine, 1983;
Pediatric Radiology CAQ, 1995

Education:
1962–65 – University of Pennsylvania
(B.A.)
1965–69 – Jefferson Medical College
(M.D.)
1970–73 – Jefferson Medical College
(Diagnostic Radiology)
1973–74 – St. Christopher's Hospital for
Childrens/Jefferson Medical
College (Pediatric Radiology)

ISS Member 1986

Spouse: Joanna

Mankin, Henry J. M.D.

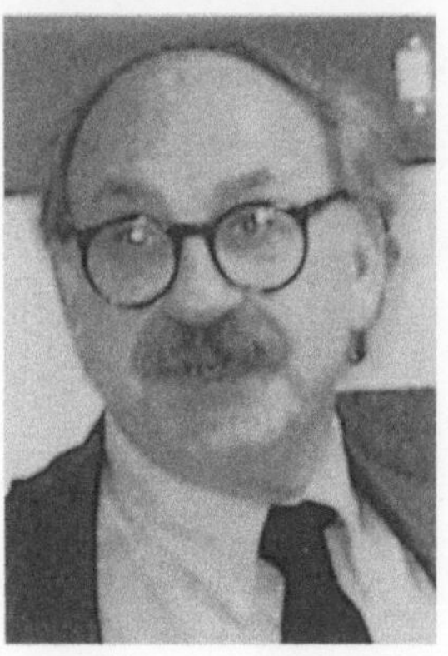

Business Address:
Harvard Medical School
Orthopaedic Department
Massachusetts General Hospital
Boston, MA 02114
U.S.A.
617-738-1541 (home)
617-726-2943 (work)
617-726-6823 (fax)

Specialty: Orthopaedic Surgery

ISS Member 1975

Spouse: Carole J.

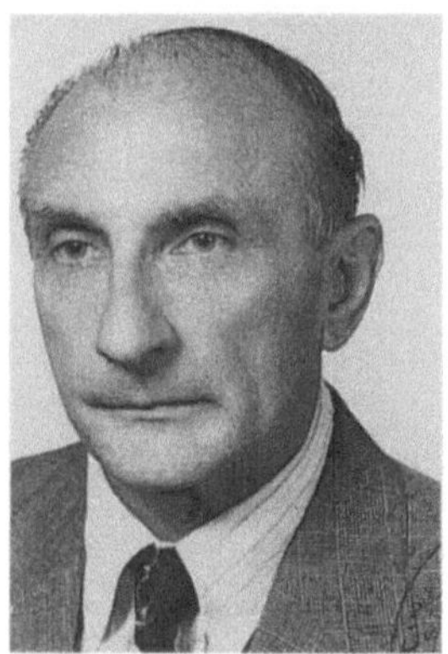

Birthdate: February 23, 1929

Academic Title: Professor

Position at Affiliation: Chief,
Department of Radiology

Business Address:
Department of Radiology
Medical University of Wroclaw
Sklodowskiej Curie 68
50-369 Wroclaw
Poland
48-71-22-61-84 (work)
48-71-21-38-96 (fax)

Home Address:
R-zyckiego 4-5
51-612 Wroclaw
Poland
48-71-48-35-48 (home)

Specialty: Radiology

Education:
1951 – Medical University Wroclaw
(M.D.)
1959–61 – Hospital of University of
Pennsylvania (Radiology residency)

ISS Member 1991

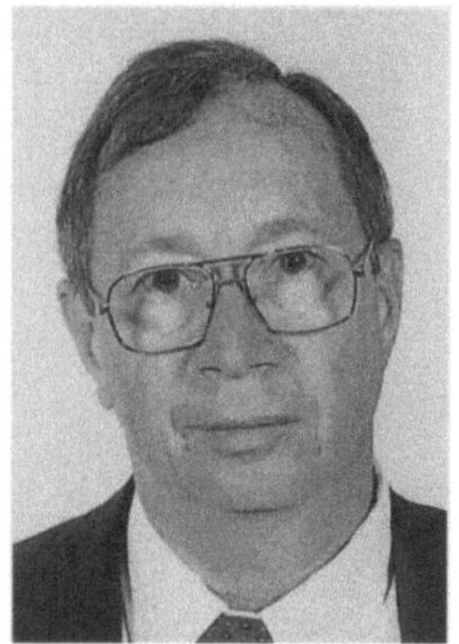

Birthdate: November 11, 1929

Academic Title: Clinical Associate
Professor of Surgery at Cornell
University Medical College

Position at Affiliation: Clinical Professor
of Orthopaedic Surgery
Columbia Presbyterian Medical Center

Business Address:
Cornell University Medical Center
517 East 71st Street
New York, NY 10021
U.S.A.
212-535-2514 (work)
212-861-6910 (fax)

Home Address:
517 East 71st Street
New York, NY 10021
U.S.A.
212-535-2514 (home)

Specialty/Certification: Orthopaedic
Surgery, 1965

Education:
1950 – Boston University, Boston, MA
(A.B.)
1954 – Boston University, Boston, MA
(M.D.)
1954–55 – University of Chicago,
Chicago, IL (rotating internship)
1957–58 – Massachusetts Memorial
Hospital, Boston, MA
(Jr. Assistant Resident)

1958 – The Hospital for Joint Diseases,
New York, NY (residency)
1959–60 – Columbia Presbyterian
Medical Center, New York, NY
(Assistant Resident)
1961 – Columbia Presbyterian Medical
Center, New York, NY (residency)
1962 – Memorial Sloan Kettering Cancer
Center, New York, NY (fellowship)

ISS Member 1978

MARTEL, WILLIAM M.D.

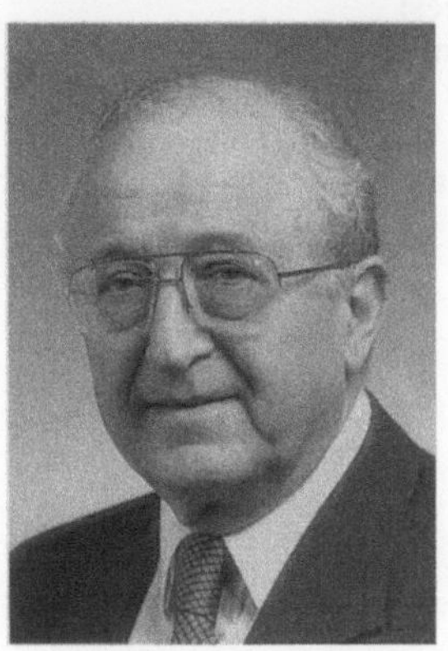

Birthdate: October 1, 1927

Academic Title: Professor of Radiology

Position at Affiliation: Professor of
Radiology

Business Address:
University of Michigan Hospitals
Department of Radiology
1500 East Medical Center Drive TC 2910
Ann Arbor, MI 48109-0326
U.S.A.
313-936-4362 (work)
313-936-9723 (fax)
martel@.umich.edu (e-mail)

Home Address:
2972 Park Ridge
Ann Arbor, MI 48103
U.S.A.
313-665-5917 (home)

Specialty/Certification: Radiology, 1957

Education:
1950 – New York University College of
Arts & Pure Science (B.S.)
1953 – New York University College of
Medicine (M.D.)
1953–54 – Kings County Hospital,
Brooklyn, NY (internship)
1954–57 – The Mt. Sinai Hospital,
New York (residency Radiology)

ISS Member Founding member

ISS Medals and Awards:
Founders' Gold Medal, Torontro, 1993

ISS Committees:
Liaison Committee
Travel Awards (grants) Committee

Spouse: Rhoda

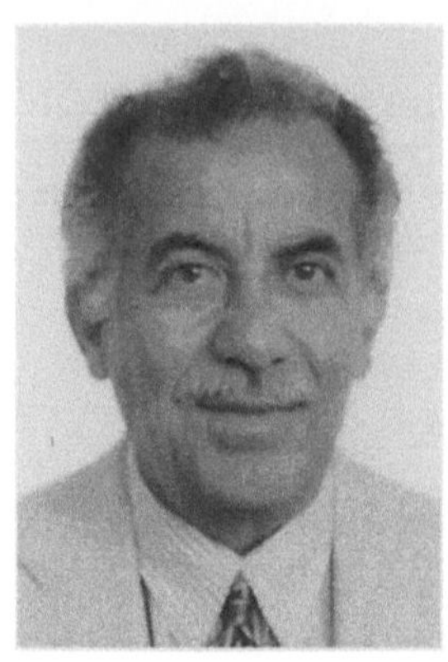

Academic Title: Professor

Position at Affiliation: Professor of
Radiology, Musculoskeletal Section

Business Address:
Duke University Medical School
Department of Radiology, Box 3169
Durham, North Carolina 27710
U.S.A.
919-684-7620 (work)
919-684-7125 (fax)
marti035@mc.duke.edu (e-mail)

Home Address:
10 Dorset Place
Durham, NC 27713
U.S.A.
919-544-6234 (home)

Specialty/Certification: Radiology, 1974

Education:
1957 – National Inst. of Secondary Edu.,
Pinar del Rio, Cuba (college)
1961 – University of Havana, Professional
School of Medicine (MD)
1971 – Specialized Training – Duke
University Medical Center

ISS Member 1991

Martinez-Tello, Francisco J. M.D., Ph.D.

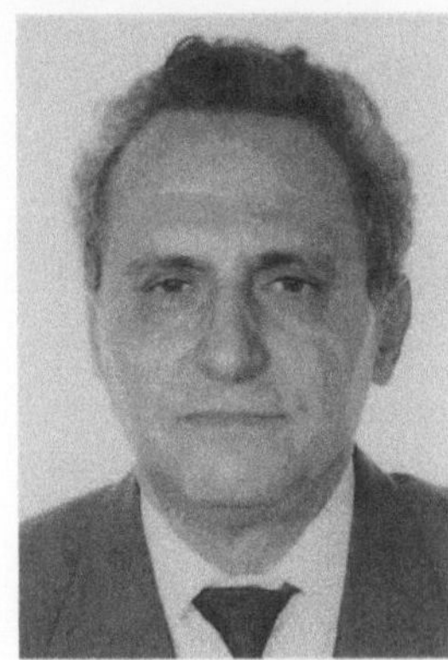

Birthdate: November 29, 1936

Academic Title: Professor

Position at Affiliation: Chief of Department

Business Address:
Department of Pathology
Hospital Universitario 12 de Octubre"
Ctra. de Andalucia km 5,400
28041 Madrid
Spain
(1) 390-82-75 and 1-390-80-68 (work)
(1) 469-57-75 (fax)

Home Address:
c/.AZOR, 7
28230 Las Rozas
Madrid
Spain
(1) 630-23-41 (home)

Specialty/Certification: Anatomic Pathology, 1968

Education:
1953 – Bachillerato
1960 – Falcultad Medicina Zaragoza (MD)
1961–66 – Pathologisches Institut der Universität Bonn (Germany) (training in Pathology)
1966–68 – University of Columbia, Babies Hospital (fellowship)

ISS Member 1987

Spouse: Demetra Rigopoulou

Masel, John Philip M.D.

Business Address:
Director of Radiology
Department of Radiology
Royal Children's Hospital
Brisbane, Qld. 4029
Australia
7-2537999 (work)
7-3695076 (home)
7-257-1768 (fax)

Specialty: Radiology

ISS Member 1988

Spouse: Margaret

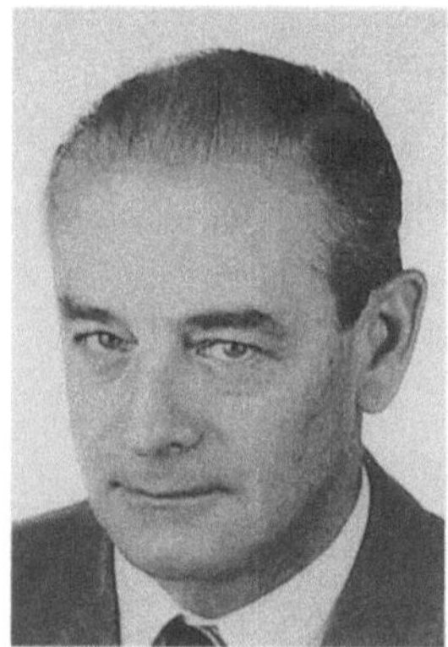

Birthdate: April 30, 1930

Academic Title: Professor of Orthopaedics

Position at Affiliation: Professor and Chairman, Orthopaedic Clinic

Business Address:
Orthopaedic Clinic
Institute for Postgraduate Studies
University Hospital Bulovka
CZ 180 81 Prague 8
Czech Republik
420-2-822 966 (work)

Home Address:
Sitkova 1
CZ 110 00 Prague 1
Czech Republik
420-2-249 15194 (home)
420-2-291 677 (fax)

Specialty/Certification: Orthopaedic Surgery, 1963

Education:
1949–55 – Faculty of General Medicine, Charles University Prague (M.D.)
1955–60 – General and Thoracic Surgery
1963 – Specialized in Orthopedic Surgery

ISS Member 1978

ISS Committees:
Membership Committee 1992–94

Spouse: Jana

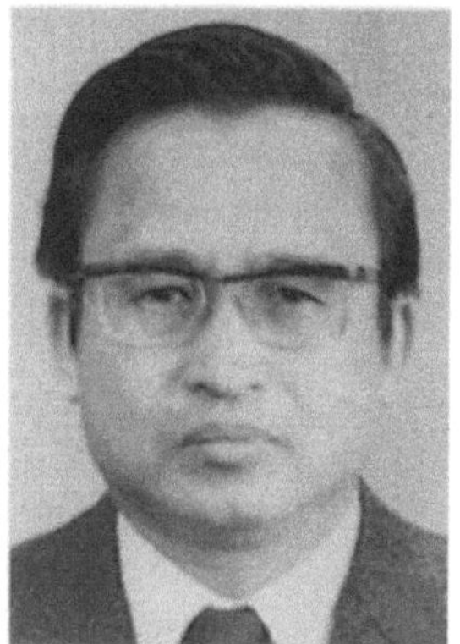

Birthdate: January 9, 1935

Academic Title: Professor

Position at Affiliation: Director, Department of Radiology

Business Address:
Department of Radiology
Kitasato University School of Medicine and Hospital
1-15-1, Kitasato, Sagamihara,
Kanagawa 228
Japan
427-78-8111 (work)
427-78-8441 (fax)
vyq0401@niftyserve.or.jp (e-mail)
matsu@raz.so-net.or.jp (e-mail)

Home Address:
25-23-2, Minami, Koenji
Suginami, Tokyo 166
Japan
3-3312-7137 (home)
3-3312-9320 (fax)
vyq04010@niftyserve.or.jp (e-mail)
matsu@raz.so-net.or.jp (e-mail)

Specialty/Certification: Radiology, 1971

Education:
School of Medicine and Graduate School of Medicine, Keio University, Tokyo, Japan (Radiology)
University of Missouri School of Medicine, Department of Radiology, Columbia, MO. USA (research fellow)

ISS Member 1975

Spouse: Noriko

Matsuno, Takeo M.D.

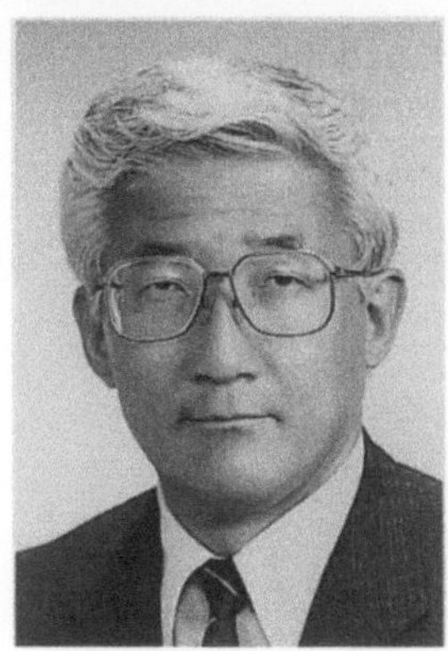

Academic Title: Professor

Position at Affiliation: Chairman and Professor

Business Address:
Department of Orthopaedics
Asahikawa Medical College
3-11 4-sen 5-goh
Nishikagura Asahikawa 078
Japan
81-11-166-65-8949 (work)
81-11-166-65-8949 (fax)

Home Address:
5-13 3-jo 12-chome Miyanomori Chuo-ku
Sapporo 064
Japan
81-11-641-3643 (home)
81-11-642-7138 (fax)

Specialty: Orthopaedic Surgery

Education:
1971–78 – Department of Patholoy.
Hokkaido University School of Medicine
1979 – Hokkaido University School of
Medicine (M.D.)
1978–97 – Department of Orthopaedics,
Hokkaido University School of Medicine
1997 – Department of Orthopaedics,
Asahikawa Medical College

ISS Member: 1982

Spouse: Yorika

Mazabraud, Andre M.D.

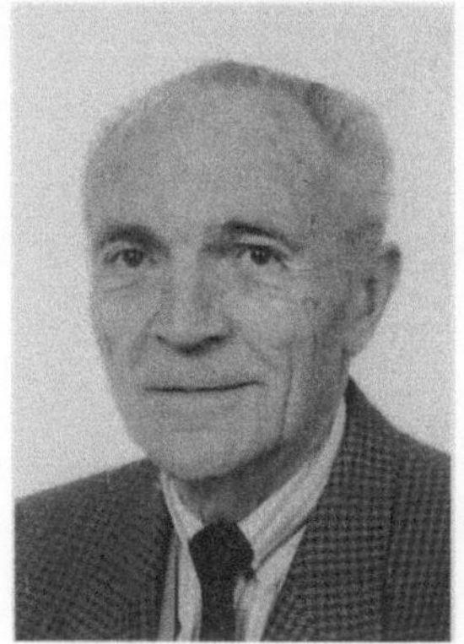

Birthdate: July 15, 1921

Home Address:
4 rue du Sud
92140 Clamart
France

Specialty: Pathology

ISS Member 1979

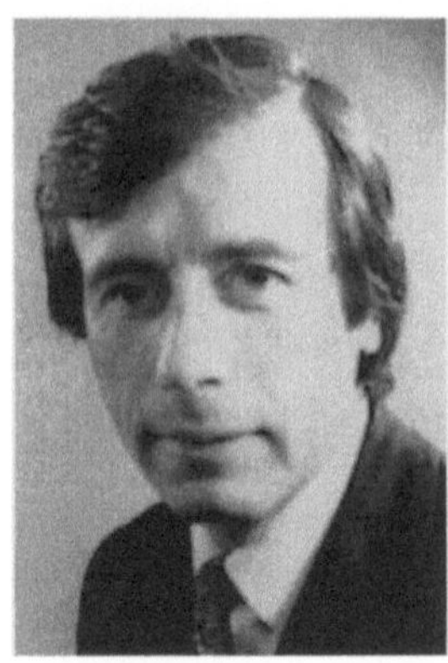

Business Address:
Department of Diagnostic Radiology
The Robert Jones and Agnes Hunt
Orthopaedic Hospital
Oswestry, SY10 7AG
United Kingdom
1691-404000 (work)
1743-81329 (home)
1691-404057 (fax)

Specialty: Radiology

ISS Member 1983

Spouse: Rosemary

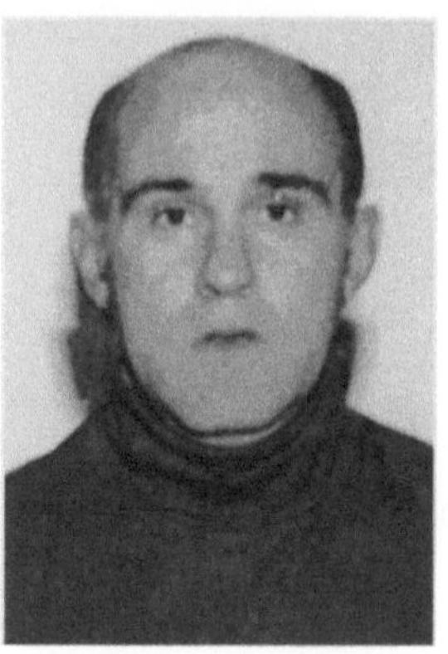

Birthdate: August 13, 1944

Business Address:
Department of Pathology and
Orthopaedic Surgery
John Hopkins Hospital
600 North Wolfe Street, Room 306
Baltimore, MD 21287
U.S.A.
410-614-3653 (work)
410-614-3766 (fax)

Home Address:
550 Springlake Way
Baltimore, MD 21212
U.S.A.
410-433-5686 (home)
410-433-0252 (fax)

Specialty: Pathology

Education:
Columbia Unviersity (AB)
University of Chicago (MD)
University of Iowa (Orthopaedics and
Pathology)

ISS Member 1984

Spouse: Lucille

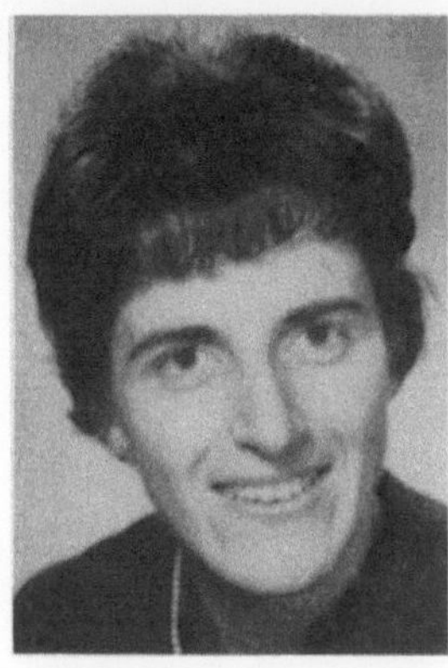

Academic Title: Dr.

Position at Affiliation: Visiting Medical Officer

Business Address:
Royal Prince Alfred Hospital
Missenden Road
Newtown, Sydney
N.S.W. 20
Australia

Home Address:
2A/27 Sutherland Crescent
Darling Point, Sydney NSW 2027
Australia
2-328-7879 (home)
2-363-9033 (fax)

Specialty: Radiology

Education:
1961 – 64 DMRD London, U.K.

ISS Member 1979

Offices Held in ISS and Dates of Service:
Member-at-Large, 1996

ISS Committees:
Conveyor of Sydney ISS Meeting, 1988
Committee member prior to 1988 – 89

Birthdate: August 4, 1956

Academic Title: Associate Professor

Position at Affiliation: Associate Professor of Orthopedic Surgery

Business Address:
St. Louis University
Department of Orthopedic Surgery
3635 Vista Blvd.
St. Louis, MO 63110
U.S.A.
314-577-8850 (work)
314-268-5121 (fax)
mcdonamj@slu.edu (e-mail)

Specialty/Certification: Orthopaedic Surgery, 1990

Education:
St. John's University, Collegeville, MN – undergraduate
University of Minnesota, Medical School
Mayo Graduate School of Medicine, Orthopedic Surgery
Instituto Orthopedico Rizzoli – Orthopedic Oncology

ISS Member 1993

Spouse: Lisa

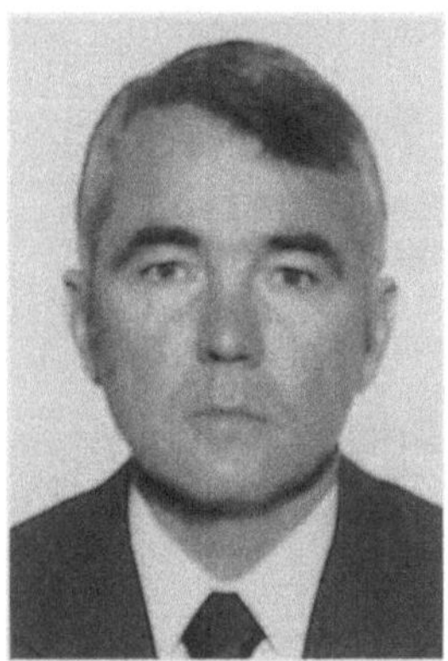

Business Address:
Mayo Clinic
Rochester, MN 55905
U.S.A.
507-753-2836 (home)
507-284-4384 (work)
507-284-8996 (fax)

ISS Member 1974

Spouse: Janet

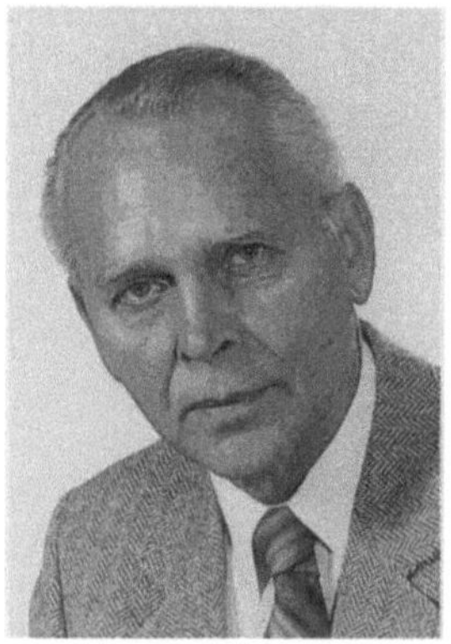

Birthdate: April 16, 1923

Academic Title: Professor Emeritus

Position at Affiliation: Consultant
Radiologist

Business Address:
Toronto Western Hospital
Department of Radiology
399 Bathurst Street
Toronto, Ontario M5T 2S8
Canada

Home Address:
38 Princess Margaret Blvd.
Islington, Ontario M9A 1Z6
Canada
416-233-7772 (home)

Specialty/Certification: Radioliogy, 1955

Education:
1950 – Graduate of Karolinska Institutet,
Stockholm, Sweden
1951 – 52 Sabbatsbergs Hospital, Stockholm, Sweden (Diagnostic Radiology)
1953 – 55 Toronto Western Hospital and
Sick Children's Hospital, Toronto,
Canada (Diagnostic Radiology)
1954 – Diploma of Medical Radiology,
University of Toronto, Canada

ISS Member 1976

Spouse: Silvia

Business Address:
Department of Pathology
Sahlgrenska University Hospital
University of Gothenburg
41345 Gothenburg
Sweden

Home Address:
Engelbrektsgatan 6
41127 Gothenburg
Sweden
46-31-603869 (work)
46-31-827194 (fax)
46-31-138584 (home)
46-31-138584 (fax)

Specialty: Pathology

Education:
1975 – Iowa State University (college)
1979 – University of Iowa (M.D.)
1984 – St. John Hospital, Detroit
(residency)
1985 – M.D. Anderson Hospital & Tumor
Institute (fellowship)

ISS Member 1993

Spouse: Lars-Gunnar Kindblom, M.D.

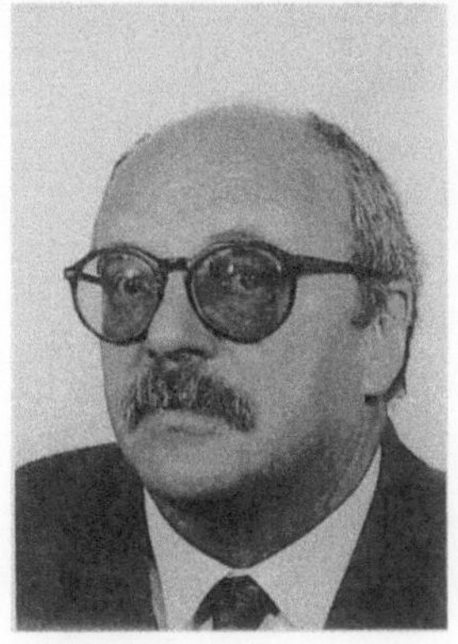

Birthdate: May 12, 1931

Academic Title: Professor

Position at Affiliation: Professor
(retired)

Business Address:
Ludwig-Maximilians-Universitat
(LMU) Munich
Germany

Home Address:
Hesseloherstrasse 8
80802 Munich
Germany
089-332703 (home)

Specialty: Pathology

Education:
University of Zurich, Switzerland (M.D.)
Cook County Hospital, Chicago, IL
(Pathology residency)

ISS Member 1975

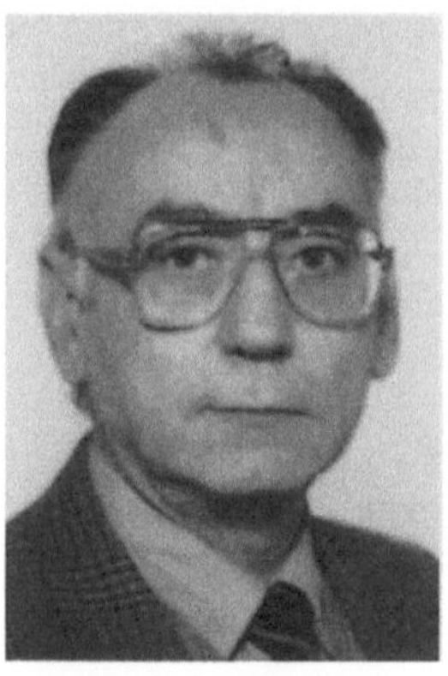

Business Address:
Cattedra di Clinica
Orthopedica e Traumatologica
Universita di Padova
C.T.O.
Vi Facciolati, 71
35100 – Padova
Italy

ISS Member 1974

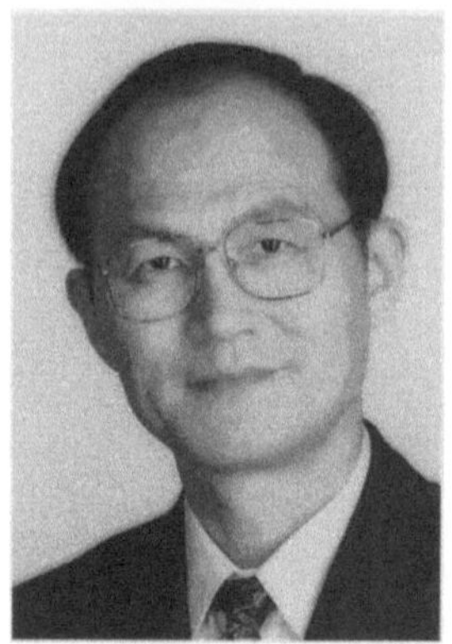

Birthdate: December 4, 1945

Academic Title: Professor

Position at Affiliation: Professor and Chairman

Business Address:
Sun Yat-Sen University of Medical
Sciences
The First Hospital
Department of Radiology
2 Zhongshan Road
Guangzhog, Guangdone 510080
P.R. of China
20-87755766 ext. 8466 (work)
20-87750632 (fax)

Home Address:
Room 901
11-2 Ma-peng Gang Road
Guangzhou, Guangdong 510080
P.R. of China
20-87614146 (home)

Specialty/Certification: Radiology, 1983

Education:
1963–69 – Beijing University of Medical
Sciences (student)
1971–75 – Lanzhou Medical College
(Radiologist training)
1980–83 – Beijing University of Medical
Sciences (Skeletal Radiologist training)

ISS Member: 1996

Spouse: Lirong He

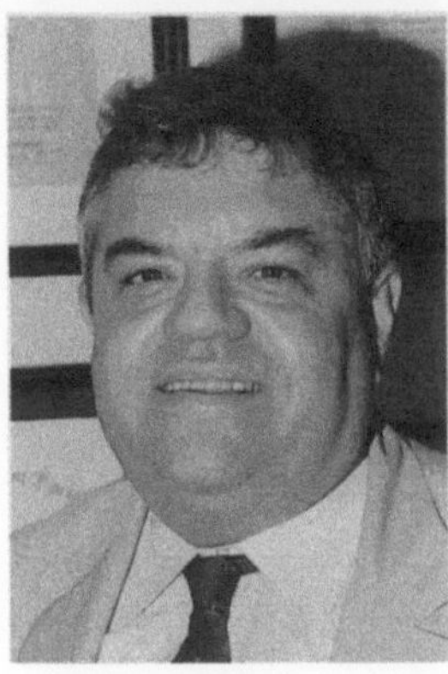

Birthdate: February 24, 1939

Academic Title: Professor

Position at Affiliation: Professor

Business Address:
Department of Orthopaedic Surgery
Northwestern University Medical School
303 East Chicago Avenue
Chicago, IL 60611
U.S.A.
312-908-7937 (work)
312-943-3888 (fax)

Home Address:
1352 Estate Lane
Lake Forest, IL 6004
U.S.A.
847-735-0055 (home)

Specialty/Certification: Orthopaedic
Surgery, 1973

Education:
1961 – Columbia College (B.A.)
1965 – John Hopkins Medical School
(M.D.)
1965 – 66 – University of Chicago
Hospital (intern, surgery)
1966 – Armed Forces Institute of
Pathology (fellow, orthopaedic)
1967 – Hospital for Joint Diseases
(residency, orthopaedic surgery)
1967 – 69 – Johns Hopkins Hospital
(resident, orthopaedic surgery)

ISS Member 1979

Spouse: Carol

Academic Title: Professor

Position at Affiliation: Professor,
Department of Orthopaedics

Business Address:
Hadassah University Hospital
Kiryat Hadassah
P.O. Box 12000
Jerusalem 91120
Israel
972 2 414762/776412 (work)
972 2 414762 (fax)
milgrim@md2.huji.ac.il (e-mail)

Home Address:
9 Gelber Street
Jerusalem
Israel
972 2 431866 (home)

Specialty: Orthopaedic Surgery

Education:
Bucham Univ., Chicago (B.S.)
Downstate SUNY, New York, NY (M.D.)
Maimonodes, Brooklyn, NY
(Orthopaedic residency)

ISS Member: 1995

Spouse: Ruth

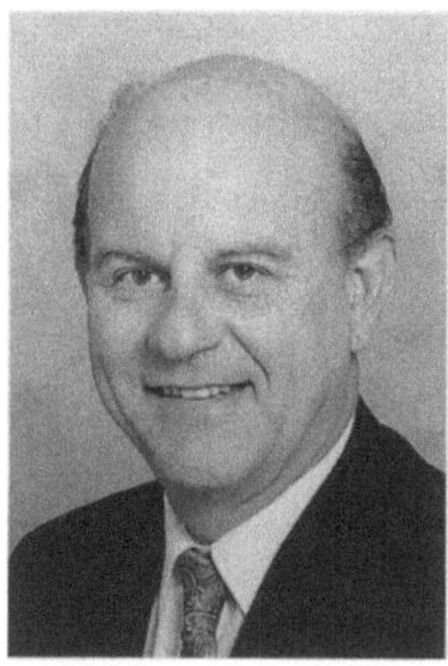

Birthdate: November 22, 1937

Academic Title: Professor of Pathology

Position at Affiliation: Chief of Pathology

Business Address:
Orthopaedic Hospital
2400 S. Flower Street
Room 524
Los Angeles, CA 90007
U.S.A.
213-742-1017 (work)
213-747-1077 (fax)

Home Address:
7301 Vista Del Mar, A112
Playa Del Ray, Ca 90293
U.S.A.
213-822-7677 (home)

Specialty/Certification: Pathology (anatomic and clinical), 1971

Education:
Columbia College
Downstate Medical Center
Kings County Hospital

ISS Member 1978

ISS Committee:
Admissions Committee, 1984–89

Spouse: Carmen

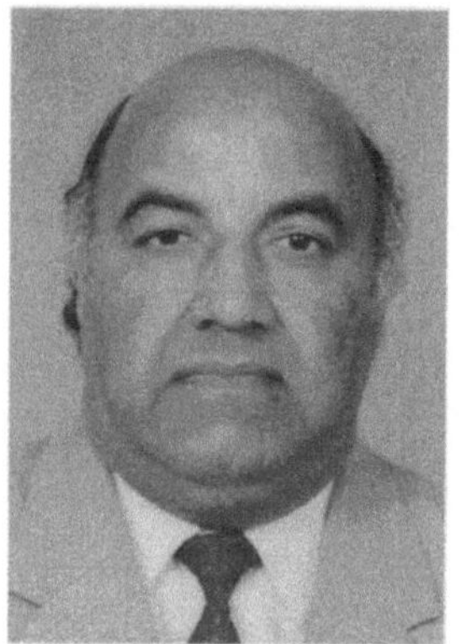

Academic Title: Professor

Position at Affiliation: Senior Consultant and Head

Business Address:
The Armed Forces Hospital, Muscat.
P.O. Box 726
CPO Seeb
Post. Code 111
Sultanate of Oman
968-617744 (work)
968-617197 (fax)

Home Address:
349-A
Shastri Nagar
Jammu Tawi-180004
J&K State
India
968-614306 (home)

Specialty: Radiology

Education:
1975 – M.D.
1980 – Ph.D.

ISS Member: 1992

Spouse: Urmil

Moncada, Rogelio M.D.

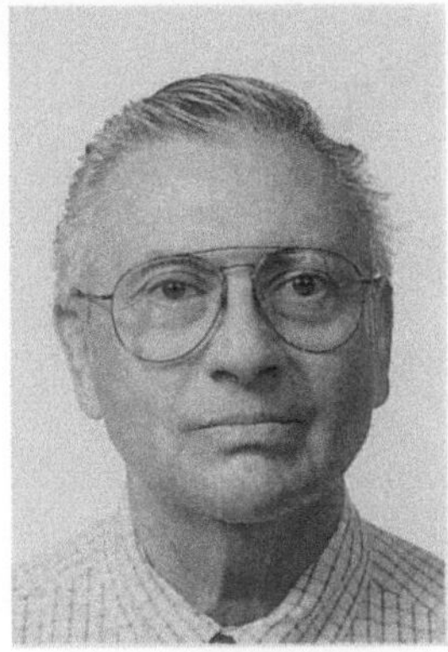

Birthdate: March 10, 1933

Academic Title: Professor of R.-LUMC

Position at Affiliation: Professor of Radiology

Business Address:
Radiology Department
Loyola University Medical Center
2160 South First Avenue
Maywood, IL 60153
U.S.A.
708-216-3919 (work)
708-216-8394 (fax)

Home Address:
306 Ottawa Lane
Oak Brook, IL 60521
U.S.A.
630-325-9150 (home)
630-325-8723 (fax)

Specialty/Certification: Radiology, 1966

ISS Member 1979

Spouse: Dolores

Moore, Timothy E. MB, ChB, FRACR

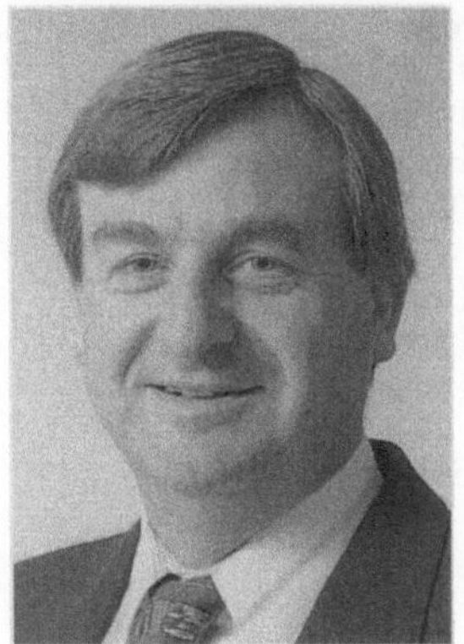

Birthdate: October 31, 1947

Academic Title: Associate Professor

Position at Affiliation: Radiologist

Business Address:
Department of Radiology
University of Nebraska Medical Center
600 South 42nd Street
Omaha, Nebraska 68198-1045
U.S.A.
402-559-9378 (work)
402-559-1011 (fax)
temoore@unmc.edu (email)

Home Address:
17798 Holly Lane
Crescent, Iowa 51526
U.S.A.
712-323-0362 (home)

Specialty/Certification: Radiology, 1977

Education:
1966–71 – University of Otago School of
Medicine, Dunedin, New Zealand
1972–73 – General internship in
New Zealand Hospitals
1974–77 – Radiology Registrar,
Auckland Hospital Board
1977 – Musculoskeletal Radiology
Fellowship, Middlemore Hospital,
Auckland, New Zealand

ISS Member 1994

Spouse: Ann

MOSER, RICHARD P. JR., M.D.

Business Address:
Department of Radiology
Penn State University Hospital
The Milton S. Hershey Medical Center
Hershey, PA 17033
U.S.A.
717-531-5596 (fax)
717-531-8039 (work)
717-566-6846 (home)

Specialty: Radiology

ISS Member 1988

MUNK, PETER L. M.D., C.M.

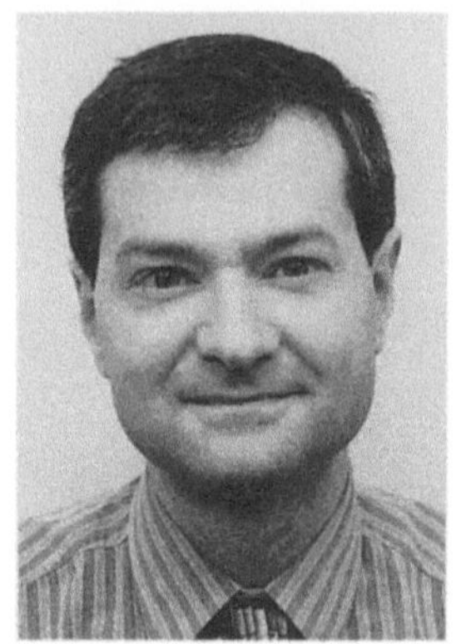

Birthdate: June 8, 1958

Academic Title: Professor, Radiology

Position at Affiliation: Staff Radiologist

Business Address:
Department of Radiology
Vancouver Hospital and Health Sciences
Centre
855 West 12th Avenue
Vancouver, British Columbia V5Z 1M9
Canada
604-875-4533 (work)
604-875-4319 (fax)
pmunk@unixg.ubc.ca (e-mail)

Home Address:
1957 Aspen Avenue
Vancouver, British Columbia V6M 1E5
Canada
604 263-9587 (home)

Specialty: Radiology

Education:
1974–76 John Abbott College
1976–83 McGill University, Montreal
1983–88 Vancouver Hospital and University of British Columbia Health
Sciences Ctr. Hosp. (residency)
1988 – Univ of CA, San Francisco,
School of Medicine

ISS Member 1994

Spouse: Maria Chung

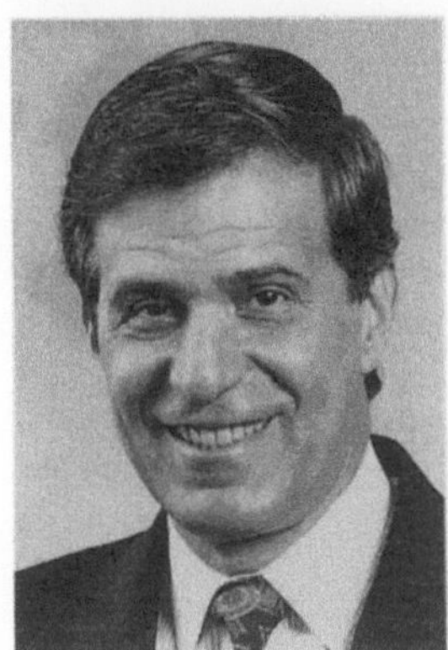

Birthdate: December 26, 1942

Academic Title: Clinical Professor of Radiology

Position at Affiliation: President

Business Address:
Educational Symposia Inc.
1527 S. Dale Mabry Highway
Tampa, FL 33627
U.S.A.
813-573-5114 (work)
813-573-5404 (fax)
edusymp@cyberspy.com (e-mail)

Home Address:
801 Bayshore Blvd.
Tampa, FL 33627
U.S.A.
813-251-2942 (home)

Specialty/Certification: Nuclear Medicine, 1973; Radiology, 1973

Education:
1964 – Dartmouth College (A.B.)
1965 – Dartmouth Medical School (B.M.S.)
1967 – Harvard Medical School (M.D.)
1973 – Columbia-Presbyterian Medical Center (Radiology residency)

ISS Member 1982

Spouse: Carol

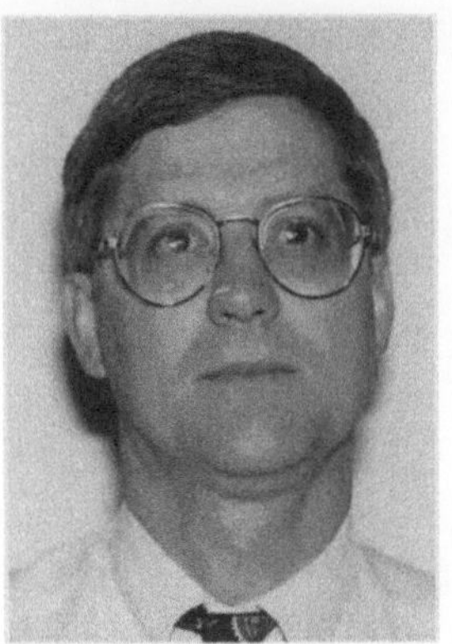

Birthdate: November 18, 1955

Academic Title: Associate Professor

Position at Affiliation: Chief, Musculo-skeletal Radiology

Business Address:
Armed Forces Institute of Pathology
Department of Radiologic Pathology
6825 16th Street, N.W.
Washington, DC 20306
U.S.A.
202-782-2162 or 2169 (work)
202-782-0768 (fax)
murphey@e-mail.afip.osd.mil (e-mail)

Home Address:
16209 Whitehaven Road
Silver Spring, MD 20906
U.S.A.
301-570-4098 (home)

Specialty/Certification: Radiology, 1986

Education:
1974–78 – Jamestown College, Jamestown, ND
1978–82 – University of Kansas Medical Center, Kansas City, KS (M.D.)
1982–86 – University of Kansas, Kansas City, KS (Radiology residency)
1985–86 – UCSD, Mallinckrodt, St. Louis, MO (Musculoskeletal training)

ISS Member: 1993

ISS Awards and Medals:
Presidents' Medal, Dublin, 1998

Spouse: Jill

MURPHY, JR., WILLIAM A. M.D.

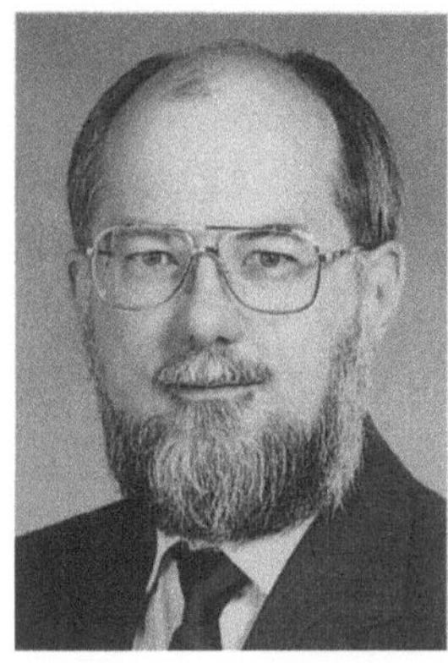

Birthdate: April 26, 1945

Academic Title: Professor and
John S. Dunn, Sr. Chair

Position at Affiliation: Head, Division
of Diagnostic Imaging, Chairman,
Diagnostic Radiology

Business Address:
Diagnostic Imaging 057
UTMD Anderson Cancer Center
1515 Holcombe Blvd.
Houston, TX 77030
U.S.A.
713-745-1149 (work)
713-745-1155 (fax)
william-murphy@diag-
imaging.mda.uth.tmc.edu (e-mail)

Home Address:
4808 Bellview Street
Bellaire, TX 77401
U.S.A.
713-63-7382 (home)

Specialty/Certification: Radiology, 1975

Education:
1967 – University of Pittsburgh (B.S.)
1971 – The Pennsylvania State University
(M.D.)
1975 – Mallinckrodt Institute of
Radiology Washington University
School of Medicine (Radiology resident)

ISS Member 1980

Spouse: Judy

MURRAY, I. PROVAN M.D.

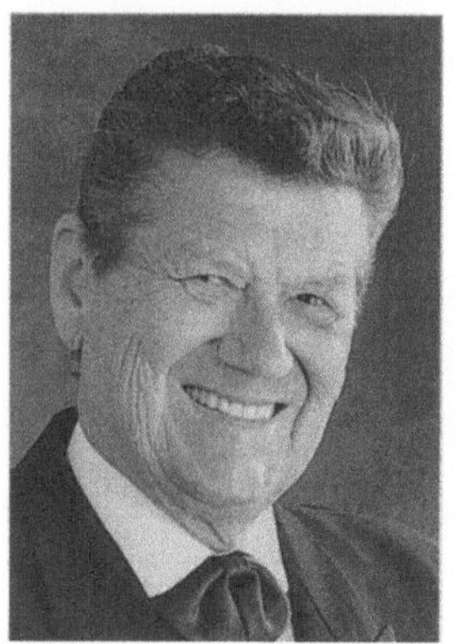

Academic Title: Professor

Position at Affiliation: Consultant
Emeritus

Business Address:
Department of Nuclear Medicine
The Prince of Wales Hospital
High Street, Randwick
NSW 2021
Australia

Home Address:
21 Gipps St.
Paddington
NSW 2021
Australia
612-9331-5651 (home)
612-9331-5651 (fax)

Specialty: Radiology

Education:
1952 – University of Glasgow (MB Ch.B)
1955 – Edinburgh (MRCP)
1962 – University of Glasgow (MD)
1964 – FRCP
1964 – MRACP

ISS Member 1977

Spouse: Margaret

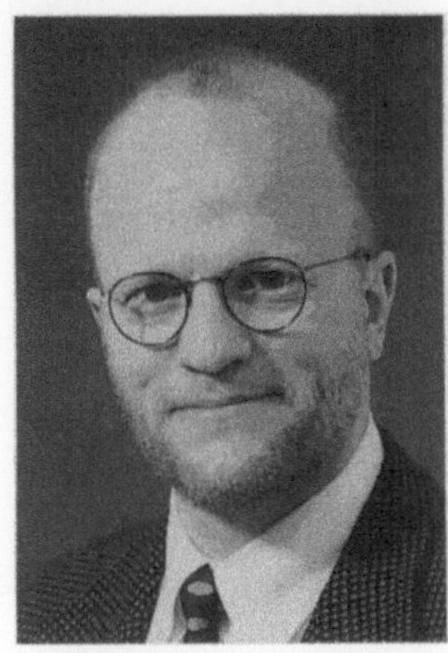

Birthdate: November 9, 1951

Academic Title: Associate Professor

Position at Affiliation: Chief Musculo-skeletal and Emergency Radiology

Business Address:
Vanderbilt University Medical Center
Department of Radiology
21st Avenue, South & Garland Street
Nashville, TN 37232-2675
U.S.A.
615-322-3357 (work)
615-322-3764 (fax)
paul.mance@mcmail.vanderbilt.edu
at tiNET (e-mail)

Home Address:
2905 Compton Road
Nashville, TN 37215
U.S.A.
615-383-6466 (home)

Specialty/Certification: Radiology, 1980

Education:
1973 – University of North Carolina,
Chapel Hill, NC (BS)
1976 – University of North Carolina,
Chapel Hill, NC (MD)
1976-80 – Vanderbilt University,
Nashville, TN (Radiology residency)

ISS Member 1984

ISS Committees:
Refresher Course Committee, 1997

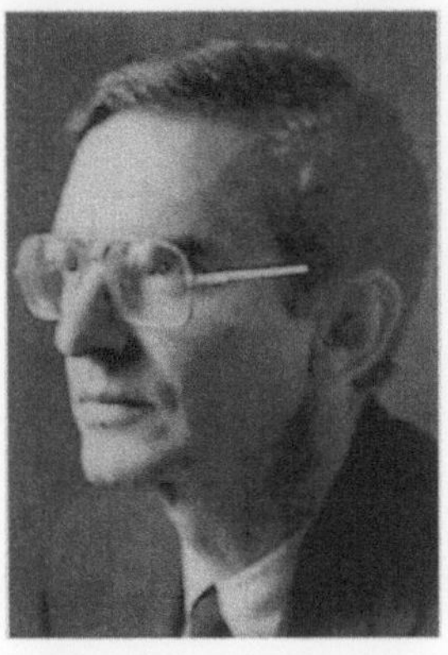

Business Address:
University of Kansas Medical Center
Department of Orthopaedics
39th and Rainbow Boulevard
Kansas City, KS 66103
U.S.A.

Specialty: Orthopaedic Surgery

ISS Member 1983

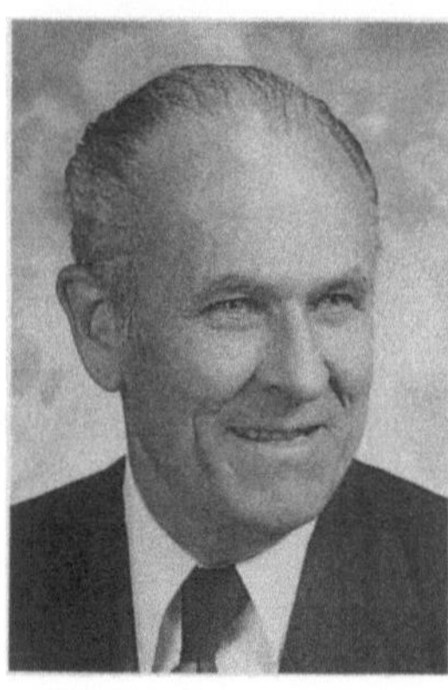

Academic Title: Clinical Professor

Position at Affiliation: Clinical Professor

Business Address:
Harborview Medical Center
Department of Radiology
325 Ninth Avenue
Seattle, WA 98104-2499
U.S.A.
206-731-3561 (work)
206-731-8560 (fax)

Home Address:
4615 – 139th Street, S.E.
Bellevue, WA 98004
U.S.A.
206-641-0738 (home)

Specialty/Certification: Radiology, 1953

Education:
1942 – University of Washington, Seattle,
WA (B.S.)
1945 – Northwestern University Medical
School, Chicago (M.D.)
1950 – 53 – University of Chicago, IL
(Radiology residency)

ISS Member Founding member

Spouse: Jeannette

Business Address:
36 Metacomet Road
Newton, MA 02168
U.S.A.
617-964-1428 (home)
617-739-5290 (work)
617-739-5291 (fax)

ISS Member 1984

Spouse: Marlene

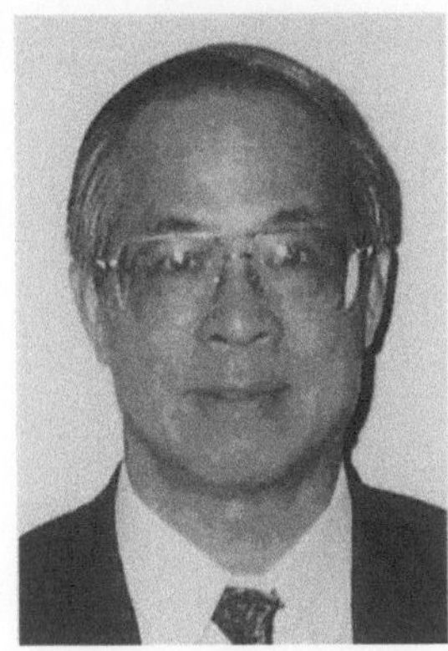

Birthdate: December 25, 1938

Academic Title: Associate Professor

Position at Affiliation: Consultant, Osteoarticular Radiology

Business Address:
The University of Texas Health Science Center nat San Antonio
7703 Floyd Curl Drive
San Antonio, TX 78284-7800
U.S.A.
210-567-6488 (work)
210-567-6418 (fax)

Home Address:
3511 Hunters Sound
San Antonio, TX 78230
U.S.A.
210-492-3593 (home)

Specialty/Certification: Radiology, 1979

Education:
1956–57 – Saigon Science Univ., VN: (physics-chemistry-biology certificate)
1957–63 – Saigon Medical School, VN: (M.D.)
1961–63 – Binhdan, Choray Hospital (intern)
1975–77 – Bexar County Hospital (Radiology residency)

ISS Member: 1993

Spouse: Quy Tran

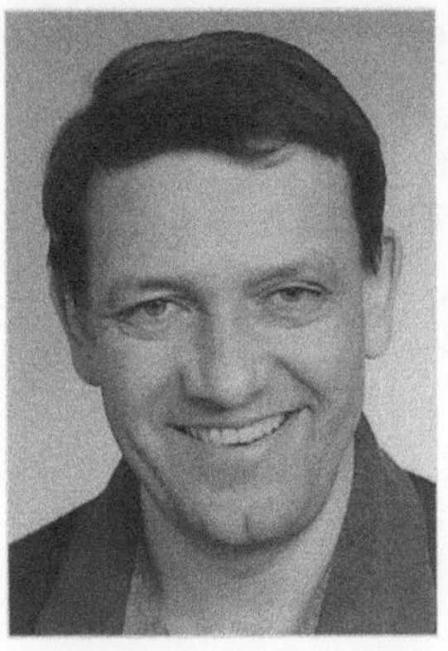

Birthdate: October 1, 1947

Academic Title: Assistant Professor

Position at Affiliation: Assistant Professor, University of Basel, Dept. of Radiology

Business Address:
Roentgen Institute
Untere Rebgasse 18
4058 Basel
Switzerland
061-681-8214 (fax)
061-681-6660 (work)
anidecker@blur.win.ch (e-mail)

Home Address:
Oberer Rheinweg 81
CH-4058 Basel
Switzerland

Specialty/Certification: Radiology, 1979

Education:
University of Toronto (residency in Radiology)
University of Basel

ISS Member 1990

Spouse: Irma

Business Address:
Department of Pathology
Hokkaido University Hospital
Nishi 5, Kita 14
Kita Ku, Sapporo 060
Japan
562-5106 (home)
716-1161 (work)
747-1622 (fax)

Specialty: Pathology

ISS Member 1989

Spouse: Keiko

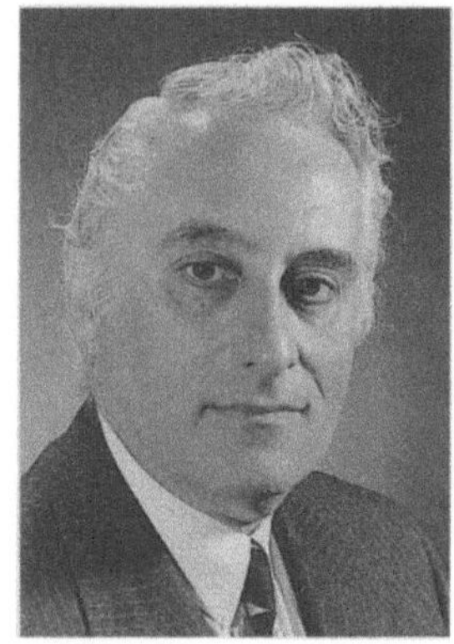

Birthdate: August 7, 1923

Academic Title: Professor of Radiology

Business Address:
Radiology Department
New York Medical College
Valhalla, NY 10595
U.S.A.
914-285-7355 (work)
914-285-7994 (fax)

Home Address:
289 Daisy Farms Drive
Scarsdale, NY 10583, U.S.A.
914-636-7158 (home)

Specialty/Certification: Radiology, 1952

Education:
1944 – New York University Heights
College (B.A.)
1948 – Chicago Medical School (M.D.)
1950 – Hospital Joint Disease, New York
(residency)
1951 – Beth Israel Hospital, New York
(residency)
1952 – National Cancer Institute/
Bellevue Hospital Medical Center
(Fellowship)

ISS Committees:
Audit Committee – 1979–80; 1984
Closed Meeting Program Committee

ISS Member Founding member

ISS Awards and Medals:
Founders' Gold Medal, Paris, 1996

Spouse: Muriel Dawn

ODITA, JOHN C. M.D.

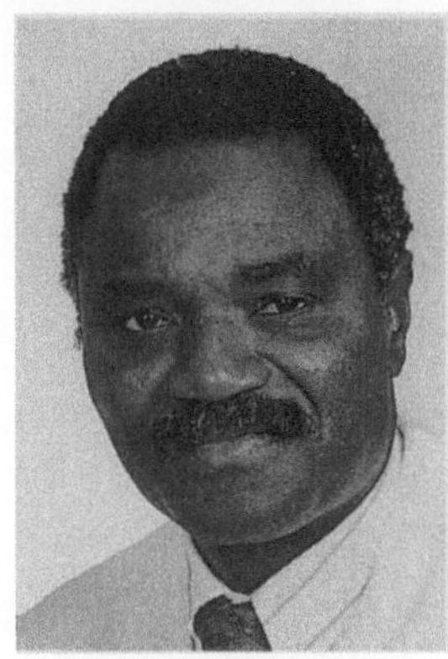

Birthdate: July 24, 1945

Academic Title: Associate Professor

Position at Affiliation: Associate Professor

Business Address:
Department of Radiology
University of Texas Medical School
6431 Fannin Street – MSB2.100
Houston, TX 77030
U.S.A.
713-704-1781 or 1784 (work)
713-704-1597(fax)
jodita@msrad3.med.uth.tmc.edu (e-mail)

Home Address:
4723 Yorkshire Street
Sugar Land, Texas 77479
U.S.A.
713-980-6110 (home)

Specialty/Certification: Pediatric Radiology, 1975

Education:
University of Ibadan Medical School/Nigeria

ISS Member 1994

ISS Committees:
Committee for the Promotion
of the Refresher Course Outside North America

Spouse: Helen

OESTREICH, ALAN E. M.D.

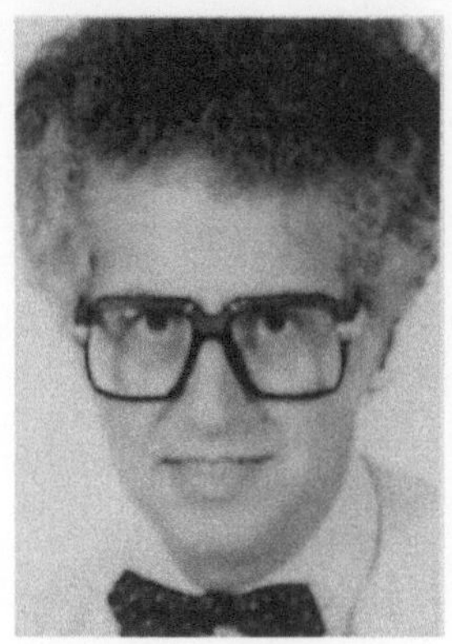

Birthdate: December 4, 1939

Academic Title: Professor

Position at Affiliation: Staff Radiologist

Business Address:
Division of Radiology
Children's Hospital Medical Center
Elland and Bethesda Avenue
Cincinnati, OH 45229-3039
U.S.A.
513-559-8552 (work)
513-636-8145 (fax)

Home Address:
340 Warren Avenue
Cincinnati, OH 45220-1135
U.S.A.
513-281-1903 (home)

Specialty: Pediatric Radiology

Education:
1961 – Princeton (AB)
1965 – Johns Hopkins (MD)
1965–66 – Baltimore City Hospitals
(intern, Internal Medicine)
1966–69 – Strong Memorial Hospital,
Rochester, NY (Radiology residency)

ISS Member 1983

ISS Committees:
Membership Committee

Spouse: Tamar Kahane Oestreich

Ogden, John A. M.D.

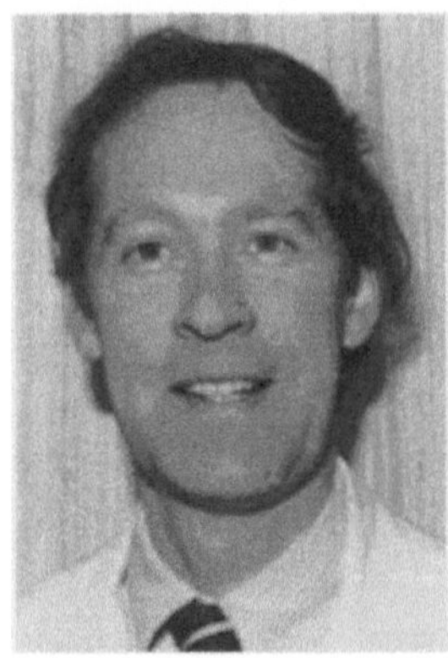

Business Address:
Shriners Hospital for Crippled Children
MDC Box 64
12901 North 30th Street
Tampa, FL 33612-4799
U.S.A.
813-972-2250 (work)
813-978-9442 (fax)

Home Address:
12502 North Pine Drive
Tampa, FL 33612-9499
U.S.A.
813-681-8194 (home)

ISS Member 1976

Spouse: Dali

Ogihara, Yoshio M.D.

Business Address:
Department of Orthopaedic Surgery
Mie University School of Medicine
Edobashi 2-174, Tsu City
Mie 514
Japan
0592-371132 (home)
0592-321111 ext. 6446 (work)
0592-315211 (fax)

ISS Member 1988

Spouse: Kurumi

Ohba, Satoru M.D.

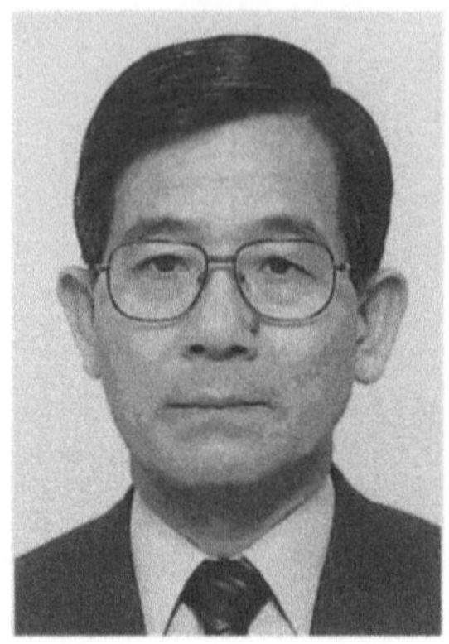

Birthdate: February 3, 1936

Academic Title: Professor

Position at Affiliation: Chairman and Professor

Business Address:
Department of Radiology
Nagoya City University School of
Medicine 1, Kawasumi, Mizuho-Cho,
Mizuho-ku
Nagoya, 467
Japan
52-853-8274 (work)
52-852-5244 (fax)
soba@cmews2.med.nagoya-cu.ac.jp
(e-mail)

Home Address:
5-205-4, Umemoridai, Nissin-SI
Aichi, 470-01
Japan
52-801-4132 (home)

Specialty/Certification: Radiology, 1971

Education:
1961 – Kanazawa University School of
Medicine (M.D.)
1962 – 66 – Postgraduate Course of
Radiology, Kanazawa University

ISS Member: 1993

Spouse: Yukiko

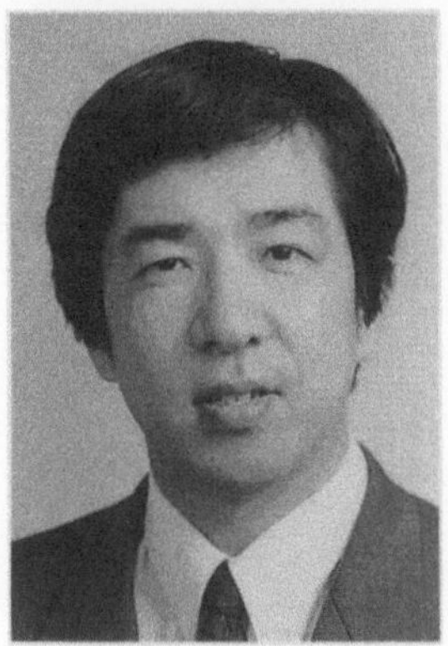

Birthdate: June 8, 1957

Academic Title: Lecturer

Position at Affiliation: Lecturer

Business Address:
Department of Orthopaedics
Akita University School of Medicine
1-1-1 Hondo, Akita, 010
Japan
81-188-34-1111 ext.2544 (work)
81-188-36-2617 (fax)

Home Address:
26-151 Omaki, Shimokitade-Matsuzaki
Akita, 010
Japan
81-188-34-5834 (home)

Specialty: Orthopaedic Surgery, 1985

Education:
1976–82 Akita University School of
Medicine, Akita, Japan

ISS Member 1995

Spouse: Hiroko

Business Address:
7480 East Holly Road
Holly, MI 48442
U.S.A.

ISS Member Founding member

ORTNER, DONALD J. PH.D, D.SC (HON.)

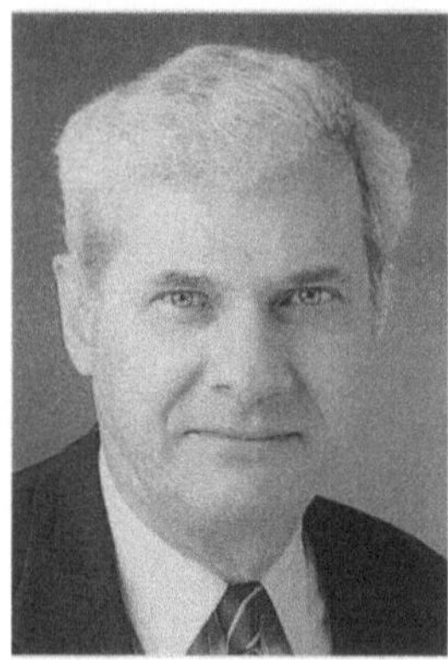

Birthdate: August 23, 1938

Academic Title: Professor

Position at Affiliation: Biological Anthropologist

Business Address:
Department of Anthropology
National Museum of Natural History
Smithsonian Institution
Washington, DC 20560
U.S.A.
202-786-2504 (work)
202-357-2208 (fax)
ortner.don@nmnh.si.edu (e-mail)

Home Address:
4510 Woodfield Road
Kensington, MD 20895
U.S.A.
301-493-8921 (home)

Specialty: Anthropology

Education:
Columbia Union College (BA)
Syracuse University (MS)
University of Kansas (Ph.D)
University of Bradford, England (D.Sc)

ISS Member 1980

Spouse: Joyce E.

OZONOFF, MAER B. M.D.

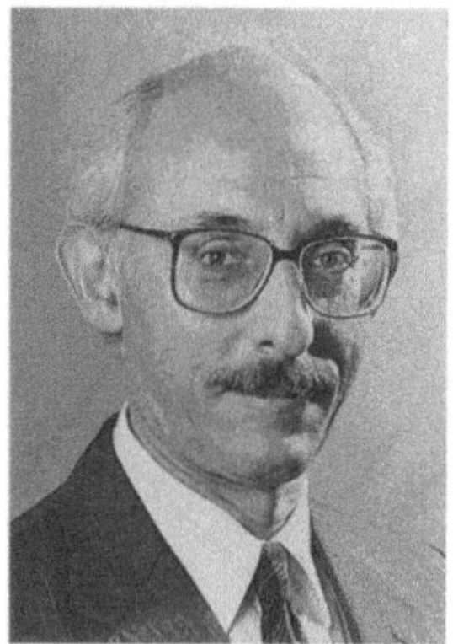

Birthdate: February 4, 1930

Academic Title: Clinical Professor of Radiology

Position at Affiliation: Honorary Staff

Business Address:
University of Connecticut School of Medicine
Radiology Department
Connecticut Children's Medical Center
Hartford, CT 06106
U.S.A.
860-233-0524 (work)

Home Address:
1043 Prospect Avenue
West Hartford, CT 06105-1103
U.S.A.
860-233-0524 (home)

Specialty/Certification: Radiology, 1963

Education:
Northwestern University Medical School (M.D.)
University California San Francisco (Radiology residency)
Karolinska Hospital Barnkliniken (fellowship Pediatric Radiology)

ISS Committees:
Nomenclature Committee
Editorial Board, Skeletal Radiology

ISS Member 1977

Spouse: Carlene

PAIS, M. JOYCE M.D., FACR

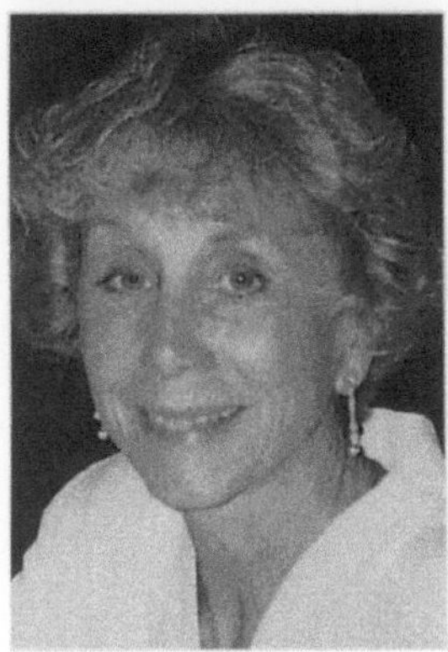

Academic Title: Professor Emeritus

Position at Affiliation: Professor

Business Address:
University of California Medical Center –
Irvine
101 City Drive South
Orange, CA 92668
U.S.A.
714-456-5033 (work)
714-675-8386 (fax)
mjpais@uei.edu (e-mail)

Home Address:
145 via Undine
Newport Beach, CA 92663
U.S.A.
714-675-9737 (home)
714-675-9737 (fax)

Specialty/Certification: Radiology, 1967

Education:
Rutgers University – Douglass College
(B.S.)
Medical College of Pennsylvania,
Philadelphia, PA (MD)
Albert Einstein Medical Center, Phila-
delphia, PA (Radiology residency)

ISS Member 1987

Spouse: Robert Chambers

PANUEL, MICHEL A. M.D.

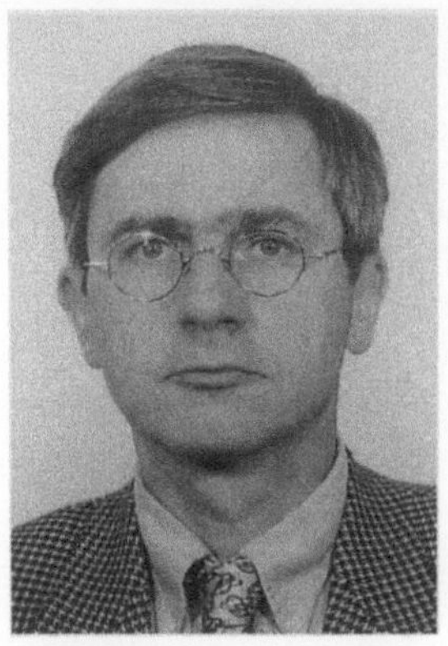

Birthdate: November 4, 1953

Academic Title: Professor

Position at Affiliation: Senior Staff

Business Address:
Service Radiologie
C.H.U. Nord
Chemin des Bourrelys
13915 Marseille Cedex 20
France
33-4-91964640 (work)
33-4-91968001 (fax)

Home Address:
8 Ter Chemin Du Pont
13007 Marseille
France
33.4.91592748 (home)
33.4.91592728 (fax)

Specialty: Radiology

Education:
Radiology 1982

ISS Member: 1993

Spouse: Nicole

PARISIEN, MAY V. M.D.

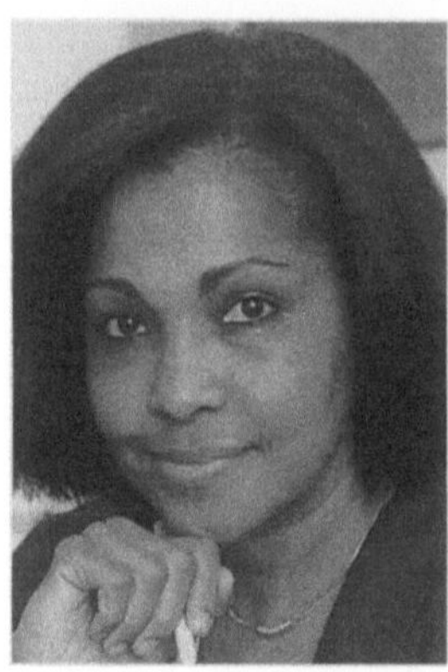

Academic Title: Associate Professor

Position at Affiliation: Associate Professor of Clinical Pathology

Business Address:
Columbia University College of
Physicians and Surgeons
1630 West 168 Street
New York, NY 10032
U.S.A.
212-305-6719 (work)
212-305-6595 (fax)

Home Address:
113 Warwick Road
Bronxville, NY 10708
U.S.A.
914-337-6848 (home)

Specialty/Certification: Anatomic and Clinical Pathology, 1976

Education:
Sante Rose deLima, Port-au-Prince, Haiti (BS)
Faculty of Medicine, State University, Port-au-Prince, Haiti (MD)
Albert Einstein Medical Center, Philadelphia, PA (internship)
New York Medical College, New York (residency)
Columbia-Presbyterian Hospital, New York (fellowship Bone Pathology)
Inserm-234, Lyon, FRANCE (research fellowship-Metabolic Bone Diseases)

ISS Member 1995

Spouse: J. Serge Parisien, M.D.

PARK, YONG-KOO M.D.

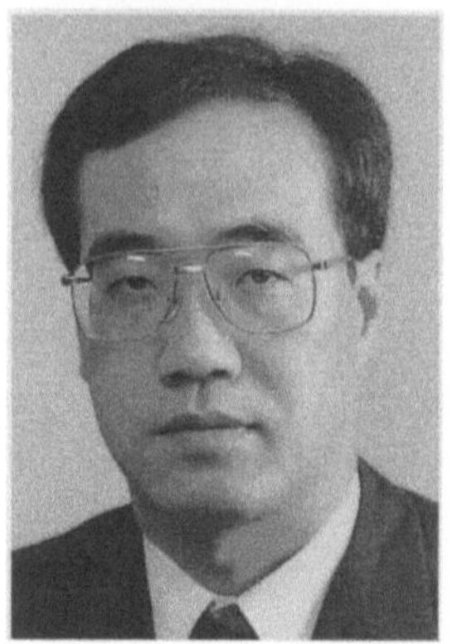

Birthdate: February 4, 1955

Academic Title: Professor

Position at Affiliation: Associate Professor

Business Address:
Kyung Hee Univ. Hospital
Department of Pathology
#1 Hoeki-Dong, Dong Dae Moon-ku
Seoul, 130-702
Korea
82-2-958-8742 (work)
82-2-957-0489 (fax)
damia@chollian.dacom.co.kr (e-mail)

Home Address:
Dong Sung Apt. #12-1905
Shin Nae Dong, Jung Rag Ku
Seoul, 131-130
Korea
82-2-207-6794 (home)

Specialty/Certification: Pathology, 1983

Education:
1979 – Kyung Hee Univ. Medical School (M.D.)
1985 – Kyung Hee Univ. Postgraduate School (Ph.D.)

ISS Member: 1996

Spouse: Dan-Young Jung

PATHRIA, MINI N. M.D.

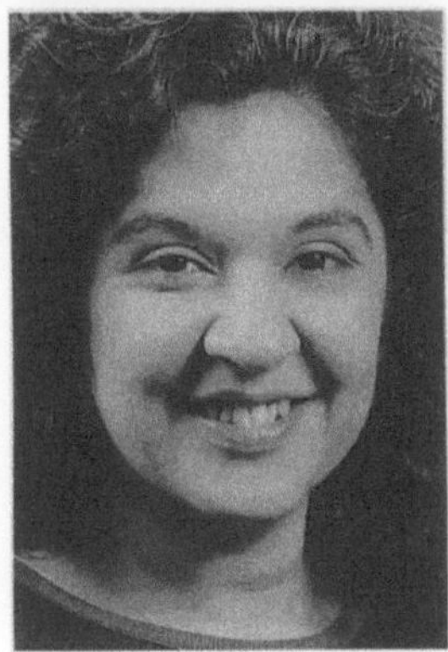

Birthdate: December 7, 1958

Academic Title: Associate Professor

Position at Affiliation: Radiologist

Business Address:
UCSD Medical Center
200 West Arbor
San Diego, CA 92103-8756
U.S.A.
619-543-6633 (work)
619-543-5345 (fax)
mpathria@ucsd.edu (e-mail)

Home Address:
2465 Avenida de la Playa
La Jolla, CA 92037
U.S.A.
619-456-8044 (home)
619-456-8045 (fax)

Specialty: Radiology

Education:
1982 – McMaster University (M.D.)
1983 – McGill University (internship)
1986 – McMaster University (Radiology residency)

ISS Member 1991

Spouse: Douglas Bates

PAVLOV, HELENE M.D.

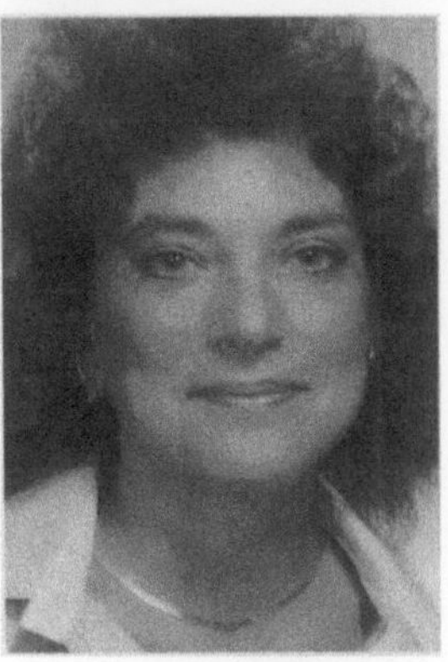

Academic Title: Professor of Radiology

Position at Affiliation: Assistant Director, Department of Radiology & Nuclear Medicine

Business Address:
Department of Radiology
Hospital for Special Surgery
535 East 70th Street
New York, NY 10021
U.S.A.
212-606-1132 (work)
212-734-7378 (fax)

Home Address:
304 East 65th Street
New York City, NY 10021
U.S.A.
212-794-3885 (home)

Specialty/Certification: Radiology, 1976

Education:
Temple University
Temple University School of Medicine (M.D.)
Germantown Hospital & Dispensary Medical Center (Radiology residency)
The Hospital for Special Surgery-Cornell Univ. Medical College (fellowship)

ISS Member 1980

ISS Committees:
Closed Program Committee, 1989
Nominating Committee – Chairman, 1995

Spouse: Harvey Zeichner

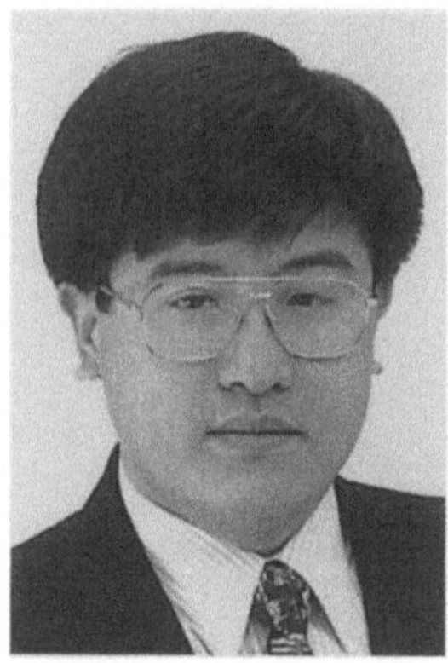

Birthdate: April 21, 1958

Academic Title: Professor

Position at Affiliation: Professor

Business Address:
The University of Hong Kong
Department of Diagnostic Radiology
Block K, Room 406
Queen Mary Hospital
Hong Kong
852-28553307 (work)
852-28551652 (fax)
wcgpeh@hkucc.hku.hk (e-mail)

Home Address:
B5 Rodrigues Court
350 Victoria Road
Hong Kong
852-28176576 (home)

Specialty/Certification: Radiology, 1990

Education:
National University of Singapore
Glasgow, U.K. and Birmingham, U.K.
(specialty training)

ISS Member 1996

Spouse: Angeline

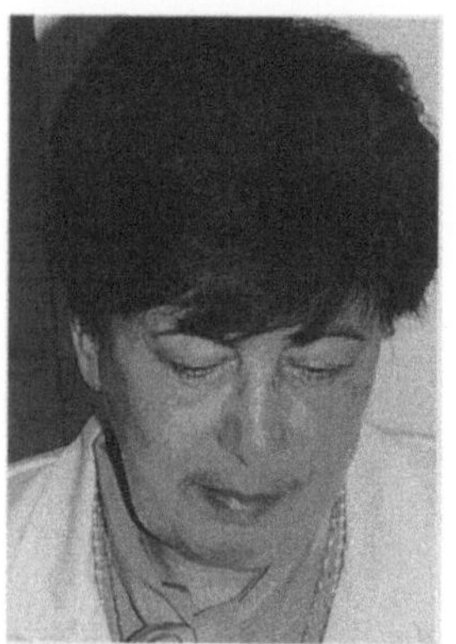

Birthdate: May 8, 1932

Academic Title: Professor

Position at Affiliation: Head of
Department

Business Address:
Hospital Universitaire des Enfants
"Reine Fabiola" U.L.B.
Av. J.J. Crocq, 15
1020 Brussels
Belgium
32-2-477-3214 (work)
32-2-478-5439 (fax)
nperlmut@resulb.ulb.ac.be (e-mail)

Home Address:
avenue du Pic-Vert, 51
1640 Rhode St. Genese
Belgium
32-2-358-2923 (home)

Specialty/Certification: Radiology, 1964

Education:
Athenee Royal D'Uccle
Universite Libre of Bruxelles

ISS Member 1987

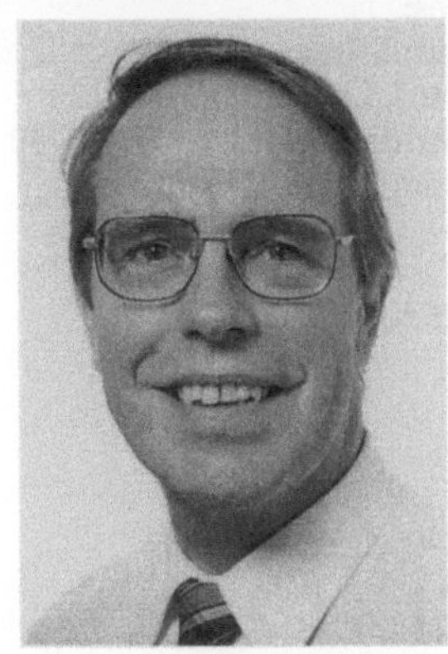

Birthdate: April 2, 1942

Academic Title: Professor of Radiology

Position at Affiliation: Deputy Medical Director, Chief County Radiologist

Business Address:
Department of Radiology
University Hospital
S-22185 Lund
Sweden
46/46-173000 (work)
46/46-2116956 (fax)
holger.pettersson@drad.lu.se

Home Address:
Trädgardsgatan 2
S-23442 Lomma
Sweden
46/40-410734 (home)
46/40-412172 (fax)

Specialty/Certification: Radiology, 1976

Education:
University of Lund – Graduate School
University of Lund – Specialty training
University of Toronto – Specialty training

ISS Member 1985

Offices Held in ISS and Dates of Service:
Executive Committee, 1992 –
President 1996 – 98

ISS Committees:
Course Chairman, 19th ISS Refresher
Course, Stockholm, 1992

Spouse: Grethe

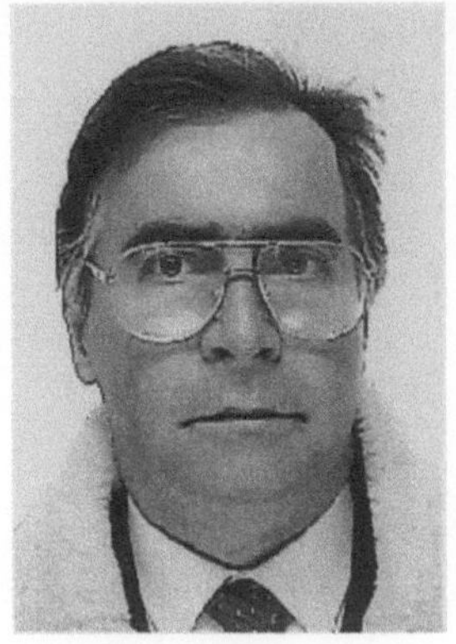

Birthdate: July 4, 1952

Position at Affiliation: Director

Business Address:
Laboratorio di Ricerca Oncologica
Instituti Orthopedici Rizzoli
Via di Barbiano 1/10
40136 Bologna
Italy
39-51-6366759 (work)
39-51-584422 (fax)
picci@oncolabrizzoli.tizeta.it (e-mail)

Home Address:
Via del Monte 9
40068 San Lazzaro, Bologna
Italy
39-51-480932 (home)

Specialty/Certification: Oncology, 1983

Education:
University of Bologna

ISS Member 1984

Spouse: Tiziana

PITT, MICHAEL J. M.D.

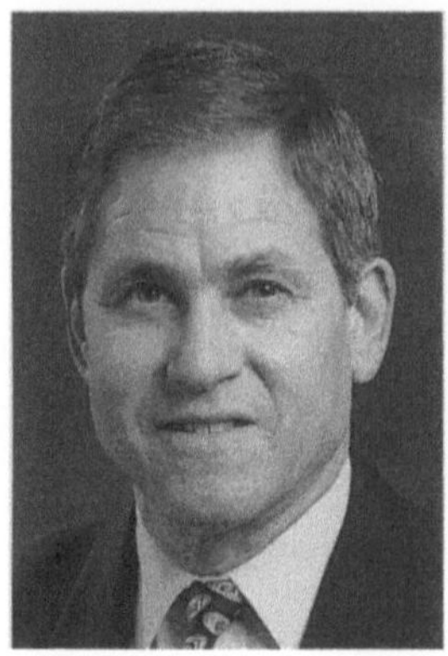

Birthdate: March 14, 1938

Academic Title: Professor of Radiology
and Orthopaedic Surgery

Position at Affiliation: Professor of
Radiology
Director of Musculoskeletal Imaging

Business Address:
Department of Radiology
University of Alabama at Birmingham
Kirklin Clinic
2000 6th Avenue South
Birmingham, AL 35233
U.S.A.
205-801-7936 (work)
205-801-8755 (fax)
mpitt@uabmc.edu (e-mail)

Home Address:
421 Vesclub Lane
Birmingham, AL 35216
U.S.A.
205-822-3719 (home)

Specialty: Radiology, 1971

Education:
1955–59 – Muhlenberg College (B.S.)
1959–63 – Jefferson Medical College
(M.D.)
1967–71 – Jefferson Medical College
(Radiology residency)

ISS Member Founding member

ISS Offices Held:
Treasurer 1992–

ISS Committees:
Endowment Fund, Treasurer, 1992–
Rules Committee, Chairman, 1988–90
Grants and Awards Committee, 1988–90
Nominating Committee, Chairman,
1983–84

Spouse: Margo Zonana

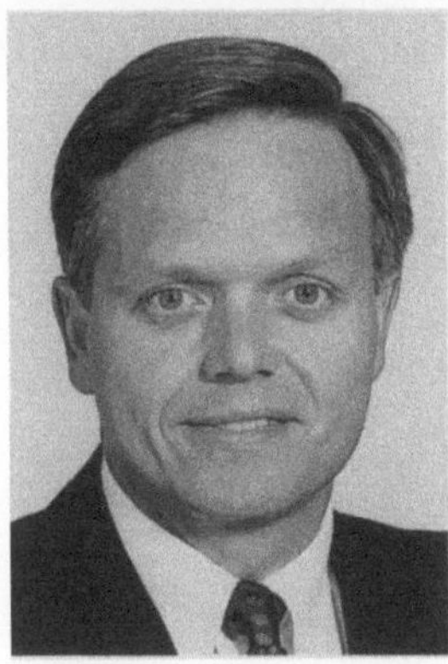

Birthdate: July 3, 1951

Academic Title: Professor of Radiology and Orthopaedics

Position at Affiliation: Professor

Business Address:
Roper Hospital
316 Calhoun St.
Charleston, SC 29401
U.S.A.
803-724-2061 (work)
803-805-6268 (fax)
vwradman@aol.com

Home Address:
22 Twin Oaks Lane
Isle of Palms, SC 29451
U.S.A.
803-886-4026 (home)

Specialty/Certification: Radiology, 1983

Education:
1973 – University of North Carolina –
Chapel Hill (AB-Religion)
1978 – University of North Carolina –
Chapel Hill (M.D.)
University of Virginia (Radiology
residency)

ISS Committees:
Refresher Course Committee
Liaison Planning Committee

ISS Member 1987

Spouse: Lou

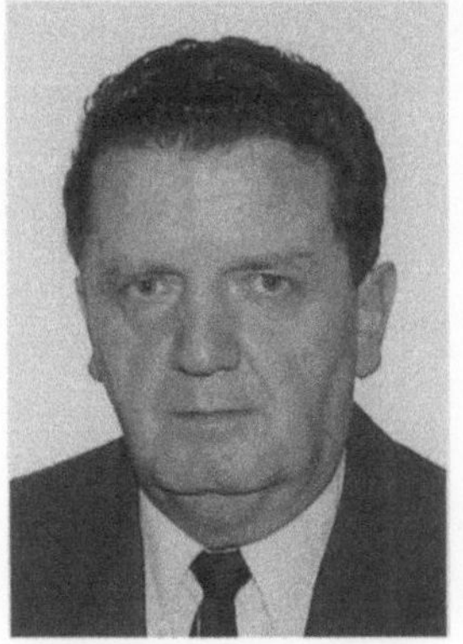

Academic Title: Professor

Position at Affiliation: Head of 2nd
Instuitute of Pathology

Business Address:
2nd Institute for Radiology, 1st Medical
Faculty Charles University
U nemocnica 4
Prague 2
Czech Repulic 128 52
42 295 572 (work)
42 2 249 15413 (fax)

Home Address:
Jablonecka 714
Prague 9
190 00
Czech Repulic
42 882 306 (home)

Specialty/Certification: Pathology, 1966,
1973, 1978

Education:
1st Medical Faculty, Charles University,
Prague
1st and 2nd Board in Pathology

ISS Member 1994

POZNANSKI, ANDREW K. M.D.

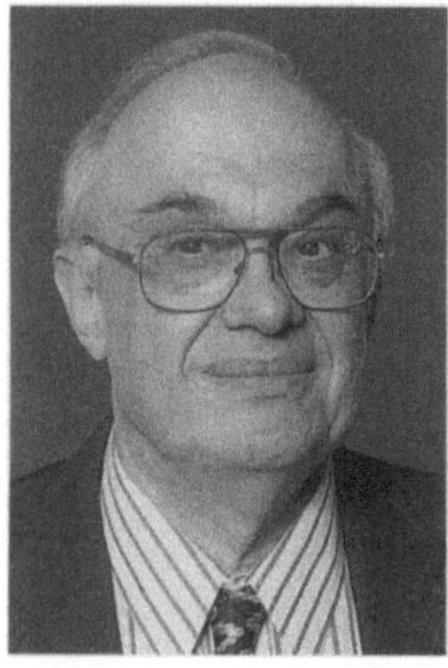

Birthdate: October 11, 1931

Academic Title: Earl J. Frederick Professor of Radiology

Position at Affiliation: Radiologist-in-Chief

Business Address:
Department of Radiology #9
The Children's Memorial Hospital
2300 Children's Plaza
Chicago, IL 60614
U.S.A.
773-880-3520 (work)
773-880-3517 (fax)
apoznanski@nwu.edu (e-mail)

Home Address:
2400 Lakeview, Apt. 2401
Chicago, Il 60614
U.S.A.
773-935-8909 (home)

Specialty/Certification: Radiology, 1961; Pediatric Radiology 1994

Education:
1949–52 – McGill University, Montreal (B. Sc.)
1952–56 – McGill University Medical School, Montreal (M. D. C. M.)
1956–57 – Montreal General Hospital (internship)
1957–60 – Henry Ford Hospital, Detroit, MI (residency in Radiology)

ISS Member Founding member

Offices Held in ISS and Dates of Service:
President-Elect, 1990–92
President, 1992–94

ISS Medals and Awards:
Founders' Medal, Santa Fe, 1997
Founders' Lecture, Santa Fe, 1997

ISS Committees:
Board of Editors, Skeletal Radiology, 1975–95
Ad Hoc Search Committee for American Assistant Chief Editor, Skeletal Radiology, 1982

Spouse: Gail Margolis

PREIN, JOACHIM M. D., D. D. S.

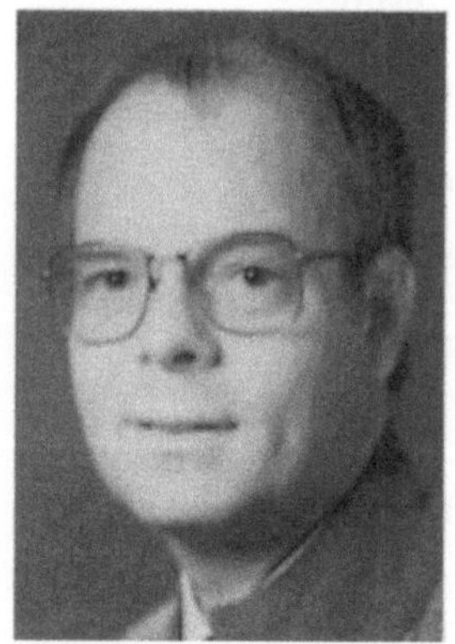

Business Address:
Kantonsspital Basel
Maxillofacial Unit Spitalstr. 21
CH-4031 Basel
Switzerland
0041-61-252525 ext. 18-386 (work)
0041-61-67-48-32 (home)

ISS Member 1983

Spouse: Elke

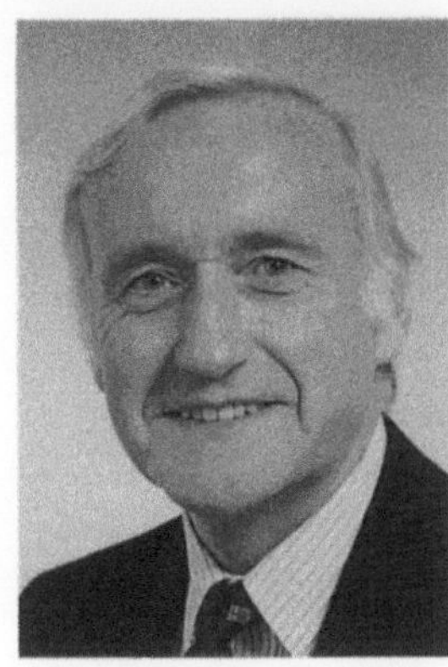

Birthdate: August 24, 1937

Academic Title: Doctor

Position at Affiliation: Consultant Radiologist

Business Address:
Radiology Department
University Hospital
Queen's Medical Centre
Nottingham NG7 2UH
England
44 0115-924-9924 ext. 43876 (work)
44 0115-970-9962 (fax)

Home Address:
124 Parkside
Wollaton
Nottingham NG8 2NP
England
44 0115-928-3650 (home)

Specialty: Radiology

Education:
London University, St. Mary's Hospital,
London, England

ISS Member 1973

ISS Committees:
Editorial Board, 1994

Spouse: Christine

Business Address:
Department of Morbid Anatomy
Institute of Orthopaedics
Royal National Orthopaedic Hospital
Brockley Hill, Stanmore
Middlesex HA7 4LP
England

ISS Member 1986

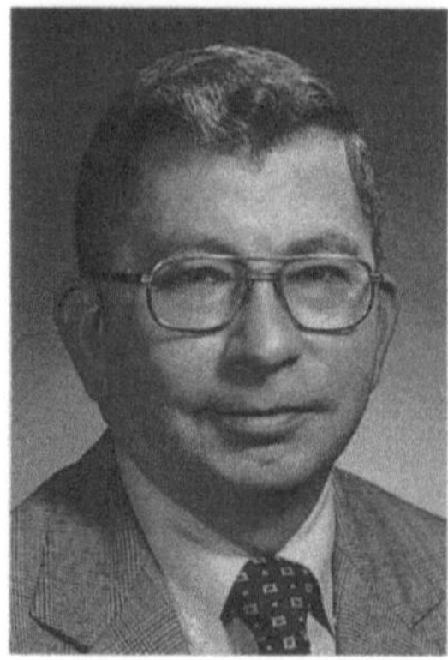

Birthdate: December 25, 1937

Academic Title: Professor of Orthopedic Surgery and Oncology

Position at Affiliation: Consultant

Business Address:
Mayo Clinic
200 First Street, S.W.
Rochester, MN 55905
U.S.A.
507-284-2511 (work)
507-284-5539 or 266-4234 (fax)
pritcharddouglas@mayo.edu. (e-mail)

Home Address:
2220 Bamber Valley Road, S.W.
Rochester, MN 55902
U.S.A.
507-288-9159 (home)

Specialty/Certification: Orthopedic Surgery, 1973

Education:
Harvard University (A.B.)
1964 – Tufts University (M.D.)
1964–66 – Hartford Hospital (internship)
1968–72 Mayo Clinic (residency)

ISS Member 1975

Spouse: Jan

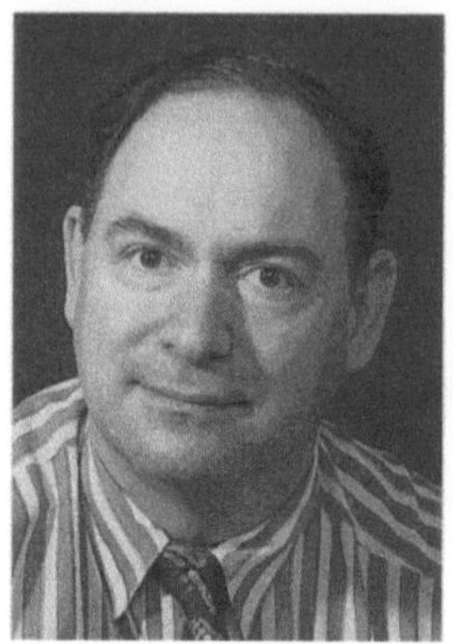

Birthdate: April 30, 1943

Academic Title: Professor

Position at Affiliation: Pathologist-in-Chief

Business Address:
Pathology and Laboratory Medicine
Mount Sinai Hospital
600 University Avenue
Toronto, Ontario M5G 1X5
Canada
416-586-4453 (work)
416-586-8589 (fax)

Home Address:
139 Glencairn Avenue
Toronto, Ontario M4R 1N1
Canada
416-486-6909 (home)

Specialty/Certification: Pathology, 1972

Education:
1969–72 – University of Toronto
(Pathology training program)
1967 – University of Toronto (MD)

ISS Member 1988

Spouse: Carol

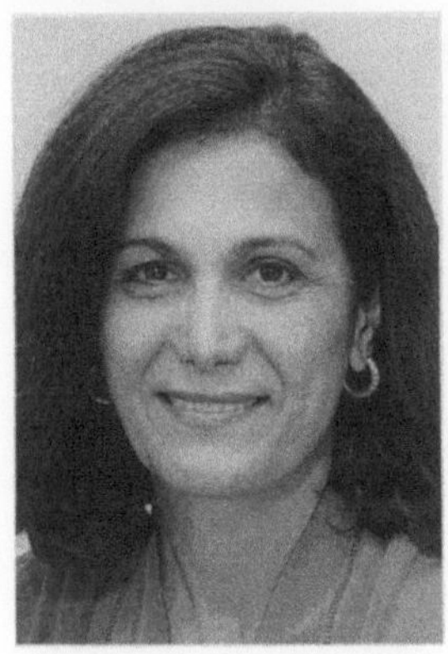

Birthdate: August 10, 1943

Academic Title: Professor of Clinical

Position at Affiliation: Attending Radiologist

Business Address:
Department of Radiology
NYU Medical Center
560 First Avenue
New York, NY 10016
U.S.A.
212-263-5941 (work)
212-263-8978 (fax)
mahvash.rafii@mctrd.med.nyu.edu
(e-mail)

Home Address:
10 Byron Lane
Great Neck, NY 11023
U.S.A.
516-487-2340 (home)

Specialty/Certification: Radiology, 1975

Education:
1969 – Tehran University School of
Medicine (M.D.)
1970–71 – New Rochelle Hospital,
New Rochelle, NY
1971–74 – New England Deaconess
Hospital, Boston, MA (Radiology
residency)

ISS Member 1989

Spouse: Daniel Abitbol

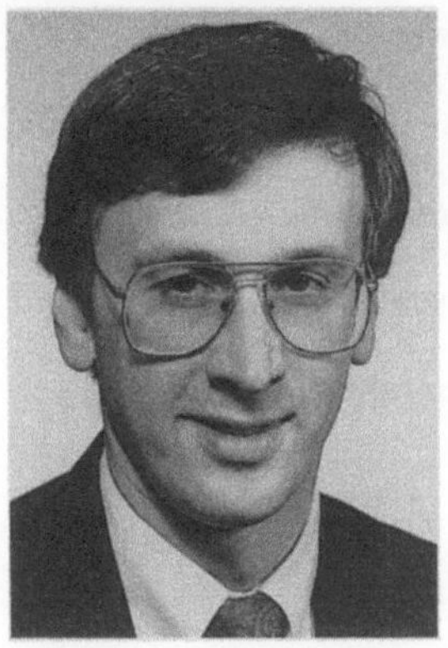

Birthdate: June 6, 1958

Position at Affiliation: Staff radiologist

Business Address:
Cleveland Clinic Foundation
Department of Radiology A21
9500 Euclid Avenue
Cleveland, OH 44195
U.S.A.
216 444-2285 (work)
216 445-9445 (fax)
recht@ccisd3.ccf.org (e-mail)

Home Address:
24025 Maidstone Lane
Beachwood, OH 44122
U.S.A.
216-464-6781 (home)

Specialty/Certification: Radiology, 1987

Education:
1979 – University of Pittsburgh (B.S.)
1983 – University of Pennsylvania (M.D.)

ISS Member 1993

Spouse: Wendy

Business Address:
Radiology Department, Room 815
University of Hawaii School of Medicine
1356 Lusitana Street
Honolulu, HI 96813
U.S.A.
808-956-5463 (work)

ISS Member Founding member

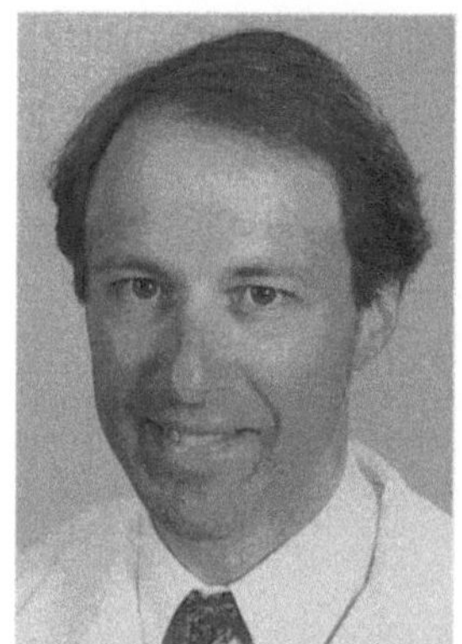

Academic Title: Associate Professor of Radiology

Position at Affiliation: Assistant Professor of Medicine

Business Address:
Mallinckrodt Institute of Radiology
Jewish Hospital
216 S. Kingshighway
St. Louis, MO 63110
U.S.A.
314 454-7399 (work)
314 454-5665 (fax)
reinus@totty.wustl.edu (e-mail)

Specialty/Certification: Radiology, 1983

Education:
1975 – Amherst College (B.S.)
1979 – NYU Medical School (M.D.)
1980 – Washington University Medicine (internship)
1983 – Mallinckrodt (Radiology)

ISS Member 1995

Spouse: Elizabeth

REISER, MAXIMILIAN F. M.D.

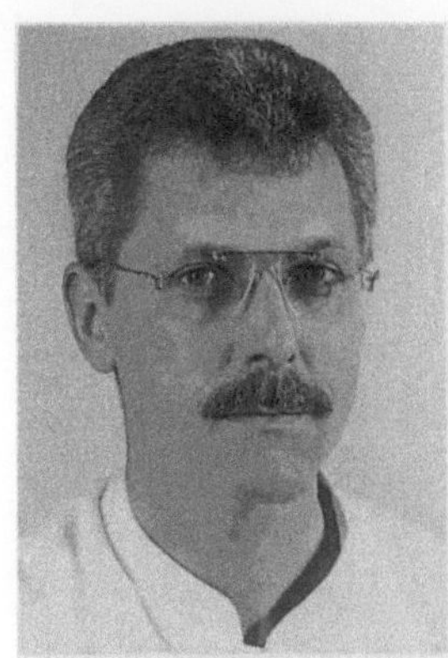

Birthdate: August 10, 1948

Academic Title: Professor of Radiology

Position at Affiliation: Chairman

Business Address:
Institut fur Radiologische Diagnostik
Klinikum GroBhadern
Ludwig-Maximilians Universität
München
Marchioninistr. 15,
81377 München
Germany
89-7095-2750 (work)
89-7095-8895 (fax)

Home Address:
Waldmüllerstr. 9
81479 München
Germany
89-7916926 (home)
89-7916869 (fax)

Specialty: Radiology

Education:
University of Munich (MD)

ISS Member 1987

ISS Committees:
Refresher Course Committee

Spouse: Elke

REMAGEN, WOLFGANG M.D.

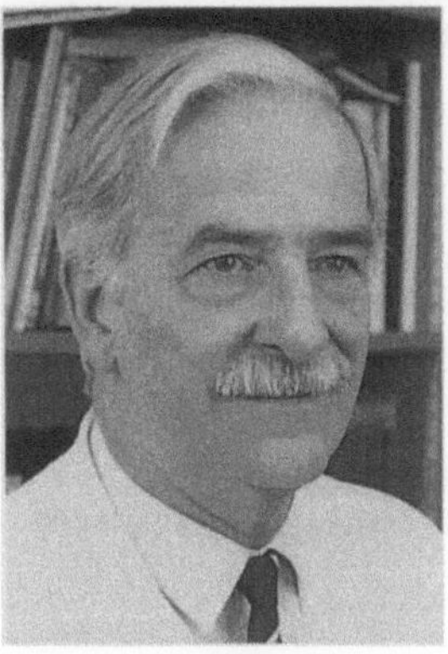

Birthdate: March 20, 1928

Academic Title: Professor of General and
Special Pathology

Position at Affiliation: Professor
Emeritus Senior Consultant

Business Address:
Division of Skeletal Pathology
Institut fuer Pathologie der
Universitaet Basel
4003 Basel, Schoenbeinstrasse 40
Switzerland
41-61-2652878 (work)
41-61-2653194 (fax)

Home Address:
Im Rapsfeld 29a
D-50933 Koeln (Cologne)
Germany
49-221-496934 (home & fax)

Specialty/Certification: Pathology, 1964

Education:
1949–54 – University of Cologne (M.D.)
1954–55 – University of Cologne,
Dept. of Pathology (internship)
1956–58 – University Geneva,
Dept. of Pathology, Geneva, Switzerland
1959 – Pasteur Institute, Division Nuclear
Medicine, Paris, France
1960–63 – University of Berlin,
Dept. of Pathology, Berlin, Germany

1964–69 – University of Kiel,
Dept. of Pathology, Kiel, Germany
1969–71 – 3rd Chair Anatomy
(bone biophysics) University Geneva,
Geneva, Switzerland

ISS Member 1978

ISS Committees:
Membership Committee
Adhoc Future Planning Committee
Closed Meeting Committee
Executive Committee

ISS Medals and Awards:
Medal of the ISS (Silver), Santa Fe, 1997

Spouse: Karin

REMBERGER, KLAUS M.D.

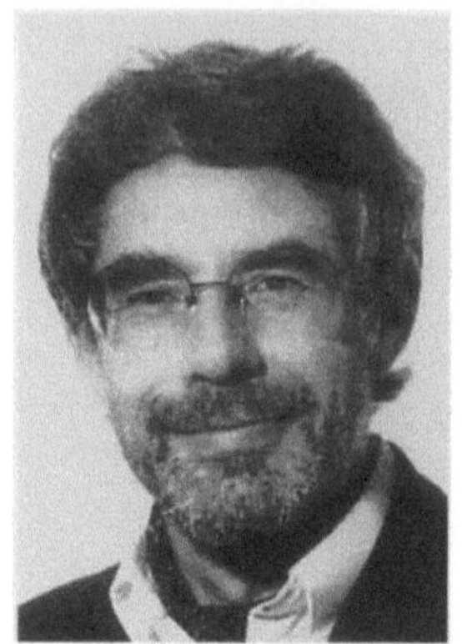

Birthdate: January 28, 1941

Academic Title: Professor

Position at Affiliation: Head of
Department

Business Address:
University of Saarland
Department of Pathology (Geb.26)
Building 26
66421 Homburg/SAAR
Germany
6841-163850 (work)
6841-163880 (fax)
pakrem@med-rz.uni-sb.de (e-mail)

Home Address:
Flotowstr. 11
D-80686 Munich
Germany
89-561-472

Specialty/Certification: Pathology, 1976

Education:
LMU – University of Munich (M.D.)

ISS Member: 1993

Spouse: Monika

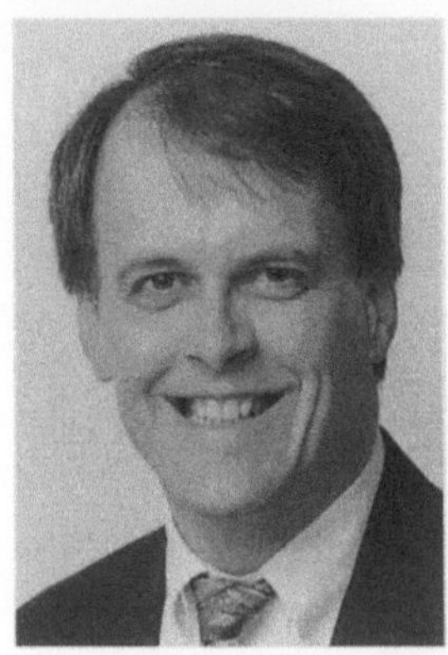

Birthdate: September 22, 1955

Academic Title: Associate Professor

Position at Affiliation: Chief of Musculoskeletal and Emergency Radiology

Business Address:
University of North Carolina School of Medicine
Department of Radiology CB 7510
Chapel Hill, NC 27599-7510
U.S.A.
919-966-2886 (work)
919-966-5934 (fax)
renner.rad@mhs.unc.edu (e-mail)

Home Address:
2526-R Sax-Beth Church Road
Graham, NC 27253
U.S.A.
910-376-0505 (home)

Specialty/Certification: Radiology, 1985

Education:
1977 – University of Virginia (B.A.)
1980 – University of Virginia (M.D.)
1981–85 – University of North Carolina (Radiology residency)
1985–86 – Duke University Medical Center (Musculoskeletal Radiology fellowship)

ISS Member 1995

Spouse: Joy J.

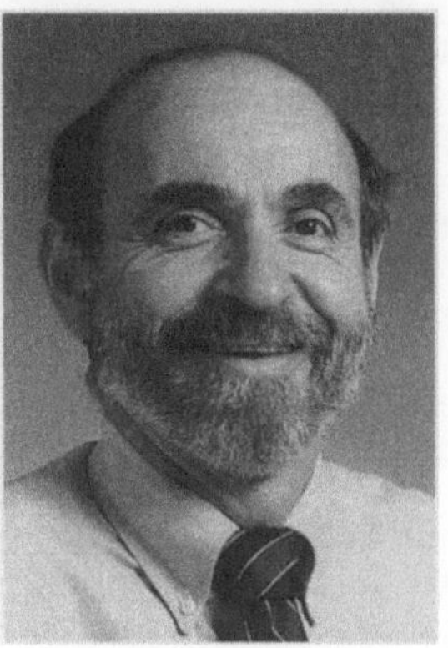

Academic Title: Professor of Radiology

Position at Affiliation: Chief, Osteoradiology

Business Address:
Radiology Department
Veterans Administration Hospital
3350 La Jolla Village Drive
San Diego, CA 92161
U.S.A.
619-552-8585 ext.3343 (work)
619-552-7452 (fax)
resnick.donald@va.gov (e-mail)

Home Address:
390 Hidden Pines Road
Del Mar, CA 92014
U.S.A.
619-755-0745

Specialty: Radiology

Education:
College – Hamilton College, Clinton, New York
Medical School – Cornell University Medical College, New York City, NY
residency – Cornell University-New York Hospital, New York, NY
Fellowship – Good Samaritan Hospital, Phoenix, AZ

ISS Member 1981

Offices Held in ISS and Dates of Service:
Assistant Secretary/Treasurer, 1987–89
Treasurer, 1989–92
Secretary, 1992–96
President-Elect, 1996–98

ISS Committees:
Continuing Education Course
Committee, 1981–82
Membership Committee, 1984–85
Executive Committee, 1985–87;
1989–present
Chairman, Awards Committee, 1996
Convention Planning Committee,
1986–present
Skeletal Committee (1983–84)
Refresher Course Committee, 1985–89;
1990–91 (Program Chairman or
Co-Chairman)

Spouse: Pauline

RESNIK, CHARLES S. M.D.

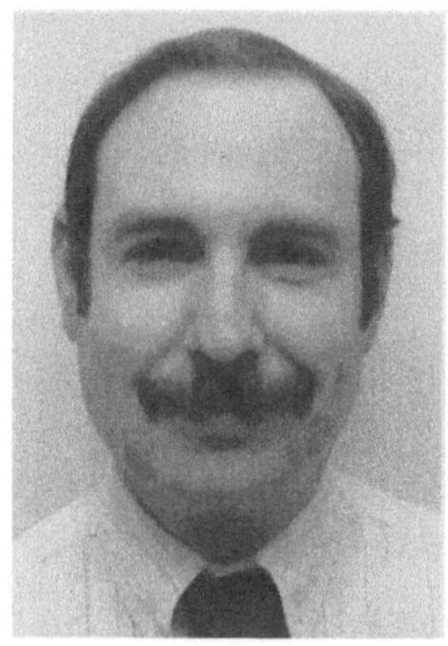

Birthdate: April 19, 1953

Academic Title: Associate Professor of
Radiology

Position at Affiliation: Director of
Musculoskeletal and Emergency
Radiology

Business Address:
Department of Radiology
University of Maryland Medical Center
22 South Greene Street
Baltimore, MD 21201
U.S.A.
410-328-2033 (work)
410 328 0641 (fax)
cresnik@radiology.ab.umd.edu (e-mail)

Specialty/Certification: Radiology, 1981

Education:
Northwestern University Medical School
(M.D.)
Medical College of Virginia (Radiology
residency)
University of California, San Diego
(Skeletal Radiology fellowship)

ISS Committees:
Evaluation of Research Grants Committee

ISS Member 1986

Business Address:
Department Histopathology
Royal Free Hospital School of Medicine
Rowland Hill Street
London NW3 2PF
United Kingdom

Specialty: Pathology

ISS Member 1986

Spouse: Margaret Ruth

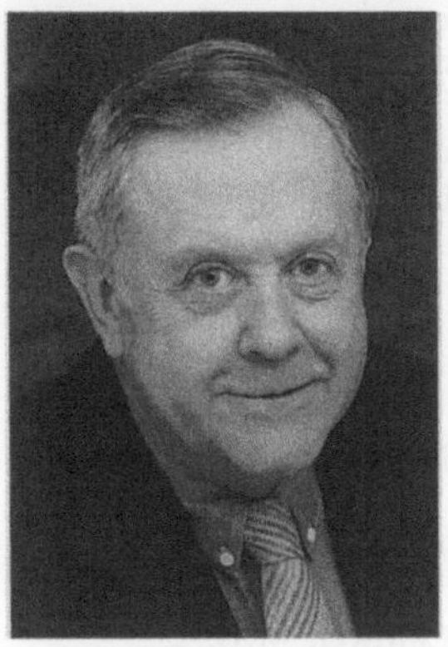

Birthdate: September 27, 1922

Academic Title: Professor

Position at Affiliation: Professor

Business Address:
Radiology Department
Univ. of Texas Southwestern Medical
Center at Dallas
5323 Harry Hines Boulevard
Dallas, TX 75235
U.S.A.
214-648-8014 (work)
214-648-2678 (fax)

Home Address:
10614 Royal Springs Drive
Dallas, TX 75229
U.S.A.
214-351-6800 (home)

Specialty/Certification: Radiology, 1957

Education:
1948 – Wesleyan University
1952 – College of Physicians & Surgeons,
Columbia Univ. NYC (M.D.)
St. Luke's Hospital, NYC (residency)

ISS Member Founding member

Spouse: Mary Jane

RICHARDSON, MICHAEL L. M.D.

Business Address:
University Hospital
Department of Radiology – SB 05
1956 NE Pacific Street
Seattle, WA 98195
U.S.A.
206-285-4673 (home)
206-543-6317 (fax)
206-543-3320 (work)

Specialty: Radiology

ISS Member 1988

Spouse: Chris Caldwell, M.D.

ROESSNER, ALBERT M.D.

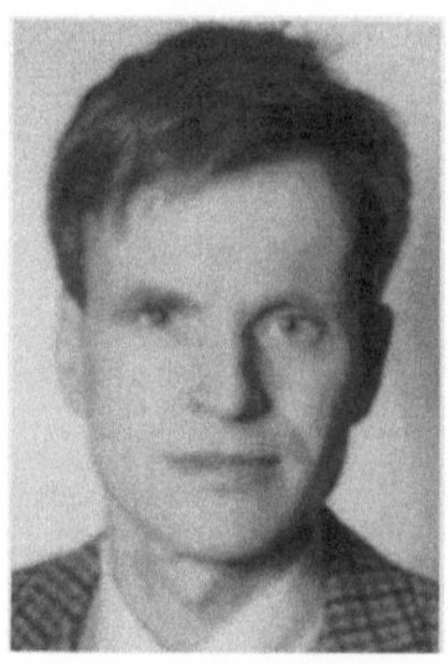

Business Address:
Bone Tumor Registry of West Phalia
Munster Institute of Pathology
Munster
Germany

ISS Member 1983

ROGERS, LEE F. M.D.

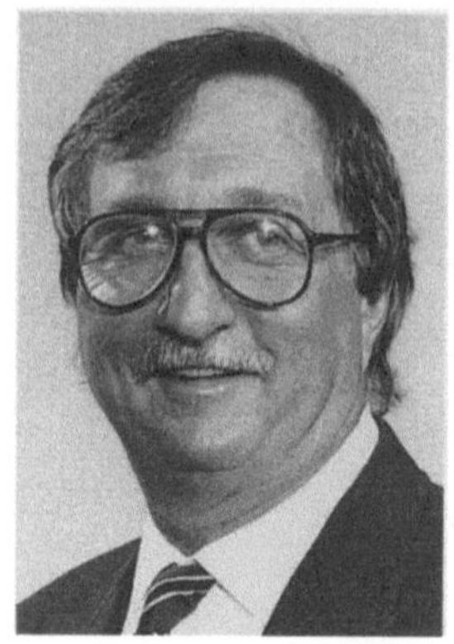

Birthdate: September 24, 1934

Academic Title: Meschan Professor

Position at Affiliation: Editor-in-Chief,
American Journal of Radiology

Business Address:
Bowman Gray School of Medicine
Wake Forest University
Medical Center Boulevard
Winston-Salem, NC 27157
U.S.A.
910-750-0123 (work)
910-750-0129 (fax)

Home Address:
4551 Chinaberry Lane
Winston-Salem, NC 27106
U.S.A.
910-924-8524 (home)
910-922-5866 (fax)

Specialty/Certification: Radiology, 1964

Education:
1956 – Northwestern University (BMA)
1959 – Northwestern University Medical
School (MD)
1959 – 60 – Walter Reed General Hospital
(internship)
1960 – 63 – Fitzsimons General Hospital,
Denver, CO (residency)

ISS Member 1986

Spouse: Donna

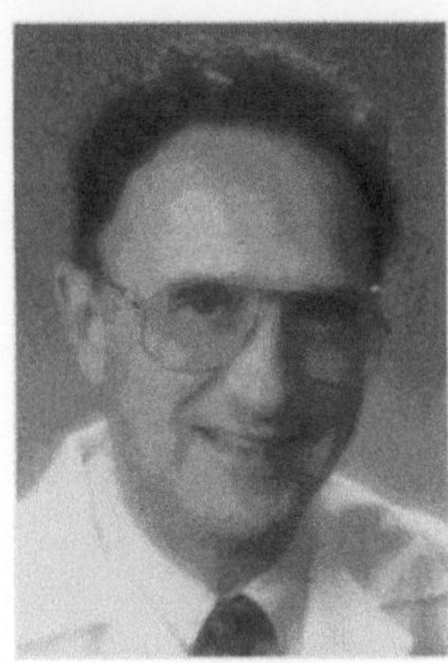

Birthdate: November 4, 1939

Position at Affiliation: Attending Physician

Business Address:
St. Vincent's Comprehensive Cancer Center
153 West 11th Street, 14th Floor
New York, NY 10011
U.S.A.
212-604-6020 (work)
mtx@ix.netcom.com

Home Address:
245 E. 58th Street, #17E
New York City, NY 10022
U.S.A.

Specialty/Certification: Medical Oncology, 1975

Education:
1961 – Massachusetts Institute of Technology (B.S.)
1966 – Stanford University School of Medicine (M.D.)

ISS Member 1986

Spouse: Elizabeth

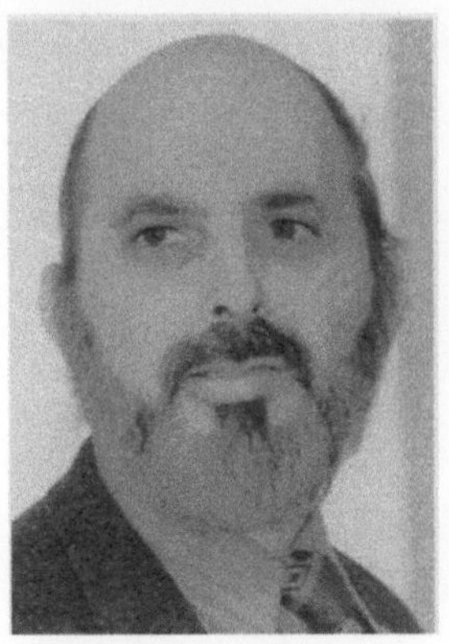

Birthdate: April 11, 1939

Academic Title: Associate Professor

Position at Affiliation: Director, Radiology

Business Address:
Bronx-Lebanon Hospital Center
1650 Grand Concourse
Bronx, NY 10457
U.S.A.
718-518-5031 (work)
718-518-5224 (fax)
rrosen@ix.netcom.com

Home Address:
55 Parkway West
Mt. Vernon, NY 10552
U.S.A.
914-699-2397

Specialty/Certification: Radiology, 1968; Nuclear Medicine, 1972

Education:
1960 – Brandeia University (B.A.)
1963 – AECOM of Yeshiva University (M.D.)

ISS Member 1973

Spouse: Phyllis

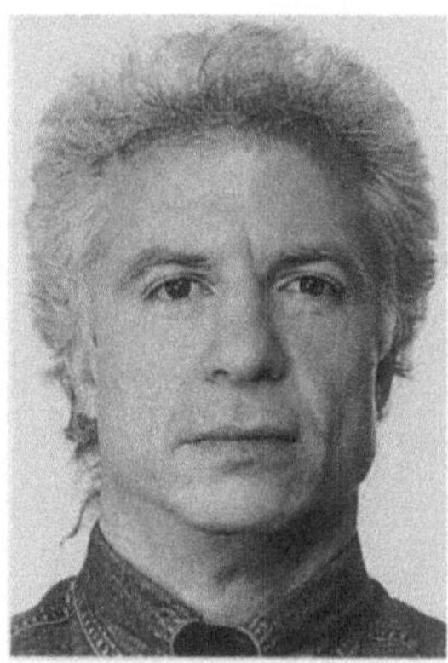

Birthdate: June 5, 1953

Academic Title: Associate Professor

Position at Affiliation: Assistant
Pathologist

Business Address:
Massachusetts General Hospital
Department of Pathology
Fruit Street
Boston, MA 02114
U.S.A.
617-726-5127 (work)
617-726-7476 (fax)
rosenberg@helix.mgh.harvard.edu
(e-mail)

Home Address:
12 Mason Terrace
Brookline, MA 02146
U.S.A.

Specialty/Certification: Pathology, 1985

Education:
1981 – Temple University School of
Medicine (M.D.)

ISS Member: 1993

Spouse: Laura

Business Address:
Department of Orthopaedic Surgery
Montefiore Hospital & Medical Center
111 East 210th Street
Bronx, NY 10467
U.S.A.
914-423-2292 (home)
212-920-4946 (work)
212-920-6373 (fax)

ISS Member 1976

ROSENBERG, ZEHAVA S. M. D.

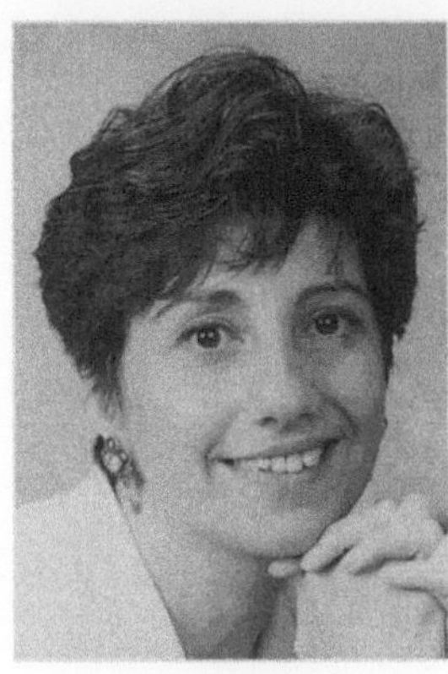

Academic Title: Associate Professor of Clinical Radiology

Position at Affiliation: Associate Professor

Business Address:
Radiology Department
Hospital for Joint Diseases
301 East 17th Street
New York, NY 10003
U.S.A.
212-598-6373 (work)
212-598-6125 (fax)

Home Address:
127 Bloomfield
Hoboken, NJ 07030
U.S.A.
201-653-7641 (home)
201-653-8716 (fax)

Specialty/Certification: Radiology, 1985

Education:
1971–74 – Tel Aviv University (B.S.)
1976–80 – Univ. of Connecticut Medical School (M.D.)
1981–84 – Albert Einstein Medical School (Radiology residency)
1984–86 – Columbia Presbyterian Hospital (Musculoskeletal fellowship)

ISS Member 1991

Spouse: Ron

ROSENTHAL, DANIEL I. M. D.

Business Address:
Harvard Medical School
Massachusetts General Hosptial
Boston, MA 02114
U.S.A.
617-726-8784 (work)
617-726-5282 (fax)
617-891-4141 (home)

Specialty: Radiology

ISS Member 1984

Spouse: Jacqueline

ROTHSCHILD, BRUCE M. M. D.

Academic Title: Professor

Position at Affiliation: Professor

Business Address:
Arthritis Center of Northeast Ohio
5500 Market St.
Youngstown, OH 44512
U.S.A.
330-783-5900 (work)
330-783-5350 (fax)
bmr@neoucom.edu (e-mail)

Home Address:
1327 Stonington
Youngstown, OH 44512
U.S.A.
330-759-3133 (home)

Specialty/Certification: Rheumatology, 1978

ISS Member 1996

Spouse: Christine

Birthdate: November 26, 1946

Academic Title: Associate Professor
(University of Toronto)

Position at Affiliation: Staff Radiologist

Business Address:
Sunnybrook Health Science Center
2075 Bayview Avenue
Toronto, Ontario M4N 3M5
Canada
416-480-4356 (work)
416-480-5855 (fax)
joel.rubenstein@sunnybrook.on.ca
(e-mail)

Home Address:
576 Briar Hill Avenue
Toronto, Ontario M5N 1M9
Canada
416-487-9931 (home)

Specialty/Certification: Radiology, 1977

Education:
University of Louisville (B. A. and M. D.)

ISS Member 1992

Spouse: Rachel

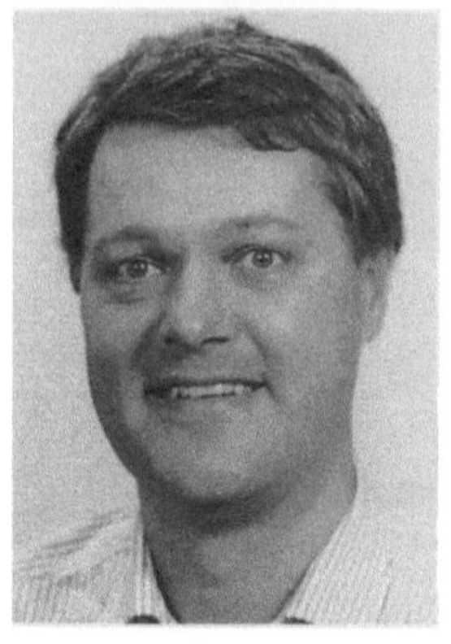

Birthdate: June 7, 1952

Position at Affiliation: Senior Consultant

Business Address:
Department of Radiology
Huddinge University Hospital
141 86 Huddinge
Sweden
46-8-585 800 00 (work)
46-8-711 48 40 (fax)
jonas.rydberg@karo.ki.se (e-mail)

Home Address:
Storgatan 20
114 55 Stockholm
Sweden
46-8-667 17 32 (home)
46-8-667 17 32 (fax)

Specialty/Certification: Radiology, 1985

Education:
1972 – 78 – Medical School
1978 – 80 – internship
1980 – 85 – Radiology residency

ISS Member 1993

Spouse: Magdalena

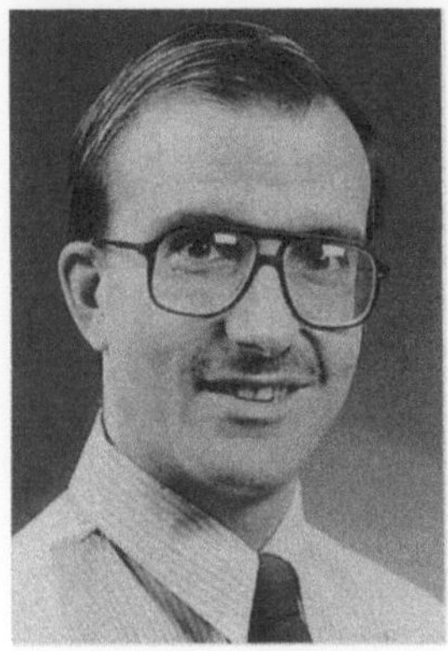

Birthdate: November 25, 1955

Academic Title: Professor of Radiology

Position at Affiliation: Chief,
Quantitative Bone Densitometry

Business Address:
CSD Medical Center Thornton Hospital
Department of Radiology
9300 Campus Point Drive
La Jolla, CA 92037
U.S.A.
619-657-6672 (work)
619-657-6699 (fax)

Home Address:
8585-24 Via Mallorca
La Jolla, CA 92037
U.S.A.
619-453-4369 (home)

Specialty/Certification: Radiology, 1984

Education:
Stanford University (B.S.)
Stanford Medical School (M.D., intern-
ship, residency)
UCSD – fellow in Osteoradiology

ISS Member 1987

ISS Committees: Nomenclature

ISS Medals and Awards:
President's Medal, New York, 1989

Spouse: Cyd

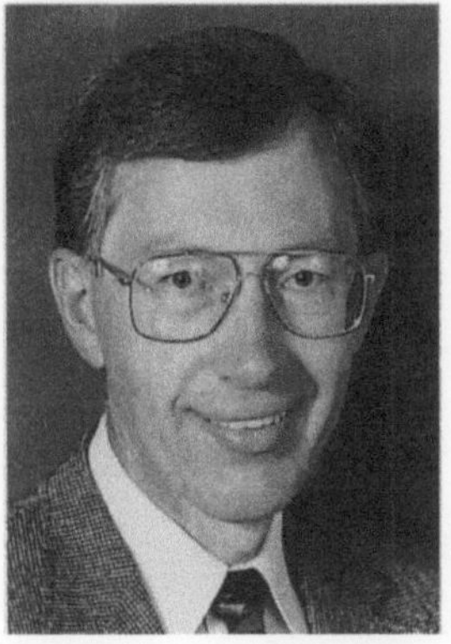

Birthdate: March 19, 1946

Academic Title: Professor of Radiology

Position at Affiliation: Vice Chairman,
Department of Radiology

Business Address:
Oregon Health Sciences University
M/S L-340
3181 S.W. Sam Jackson Park Road
Portland, Oregon 97201
U.S.A.
503-494-4511 (work)
503-494-4982 (fax)

Home Address:
8696 S.E. 141st Court
Portland, Oregon 92373
U.S.A.
503-760-8911 (home)

Specialty/Certification: Radiology, 1975

Education:
Union College
Loma Linda University, School of
Medical (MD)
Loma Linda University, (Diagnostic
Radiology residency)
The Hospital for Special Surgery,
(Musculoskeletal Radiology fellowship)

ISS Member 1984

Spouse: Mary Jo

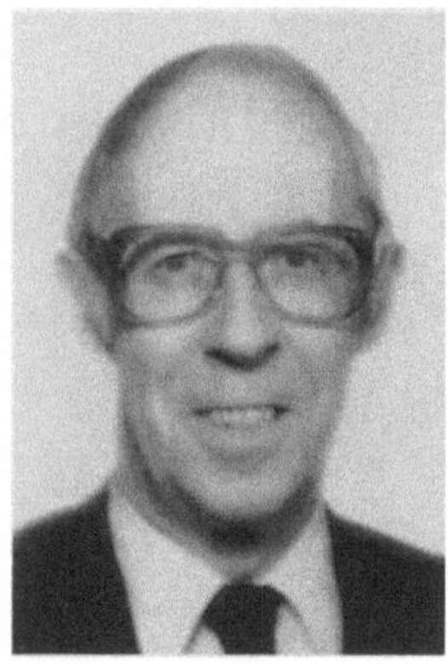

Business Address:
Nordostpassagen 41
S-413 11 Goteborg
Sweden

ISS Member Founding member

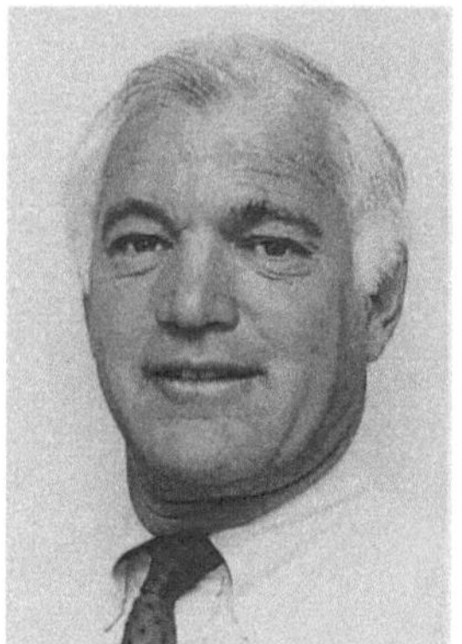

Birthdate: February 12, 1943

Academic Title: Irene Heinz Given &
John LaPorte Given, Professor of
Pathology

Position at Affiliation: Chairman

Business Address:
Department of Pathology/Box 1194
Mount Sinai Medical Center
One Gustave L. Levy Place
New York, NY 10029-6574
U.S.A.
212-241-8014 (work)
212-426-5129 (fax)

Home Address:
18 Stoneleigh Road
New Canaan, CT 06840
U.S.A.
203-972-7569 (home)
203-972-7569 (fax)

Specialty/Certification: Anatomic
Pathology, 1973

Education:
1963 – Bowdoin College, Brunswick, ME
1967 – The Chicago Medical School,
Chicago, IL (M.D.)
Harvard Medical School, Boston, MA
(Pathology residency)

ISS Member 1980

Spouse: Regina

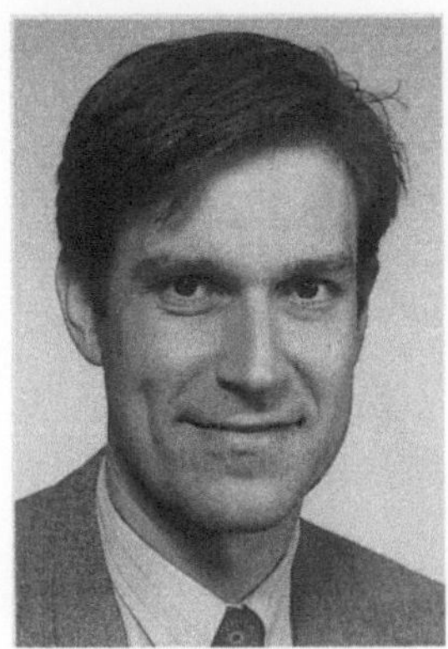

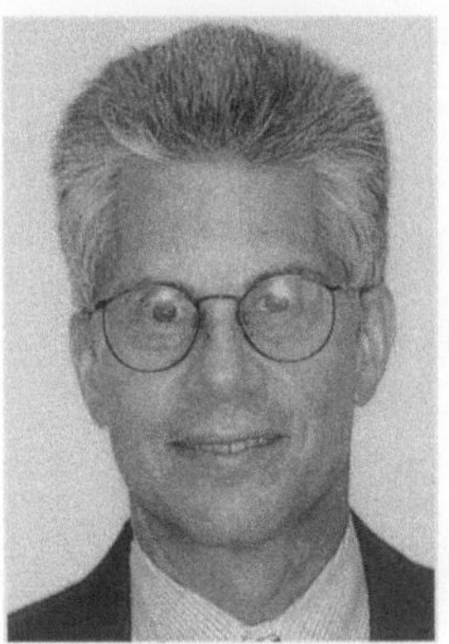

Birthdate: May 22, 1954

Position at Affiliation: Musculoskeletal Radiologist

Business Address:
Cleveland Clinic Foundation
9500 Euclid
Cleveland, OH 44195
U.S.A.
216-444-0775 (work)
216-445-9445 (fax)

Home Address:
3119 Montgomery
Shaker Heights, Ohio 44122
U.S.A.
216-491-9539 (home)

Specialty/Certification: Radiology, 1980

Education:
Universite Libre de Bruxelles, Brussels, Belgium

ISS Member 1991

Spouse: Debbie DeJoseph, M.D.

Birthdate: November 4, 1942

Academic Title: Associate Professor of Radiology

Position at Affiliation: Attending Radiologist

Business Address:
The Hospital for Special Surgery
535 East 70th Street
New York, NY 10021
U.S.A.
212-606-1187 (work)
212-734-7475 (fax)

Home Address:
184 Hickory Grove Drive East
Larchmont, NY 10538
U.S.A.
914-834-1253 (home)

Specialty/Certification: Radiology, 1974; Nuclear Medicine, 1976

Education:
Columbia University (A.B.)
New York Medical College (M.D.)
New York Hospital – Cornell University Medical College (Radiology residency)

ISS Member 1989

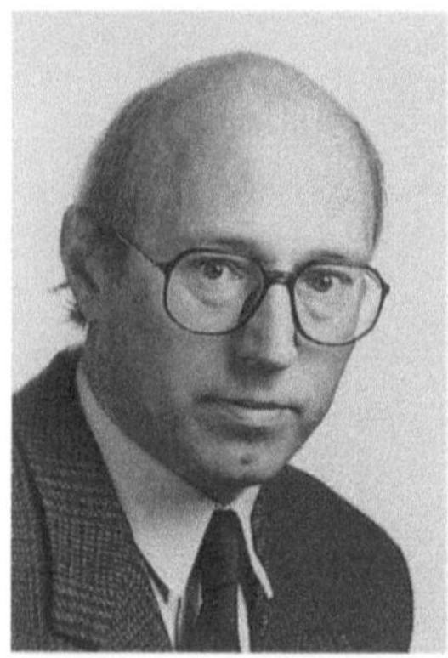

Birthdate: June 25, 1943

Academic Title: Professor

Position at Affiliation: Chairman

Business Address:
Institut fuer Pathologie der
Justus-Liebig-Universitaet
Langhansstr. 10
D-35385 Giessen
Germany
49 641 99-41100 (work)
49 641 99-41109 (fax)
andreasschulz@patho.med.uni-giessen.de
(e-mail)

Home Address:
Geranienweg 9
D-35396 Giessen
Germany
49 641 33622 (home)

Specialty/Certification: Pathology, 1976

Education:
1969 – University of Kiel (M.D.)
1978 – University of Hamburg
(residency and fellowship)

ISS Member 1990

ISS Committees:
Membership Committee

Spouse: Susanne

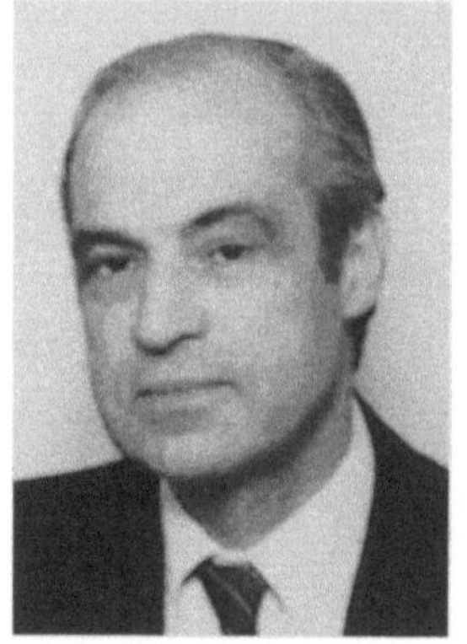

Business Address:
Radiology Department
University Hospital Dijkzigt
Dr. Molewaterpl. 40
3015 GD Rotterdam
The Netherlands

Specialty: Radiology

ISS Member 1978

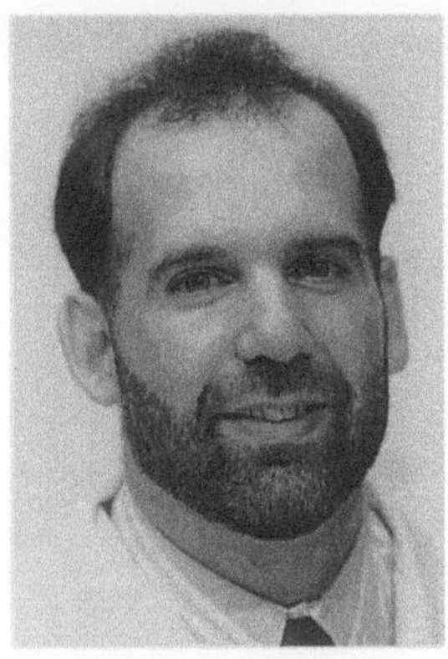

Birthdate: June 9, 1962

Academic Title: Associate Professor of Radiology and Orthopedics

Position at Affiliation: Musculoskeletal Radiologist

Business Address:
Thomas Jefferson University Hospital
Department of Radiology
132 South 10th Street,
1096 Main Building
Philadelphia, PA 19107
U.S.A.
215-955-7294 (work)
215-955-5329 (fax)

Home Address:
306 Monmouth Drive
Cherry Hill, NJ 09002
U.S.A.
609-667-7710 (home)

Specialty/Certification: Radiology, 1990

Education:
1984 – City College of New York (B.S.)
1986 – State of New York at Buffalo (M.D.)
1990 – SUNY/Stony Brook/NCMC
(Diagnostic Radiology residency)
1991 – CSD, San Diego (Osteoradiology
fellowship)

ISS Member 1995

Spouse: Sheryl

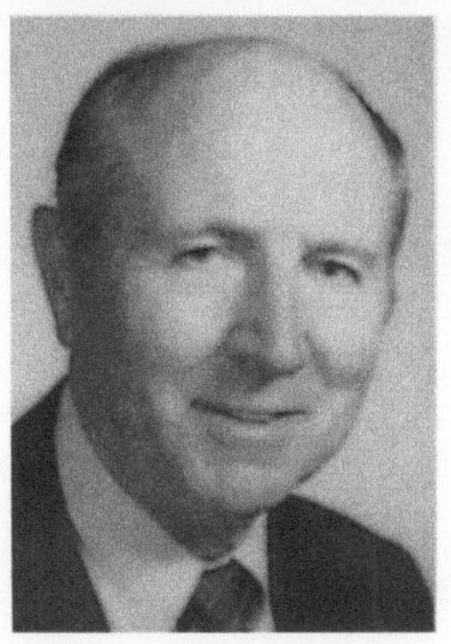

Business Address:
Pathology Department
LAC-USC Medical Center
1200 North State Street
Los Angeles, CA 90033
U.S.A.

Specialty: Pathology

ISS Member 1977

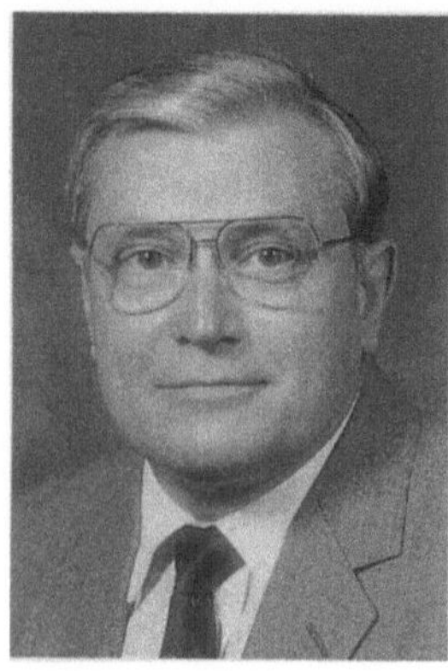

Birthdate: May 14, 1935

Academic Title: Professor of Radiology

Position at Affiliation: Professor

Business Address:
Department of Radiology
University of Tennessee
College of Medicine
800 Madison Avenue
Memphis, TN 38163
U.S.A.
901-448-6111 (work)
901-448-5352 (fax)

Home Address:
2029 Quail Creek Cove
Memphis, TN 38119
U.S.A.
901-761-3308 (home)

Specialty/Certification: Radiology, 1972

Education:
Southwestern of Memphis (Rhodes),
Memphis, TN (M.D.)
University of Tennessee, Memphis, TN
(Diagnostic Radiology residency)

ISS Member 1990

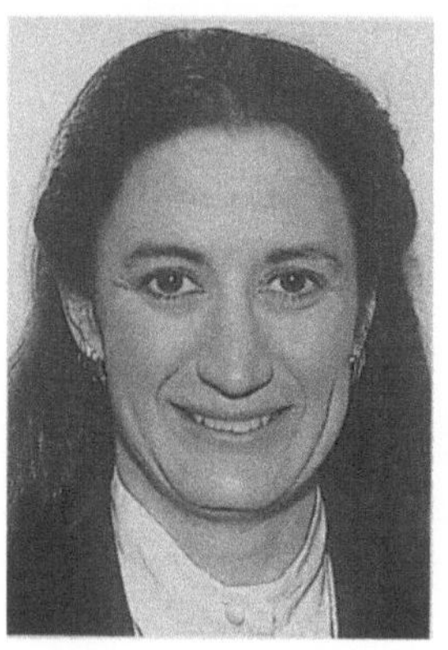

Birthdate: April 27, 1951

Academic Title: Associate Professor

Position at Affiliation: Chief, Musculoskeletal Radiology

Business Address:
UCLA Dept. of Radiological Sciences
200 UCLA Medical Plaza, Suite 165-59
Los Angeles, CA 90095-6952
U.S.A.
310-794-1499 (work)
310-794-1428 (fax)
lseeger@mail.rad.ucla.edu (e-mail)

Home Address:
3908 Carpenter Avenue
Studio City, CA 91604-3731
U.S.A.
818-766-9597 (home)

Specialty/Certification: Radiology, 1987

Education:
1973 – University of Washington, Seattle,
WA (B.S. & M.A. Nursing)
1982 – University of Washington, Seattle,
WA (M.D.)
1982–83 – Virginia Mason Hospital,
Seattle, WA (internship)
1983–87 – UCLA School of Medicine,
Los Angeles, CA (Radiology residency)

ISS Member 1992

Spouse: Rudi R. Foorman

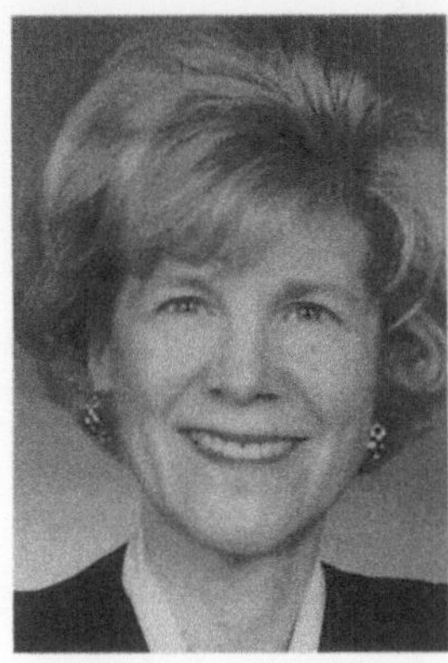

Academic Title: Associate Professor of Radiology

Position at Affiliation: Chief, Musculo-skeletal Radiology, Walter Reed Army Medical Center, Washington, DC

Business Address:
Department of Radiology, USUHS
4301 Jones Bridge Road
Bethesda, MD 20814-4799
U.S.A.
202-782-1628 (work)
202-782-0625 (fax)

Home Address:
10301 Grosvenor Place
North Bethesda, MD 20852
U.S.A.
301-493-4512 (home)

Specialty: Radiology

Education:
University of California, Berkeley
University of California School of Medicine, San Francisco (M. D.)
Hospital of the University of Pennsykvania, Philadelphia, PA
(Diagnostic Radiology residency)
Royal National Orthopaedic Hospital-Institute of Orthopaedics, London
(bone fellowship)

ISS Member 1993

ISS Committees:
Liaison Committee

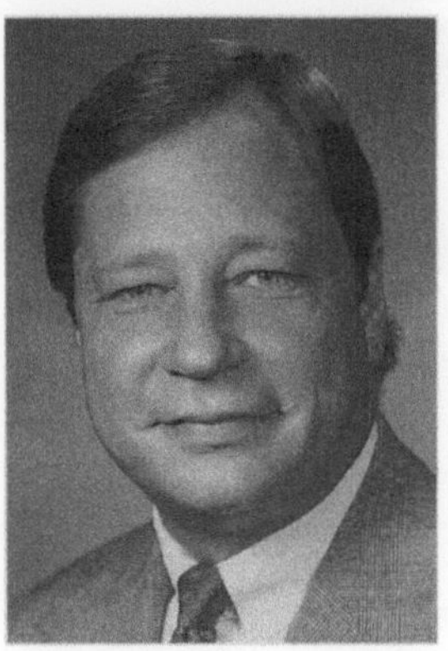

Birthdate: December 28, 1947

Academic Title: Associate Professor

Position at Affiliation: Orthopedic Surgeon

Business Address:
Department of Orthopedic Surgery
Mayo Clinic
200 First St. SW, W14A
Rochester, MN 55905
U.S.A.
507-284-8531 (work)
507-266-4234 (fax)
shives,thomas@may.edu (e mail)

Home Address:
Route 8, Box 38
Rochester, MN 55902
U.S.A.
507-282-0958 (home)

Specialty/Certification: Orthopedic Surgery, 1980

Education:
Cornell College, Mount Vernon, IA
University of Iowa, School of Medicine, Iowa City, IA (M. D.)
Orthopedic Surgery residency and Oncology Fellowship, Mayo Clinic, Rochester, MN

ISS Member 1992

Spouse: Kula

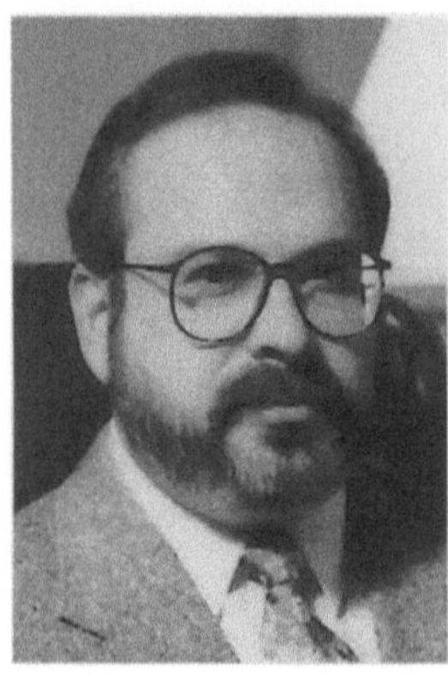

Birthdate: November 16, 1948

Academic Title: Professor

Position at Affiliation: Director of Anatomic Pathology

Business Address:
University of Alabama at Birmingham
Department of Pathology, KB 506
619 South 19th Street
Birmingham, AL 35233, U.S.A.
205-934-6608 (work)
205-975-7284 (fax)
pam@lh.path.uab.edu (e-mail)

Home Address:
4927 Cold Harbor Drive
Mountain Brook, AL 35223, U.S.A.
205 956-6199 (home)

Specialty/Certification: Anatomic Pathology, 1978

Education:
1974 – University of Louisville,
Louisville, KY (M.D.)
1979 – University of Minnesota,
Minneapolis, MN (Ph.D.)
1975–79 – Mayo Graduate School of Medicine (resident in Pathology)
1979–81 – National Cancer Institute, NIH (research associate)
1981–82 – University of Minnesota, Minneapolis (fellow in Surgical Pathology)

ISS Member 1994

ISS Committees:
Corinne Farrell Prize Committee

Spouse: Sandra

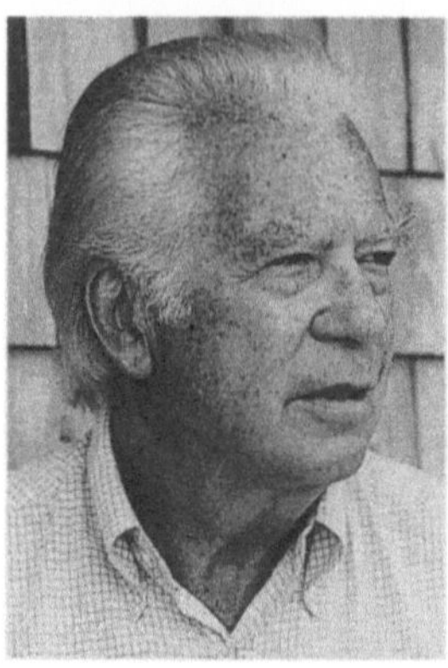

Birthdate: June 16, 1918

Academic Title: Professor

Position at Affiliation: Distinguished Service Professor

Business Address:
Mt. Sinai School of Medicine
Department of Orthopedics
New York, NY 10028
U.S.A.
212-288-7900 (work)
212-879-6742 (fax)

Home Address:
45 East 85th Street
New York, NY 10028
U.S.A.
212-288-2515 (home)

Specialty/Certification: Orthopaedic Surgery, 1952

Education:
NYU School of Medicine

ISS Member 1978

Spouse: Miriam

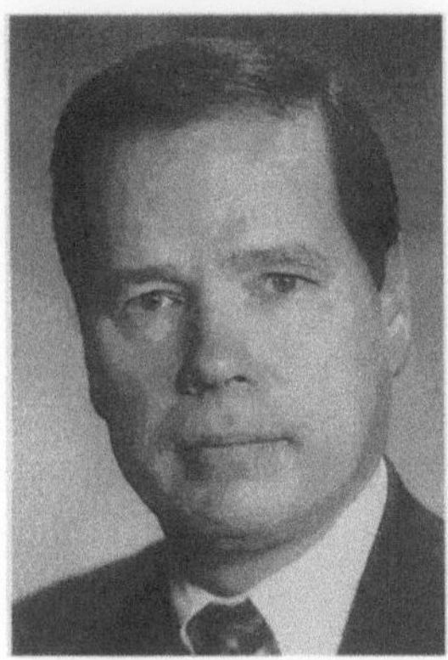

Birthdate: September 2, 1940

Academic Title: Professor of Orthopedic Surgery

Position at Affiliation: Orthopedic Surgeon

Business Address:
Department of Orthopedic Surgery
Mayo Clinic
200 First Street, S.W.
Rochester, MN 55905
U.S.A.
507-284-8314 (work)
507-266-4234 (fax)
sim.franklin@mayo.edu (e-mail)

Home Address:
1303 Woodland Drive, S.W.
Rochester, MN 55902
U.S.A.
507-289-8121 (home)

Specialty/Certification: Orthopedic Surgery, 1972

Education:
Dalhousie University
Dalhousie University Medical School (M.D.)
Mayo Graduate School (Orthopedic surgeon)

ISS Member 1983

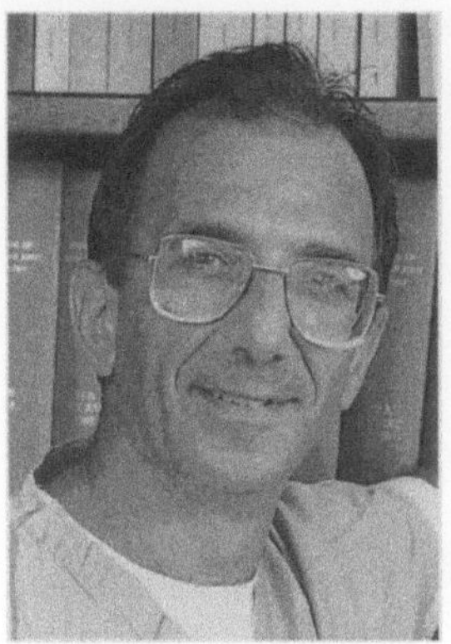

Birthdate: January 13, 1943

Academic Title: Professor

Position at Affiliation: Chair, Orthopaedic Surgery & Rehabilitation Medicine

Business Address:
University of Chicago
5841 S. Maryland MC3079
Chicago, IL 60637
U.S.A.
773-702-6144 (work)
773-702-4384 (fax)
msimon@surgery.bad.uchicago.edu

Home Address:
5641 S. Drexel
Chicago, IL 60637
U.S.A.
773-947-8878 (home)

Specialty/Certification: Orthopaedic Surgery, 1975

Education:
1960 – 63 – University of Michigan
1963 – 67 – University of Michigan (M.D.)
1967 – 69 – University of Michigan (surgery)
1971 – 74 – Orthopaedic Surgery

ISS Member 1994

Spouse: Barbara

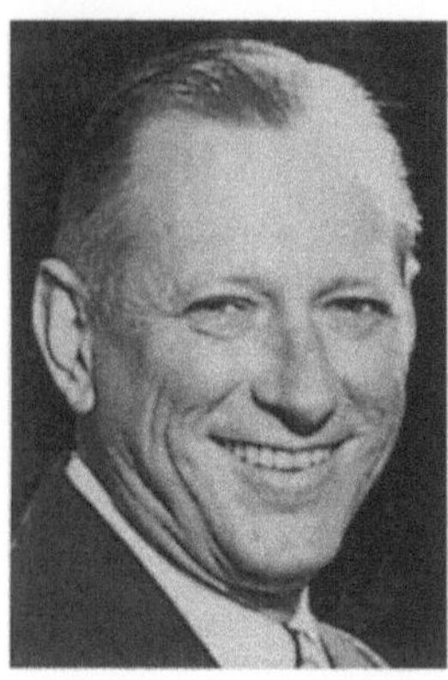

Business Address:
Texas Children's Hospital
6621 Fannin, 4-280
Houston, TX 77030
U.S.A.

Specialty: Pediatric Radiology

ISS Member 1984

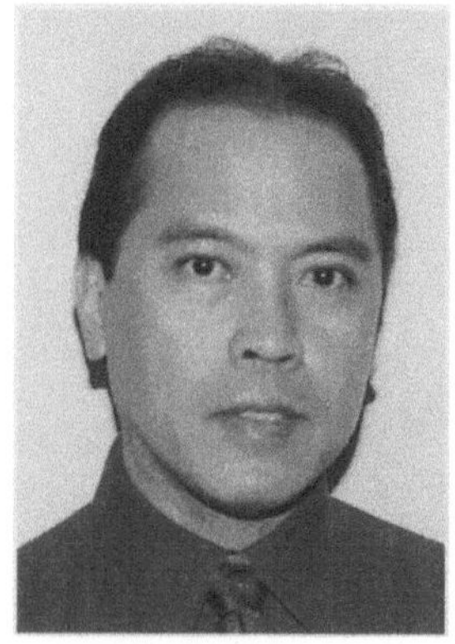

Birthdate: May 17, 1946

Academic Title: Associate Professor

Position at Affiliation: Senior Attending

Business Address:
St. Luke's/Roosevelt Hospital Center
1000 10th Avenue
New York, NY 10019
U.S.A.
212-523-7051 (work)
212-523-6019 (fax)

Home Address:
1160 3rd Avenue
New York, NY 10021
U.S.A.
212-734-0131 (home)

Specialty/Certification: Radiology, 1976

Education:
1965 – B.S.
1970 – M.D.

ISS Member 1996

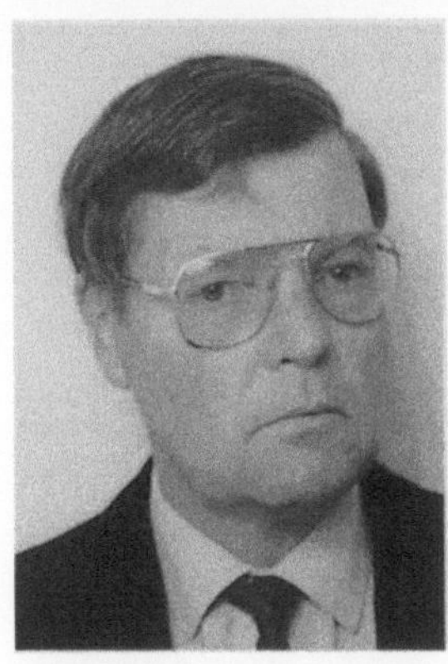

Birthdate: May 2, 1933

Academic Title: Professor

Business Address:
avenue du Prince de Ligne 116
1180 Bruxelles .
Belgium
32 2 373 99 22 (work)
32 2 373 99 33 (fax)

Home Address:
62 A Mont-Lassy
1380 Lasne
Belgium
32 2 353 09 56 (home)

Specialty/Certification: Radiology, 1965

Education:
1958 – Medical School of Free University
of Brussels ULB (M.D.)
1994 – Ph.D.

ISS Member 1987

ISS Committees:
Foreign Committee

Spouse: Claude Boels

Business Address:
Academic Hospital St. Radboud
Post Box 9101
6500 HB Nijmegen
The Netherlands
08858-4390 (home)
080-513974 (work)
080-540555 (fax)

ISS Member 1984

Spouse: Mrs. Slooff-Defoer

Smith, Chadwick F. M.D.

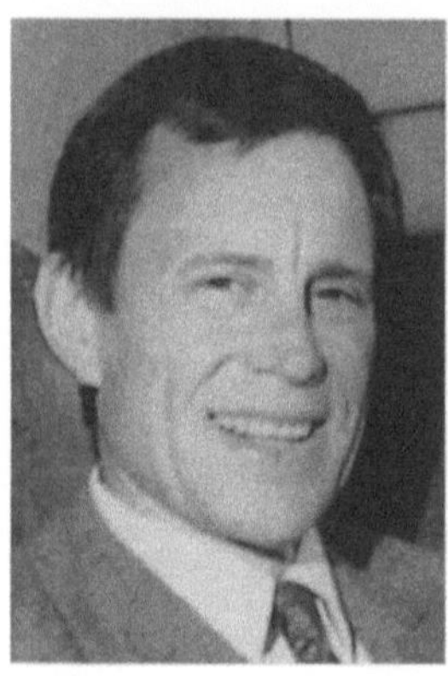

Birthdate: February 28, 1934

Academic Title: Clinical Professor of Orthopaedic Surgery

Business Address:
University of Southern California School of Medicine
1127 Wilshire Boulevard
Ste. 1008
Los Angeles, CA 90017, U.S.A.
213-481-1122 (work)
213-482-8094 (fax)

Home Address:
932 Via Del Monte
Palos Verdes Estates, CA 90274, U.S.A.
310-378-0817 (home)
310-373-9197 (fax)

Specialty/Certification: Orthopaedic Surgery, 1968, 1983, 1995

Education:
1954 – North Texas State University; Southern Methodist University (B.A.)
1958 – University of Texas Medical Branch (M.D.)
1959 – Harbor General Hospital, Los Angeles (internship)
1965 – Orthopaedic Hospital, Los Angeles (residency in Orthopaedic Surgery)
1966 – Orthopaedic Hospital, Los Angeles (fellowship)

ISS Member 1985

Spouse: Corinna

Smith, Julius M.D.

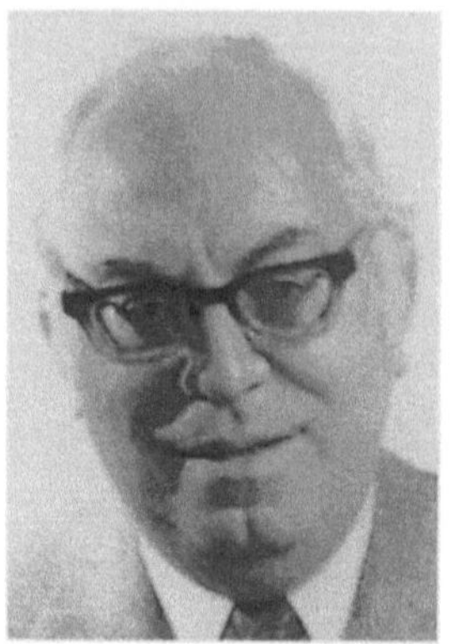

Birthdate: May 21, 1932

Academic Title: Clinical Associate Professor of Radiology (C.U.M.C.)

Position at Affiliation: Staff Radiologist

Business Address:
National Cancer Institute
Rio de Janeiro
Ed Serramar
R. Humberto de Campos, 974/1301
Leblon – Rio de Janeiro
Brazil
21-217-4124 or 4129 (work)
21-232-9657 (fax)
21-512-5690 (home and fax)

Specialty: Radiology

ISS Committees:
Committee of the Promotion of Refresher Course outside North America

Spouse: Mary

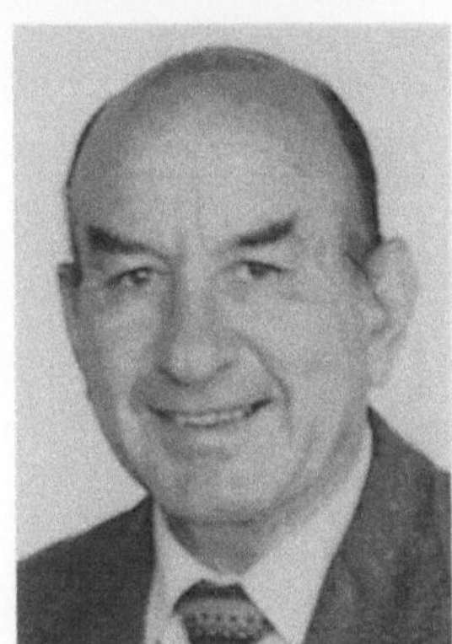

Business Address:
Orthopaedic Surgery
Bristol Royal Infirmary
University of Bristol
Bristol BS2 8HW
England
(0272) 741107 (home)
(0272) 213449 (work)
(0272) 252736 (fax)

Specialty: Orthopaedic Surgery

ISS Member 1980

Spouse: Joan

Birthdate: July 2, 1945

Academic Title: Associate Professor

Position at Affiliation: Associate
Professor

Business Address:
Kochi Medical School
Department of Pathology
Kohasu, Okoh, Nankoku, Kochi 783
Japan
81-888-80-2336 (work)
81-888-80-2336 (fax)

Home Address:
587-75, A506 Kamohara, Okoh
Nankoku, Kochi 783
Japan
81-888-66-0763 (home)
81-888-66-0763 (fax)

Specialty/Certification: Pathology, 1970

Education:
Okayama University (M.D.)
Okayama University Medical School
(post graduate course Surgical Pathology)

ISS Member: 1996

Spouse: Noriko

SOSMAN, J. LELAND M.D.

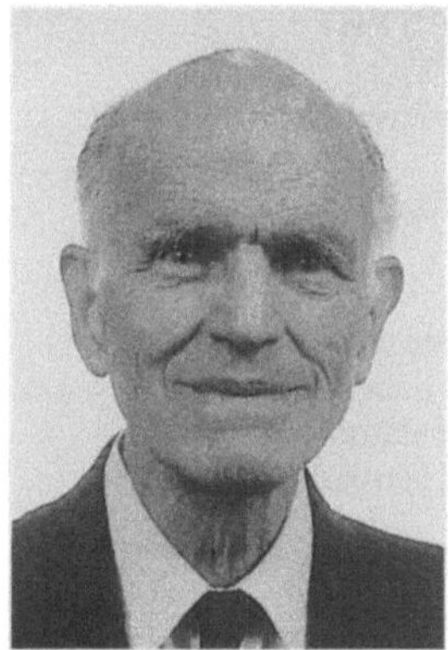

Birthdate: September 15, 1920

Academic Title: Assistant Professor

Position at Affiliation: Musculoskeletal Radiologist

Business Address:
Radiology Department
Brigham and Women's Hospital
75 Francis Street
Boston, MA 02115
U.S.A.
617-732-6295 (work)
617-732-6336 (fax)

Home Address:
648 Lowell Road
Concord, MA 01742
U.S.A.
798-369-4072 (home)

Specialty: Radiology

Education:
1943 – Harvard College (A.B.)
1946 – John Hopkins Medical School (M.D.)
1946–47 – Peter Bent Brigham Hospital (Surgery intern)
1947–49 – Army of U.S. (Pathology)
1948–49 – University of Munich (Pathology)
1949–52 – Massachusetts General Hosptial (Radiology resident)
1952 – Children's Medical Center (Pediatric Radiology)

ISS Member Founding member

SPANIER, SUZANNE STAPLES M.D.

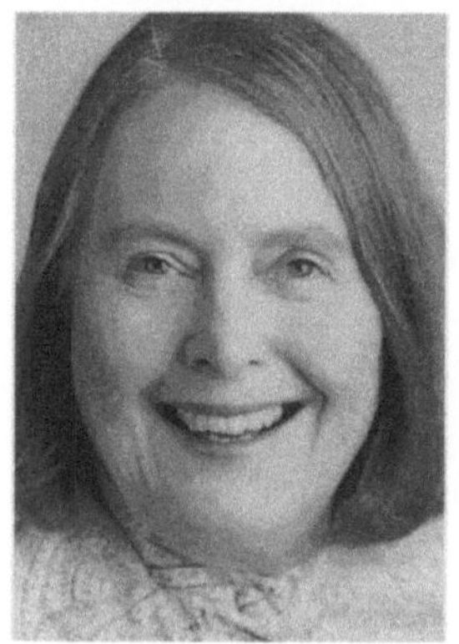

Academic Title: Associate Professor

Position at Affiliation: Associate Professor

Business Address:
Department of Orthopaedics & Pathology
Box 100-246
Health Science Center
Gainesville, FL 32610
U.S.A.
352-392-4295 (work)
352-392-8637 (fax)
suzanne-spanier@ufl.edu (e-mail)

Home Address:
1712 N.W. 63rd Street
Gainesville, FL 32605
U.S.A.
352-331-6823 (home)

Specialty/Certification: Anatomic Pathology, 1975

Education:
University of Florida (B.S. Chemistry)
1964 – University of Florida (M.S. Biology)
1969 – University of Florida (M.D.)

ISS Member 1983

Spouse: John

SPEER, DONALD P. M.D.

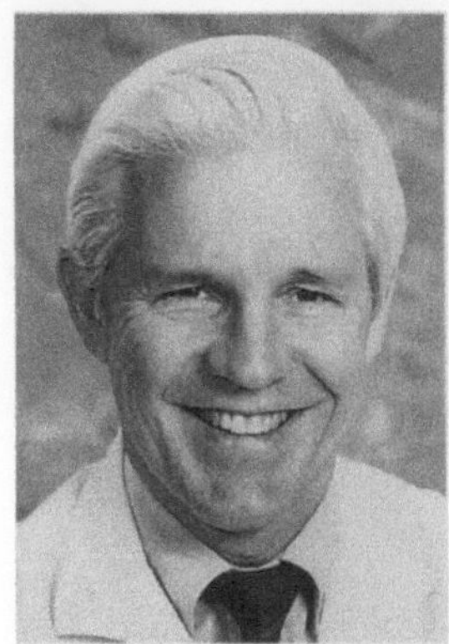

Birthdate: June 18, 1937

Academic Title: Professor of Surgery and Anatomy

Position at Affiliation: Attending Physician, Professor of Surgery and Anatomy

Business Address:
Orthopaedics Section
Arizona Health Sciences Center
P.O. Box 245064
Tucson, AZ 85724-5064
U.S.A.
520-626-6607 (work)
520-626-2668 (fax)
dspeer@aruba.ccit.arizona.edu (e-mail)

Home Address:
18695 Cactus Hill Road
Vail, AZ 85641
U.S.A.
520-647-6839 (home)
520-647-6839 (fax)

Specialty/Certification: Orthopaedic Surgery, 1974

Education:
Stanford University (B.S.)
University of California, Los Angeles
(graduate school)
University of Southern California (M.D.)
University of California, LA Hospital,
Los Angeles (Surgery internship)
University of California, LA
(General Surgery residency)
University of Kansas Hospital and
University of Arizona Health Sciences
Center (residency-Orthopaedic Surgery)

ISS Member 1983

Spouse: Isabell Speer, M.D.

Spjut, Harlan J. M.D.

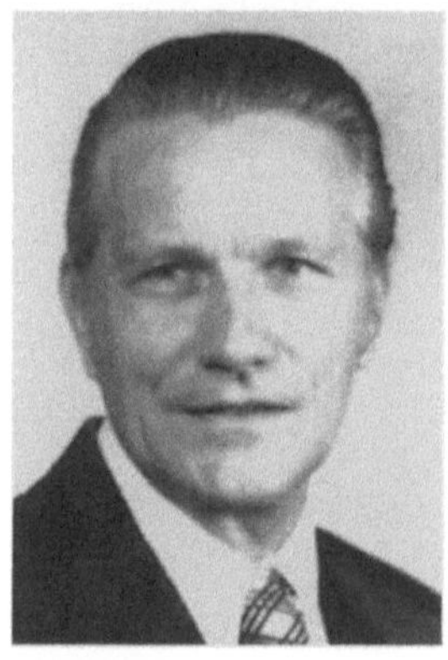

Birthdate: May 3, 1922

Academic Title: Professor

Position at Affiliation: Professor of Pathology

Business Address:
Pathology Department
Baylor College of Medicine
One Baylor Plaza
Houston, TX 77030
U.S.A.
713-798-4661 (work)
713-798-5838 (fax)

Home Address:
2001 Sunset Blvd.
Houston, TX 77005
U.S.A.

Specialty/Certification: Pathology, 1954

Education:
University of Utah (college)
University of Utah School of Medicine (M.D.)
University of Utah and Washington University St. Louis (Pathology residency)

ISS Member Founding member

Spouse: Madeleine

Sprague, Paul L. MB, BS, FRACR, FRCR, FRACP

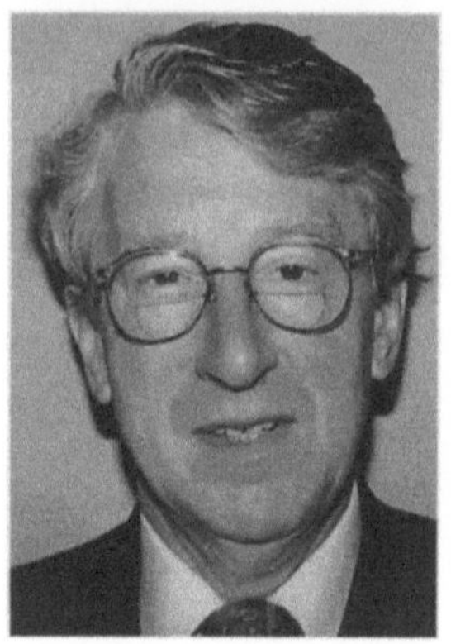

Academic Title: Dr.

Position at Affiliation: Radiologist

Business Address:
Sprague Kam Glancy
P.O. Box 24
West Perth 6005
Australia
61-9-322-4966 (work)
61-9-321-2056 (fax)
psprague!iinet.net.all (e-mail)

Home Address:
16 Saunders Street
Mosman Park 6012
Australia
61-9-384-3860 (home)
61-9-384-5790 (fax)

Specialty: Radiology

Education:
Melbourne University
Harvard Medical School (M.D.)

ISS Member 1983

Spouse: Beverley

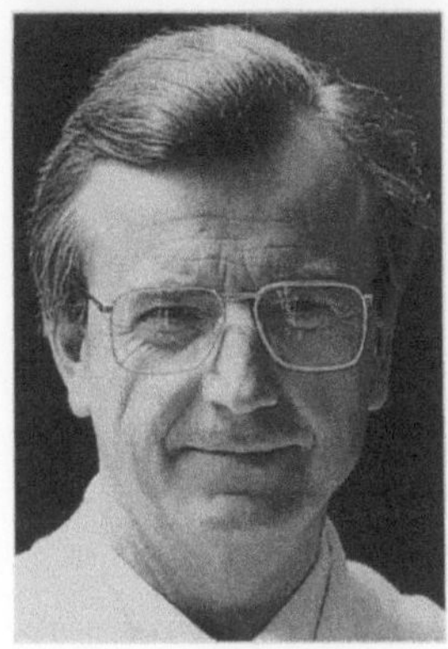

Birthdate: January 1, 1931

Academic Title: Professor of Pediatrics

Position at Affiliation: Professor of
Pediatrics

Business Address:
Children's Hospital
University of Mainz/Germany
Langenbeckstr. 1
D-55131 Mainz
Germany
49-6131-17-7325 (work)
49-6131-17-6608 (fax)

Home Address:
Sickingenstr. 1
D-55278 Köngernheim
Germany

Specialty/Certification: Pediatrics, 1963

Education:
Medical Schools Tübingen, Freiburg,
Heidelberg
Research fellow Sloan-Ketering Institute
N.Y.
Boston Children's Hospital

ISS Member 1975

Spouse: Anita

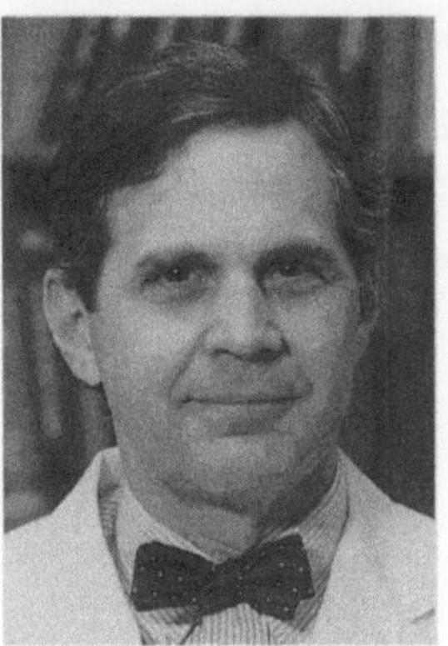

Academic Title: Professor

Position at Affiliation: Chairman,
Department of Orthopaedics

Business Address:
Mt. Sinai Medical Center
One Gustave L. Levy Place
New York, NY 10029
U.S.A.
212-241-8311 (work)
212-534-6091 (fax)
msss36a@prodigy.com (e-mail)

Home Address:
1212 5th Avenue, Apt. 12-D
New York, NY 10029
U.S.A.
212-241-7153 (home)

Specialty/Certification: Orthopaedic
Surgery, 1977

Education:
Emory University (BA)
University of Florida (MD)
University of Florida (Orthopaedic
residency)
University of Florida (Orthopaedic
Oncology)

ISS Member 1984

Spouse: Deanna

STAMP, TREVOR C. M.D.

Birthdate: September 18, 1935

Position at Affiliation: Director, Division of Bone & Mineral Metabolism

Business Address:
Royal National Orthopaedic Hospital
Brockley Hill
Stanmore
Middlesex HA7 4LP
England
181-954-2300 (work)

Home Address:
15 Ceylon Road
London W-14 OPY
England
171-603-0487 (home)

Education:
Cambridge University
St. Mary's Hospital Medical School,
London

ISS Member 1978

STAPLE, TOM W. M.D.

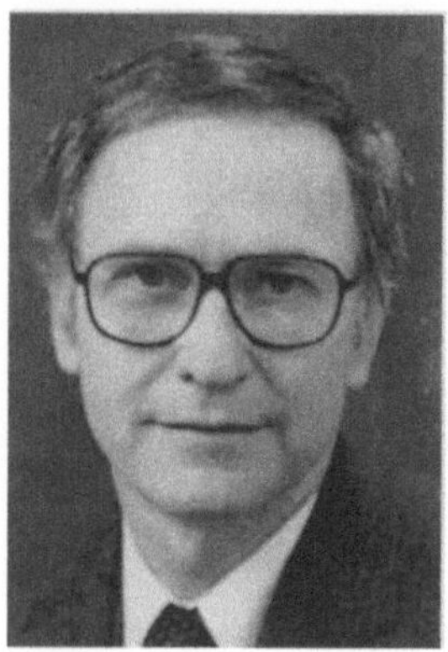

Birthdate: May 6, 1931

Home Address:
123 Via Orvieto
Newport Beach, CA 92663-4922
U.S.A.
714-723-9083 (home)
714-723-9083 (fax)

Specialty/Certification: Radiology, 1963

Education:
University of Illinois (college)
University of Illinois (M.D.)
Mallnkrodt Institute of Radiology
Washington University School
of Medicine, St. Louis, MO
(Radiology residency)

ISS Member Founding member

Spouse: Shirley

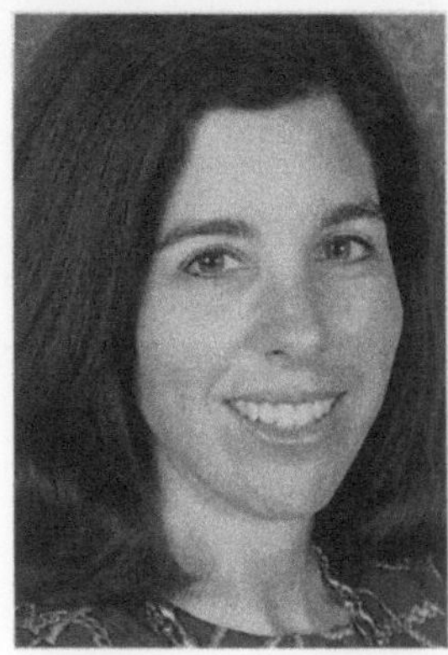

Birthdate: December 28, 1953

Academic Title: Professor

Business Address:
University of California San Francisco
Medical Center
Department of Radiology – Box 0628
San Francisco, CA 94143-0628, U.S.A.
415-476-1451 (work)
415-476-8550 (fax)
lynne_steinbach@radmac1.ucsf.edu
(e-mail)

Home Address:
6 Burrell Court
Tiburon, CA 94920, U.S.A.
415-388-7840 (home)

Specialty/Certification: Radiology, 1983

Education:
1972–75 Stanford University (B.A.)
1975–79 Medical College of
Pennsylvania (M.D.)
1980–83 New York Hospital-Cornell
Medical Ctr. (Radiology residency)
1983–84 HSS-Cornell Med. Ctr.
(Musculoskeletal fellowship)

ISS Member 1990

ISS Medals and Awards:
President's Medal, Paris, 1996

ISS Committees:
Membership Committee, 1995–

Spouse: Eric F. Tepper, M.D.

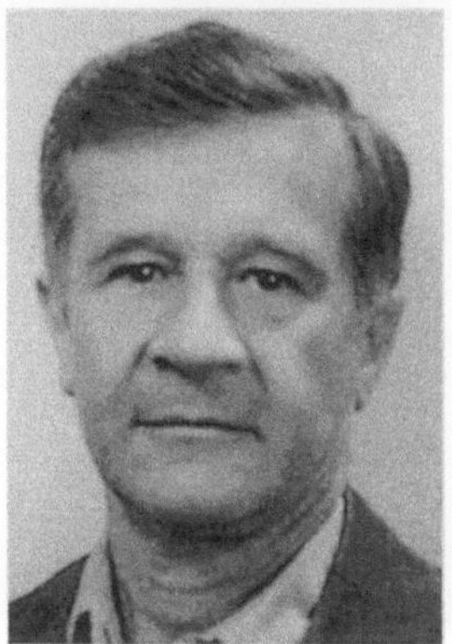

Academic Title: Professor

Position at Affiliation: Chairman of
Pathology Department

Business Address:
Pathology Department
Hospital for Joint Diseases
Orthopedic Institute
301 East 17th Street
New York, NY 10003
U.S.A.
212-598-6231 (work)
212-598-6057 (fax)

Home Address:
400 E. 56th Street, Apt. #7N
New York, NY 10022
U.S.A.
212-223-2866 (home)

Specialty: Pathology

Education:
University of Buenos Aires Medical
School, Argentina

ISS Member 1977

Spouse: Mercedes

STOKER, DENNIS J. FRCP, FRCR, FRCS

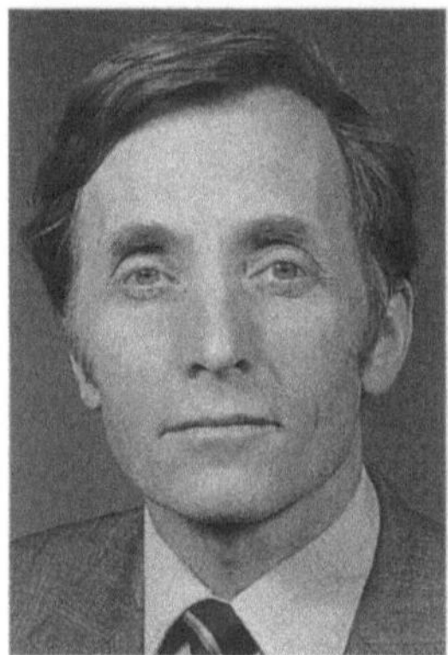

Birthdate: March 22, 1928

Academic Title: Dr.

Position at Affiliation: Consultant Radiologist

Business Address:
Radiology Department
Royal National Orthopaedic Hospital
45-51 Bolsover Street
London W1P 8AQ
England
dennis_stoker@crowthorne.demon.
com.uk (e-mail)

Home Address:
18, Llangar Grove
Crowthorne
Berks R945 6EA
England
44 1344 777 948 (home)
44 1344 777 948 (fax)

Specialty/Certification: Radiology, 1971;
Internal Medicine, 1958

Education:
Guys Hospital Medical School University
of London
Radiology Specialty training, St. George's
Hospital, London

ISS Member Founding member

ISS Medals and Awards:
Medal of the ISS (Silver), Toronto, 1993

ISS Committees:
Editorial Committee
Editor, Skeletal Radiology, 1984–96

SUBBARAO, KAKARLA M.D.

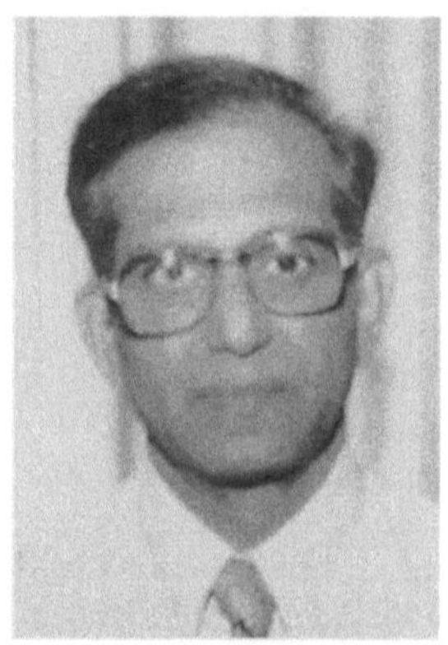

Business Address:
Nizam's Institute of Medical Science
4-1-371- ABIDS Hyderabad
500001 AP
India

Specialty: Radiology

ISS Member 1976

SUGIMOTO, HIDEHARU M.D.

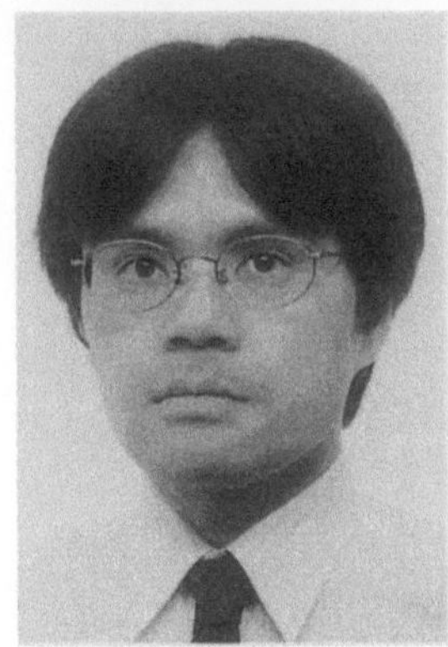

Birthdate: October 11, 1954

Position at Affiliation: Assistant Professor

Business Address:
Department of Radiology, Jichi Medical School
3311 Minamikawachi-machi, Kawachi-gun
Tochigi-ken 329-04
Japan
0285-44-2111, ext. 3413 (work)
0285-44-4296 (fax)
hideharu@jichi.ac.jp (e-mail)

Home Address:
Midori 3-3-11
Minamikawachi-machi, Kawachi-gun,
329-04 Tochigi-ken
Japan
0285-44-0723 (home)

Specialty/Certification: Radiology, 1987

Education:
1980 – Hokkaido University (M.D.)
1983–87 – Medical College of Wisconsin
(resident and fellow, Radiology)

ISS Member 1996

Spouse: Sachie

SUGIURA, ISAO M.D., D.M.SC.

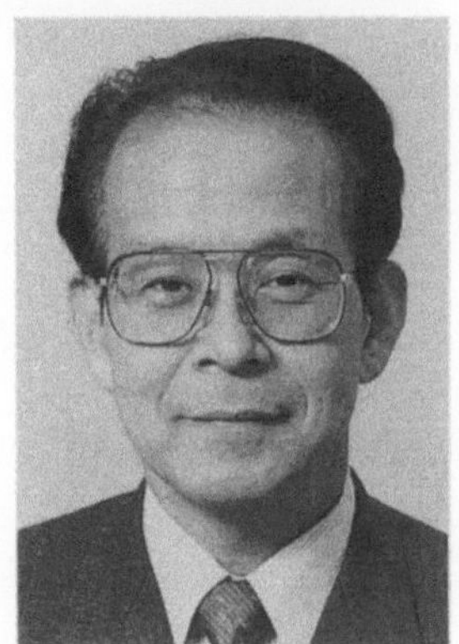

Birthdate: August 9, 1934

Academic Title: Guest Professor

Position at Affiliation: Director of
Orthopaedic Surgery

Business Address:
SL Medical Center Nagoya
1-3 Shinsakae-Machi, Naka-ku
Nagoya 460
Japan
52-953-6022 (work)
52-953-6044 (fax)

Home Address:
2-17-15 Nishi Shiro, Moriyama-Ku
Nagoya 463
Japan
52-794-8845 (home)
52-795-6577 (fax)

Specialty/Certification: Orthopaedic
Surgery, 1960

Education:
1959 – Nagoya University School of
Medicine (M.D.)
1966 – Nagoya University (D.M.Sci.)

ISS Member 1982

Spouse: Tomomi

Suh, Jin-Suck M.D.

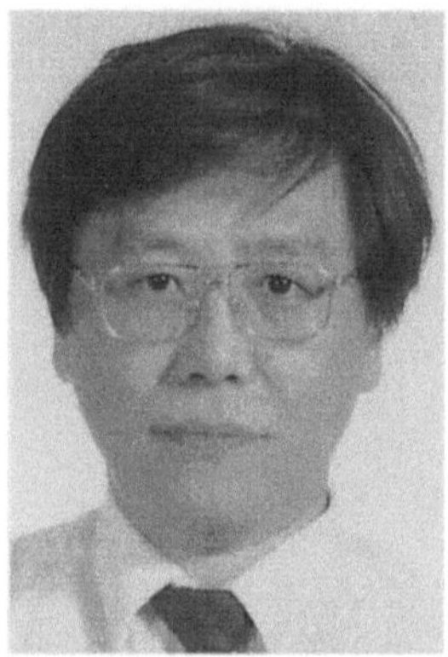

Birthdate: March 23, 1954

Academic Title: Associate Professor

Position at Affiliation: Associate Professor

Business Address:
Department of Diagnostic Radiology
Yonsei University College of Medicine
134 Shinchon-dong Seodaemoon-ku
Seoul 120-752
Korea
82-2-361-5840 (work)
82-2-393-3035 (fax)
jss@yumciris.yonsei.ac.kr (e-mail)

Home Address:
102-503 Woosung Apt. Seocho-dong
Seocho-ku
Seoul
Korea
82-2-523-8119 (home)

Specialty/Certification: Radiology, 1983

Education:
1979 – College of Medicine

ISS Member 1993

Spouse: Myeong-Ryang Shin

Sundaram, Murali M.D., FRCR

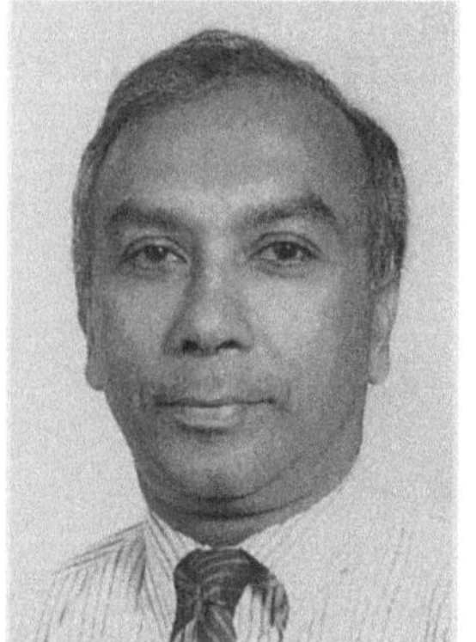

Academic Title: Professor

Position at Affiliation: Chief of
Diagnostic Radiology

Business Address:
Radiology Department
St. Louis University Medical Center
3635 Vista at Grand
St. Louis, MO 63110-0250
U.S.A.
314-268-5780 (work)
314-268-5116 (fax)
sundarm@slucarel.sluh.edu (e-mail)

Home Address:
11636 Larkridge Lane
St. Louis, MO 63126
U.S.A.
314-849-3533 (home)
Speciality: Radiology, 1972

ISS Member 1978

ISS Committees:
Editorial Board Skeletal Radiology,
1987 – present
Refresher Course Committee, 1986 – 88
Membership Committee, 1988 – 90
Liaison & Planning Committee, 1988 – 90
Audit Committee, 1994 – present
Nomenclature committee – 1994 –
present
Closed Program Committee – 1995 –
present
Editor, Skeletal Radiology – 1997 –

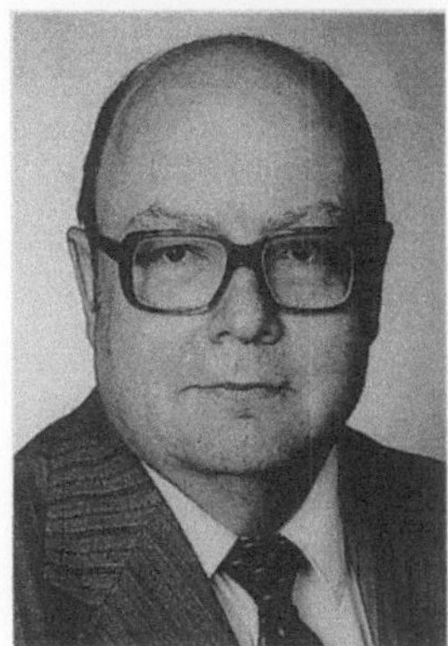

Academic Title: Clinical Professor & Associate Professor

Position at Affiliation: Chairman, Department of Orthopedic Pathology

Business Address:
Department of Orthopedic Pathology
Armed Forces Institute of Pathology
Washington, DC 20306
U.S.A.
202-782-2850 (work)
202-782-3149 (fax)
sweet@e-mail.afip.050.mil (e mail)

Home Address:
17532 Shenandoah Ct.
Ashton, MD 20861
U.S.A.
301-774-0433 (home)

Specialty/Certification: Anatomic Pathology, 1969

Education:
1959 – Fairfield University, Fairfield, CT
(B.S.)
1963 – Georgetown University,
Washington, DC (M.D.)

ISS Member 1984

Spouse: Elizabeth

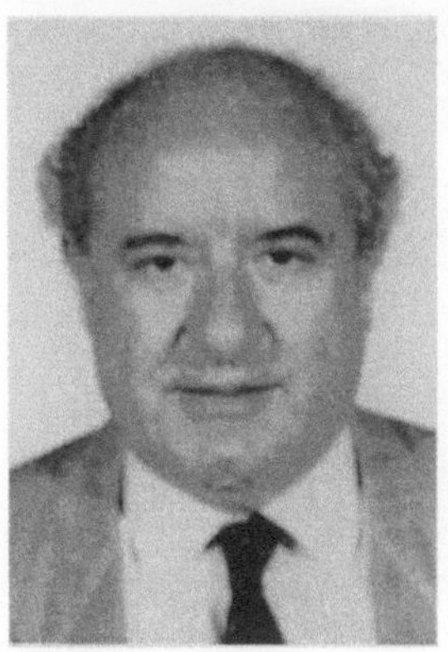

Business Address:
Attending Orthopaedic Surgeon
The Children's Memorial Hospital
2300 Children's Plaza
Chicago, IL 60614
U.S.A.

Specialty: Orthopaedic Surgery

ISS Member 1985

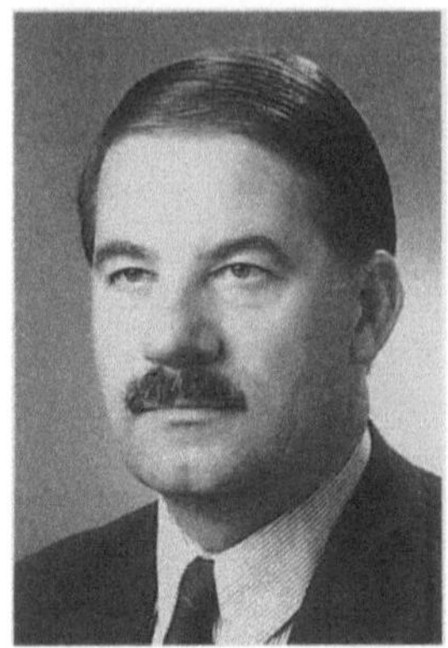

Birthdate: January 5, 1940

Position at Affiliation: Consultant Radiologist

Business Address:
Department of Radiology
Onze Lieve Vrouwe Gasthuis
1e Oosterparkstr. 179
1091 HA Amsterdam
The Netherlands
20-5993323 (work)
20-5992297 (fax)

Home Address:
Koninginneweg 24-hs.
1075 CX Amsterdam
The Netherlands
20-6754753 (home)

Specialty/Certification: Radiology, 1975

Education:
1958–66 University of Leyden, Med. Facult.
1968–71 Internal Medicine
1971–75 Radiology

ISS Member 1983

ISS Medals and Awards:
Corinne Farrell Award, 1989

Spouse: Annet

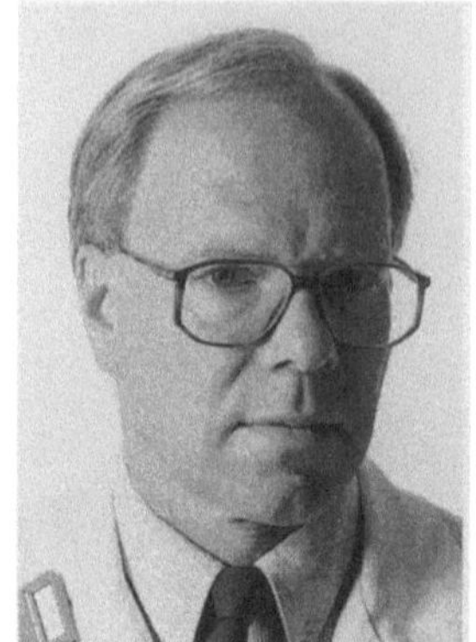

Birthdate: April 24, 1940

Academic Title: Associate Professor

Position at Affiliation: Head of Department of Radiology

Business Address:
ORTON Orthopaedic Hospital, Invalid Foundation
Department of Radiology
Tenalavagen 10
00280 Helsinki
Finland
358-9-4748396 (work)
358-9-2416 415 (fax)
kaj.tallroth@invalidisaatio.fi

Home Address:
Mellstensvagen 17 B 14
02170 Esbo
Finland
358-9-422 598 (home)

Specialty/Certification: Radiology, 1973; Nuclear Medicine, 1981

Education:
1967 – Helsinki Unversity (M.D.)
1976 – Helsinki Unversity (Ph.D.)
1969–74 – Helsinki University Hospitals (Radiology training)

ISS Member 1988

Spouse: San

Tarleton, Gadson J. Jr., M.D.

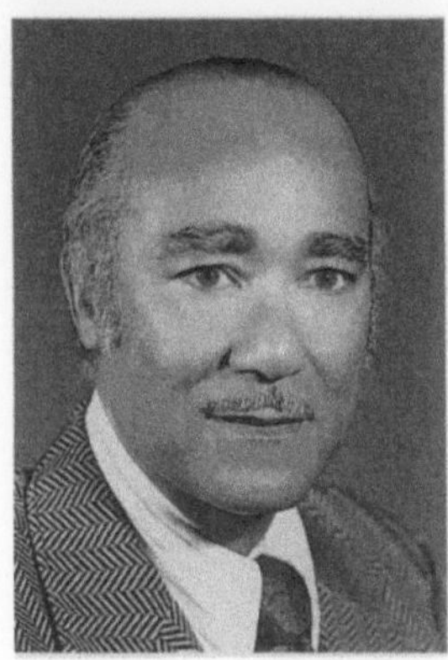

Birthdate: April 29, 1920

Academic Title: Clinical Professor

Position at Affiliation: Clinical Professor

Home Address:
1714 Windover Drive
Nashville, TN 37218-2411
U.S.A.
615-244-0894 (home)
615-893-1360 ext. 3135 (work)

ISS Member Founding member

Spouse: Rhea T.

Tehranzadeh, Jamshid M. M.D.

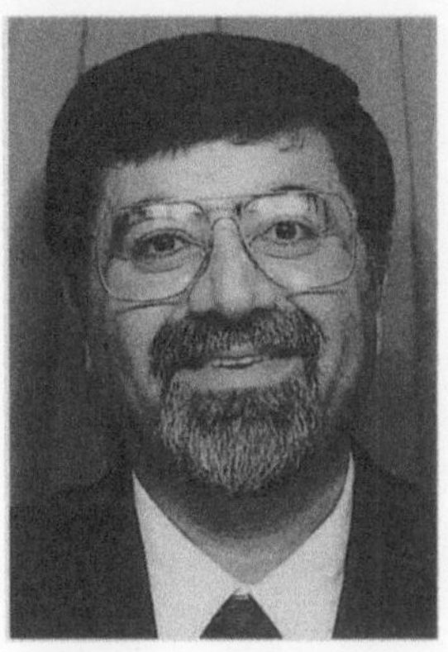

Birthdate: November 14, 1947

Academic Title: Professor of Radiology
and Orthopaedics

Position at Affiliation: Professor of
Radiology and Orthopaedics; Vice
Chair, Department of Radiology

Business Address:
Department of Radiology, R. 140
UCI Medical Center
101 The City Drive
Orange, CA 92868-3268, U.S.A.
714-456-6921 (work)
714-456-8386 (fax)
jtehranz@uci.edu (e-mail)

Home Address:
19181 Edgehill
Irvine, CA 92612, U.S.A.
714-725-9500 (home)

Specialty/Certification: Radiology, 1979

Education:
Pahlavi University Medical School,
Shiraz, Iran (MD)
Yale-New Haven Hospital, New Haven,
CT (Radiology residency)
The Hospital for Special Surgery,
New York, NY (Fellowship in
Musculoskeletal Radiology)

ISS Member 1987

ISS Committees:
Awards Committee, 1995–96

Spouse: Shahla

Thijn, Cornelius J. P. M. D.

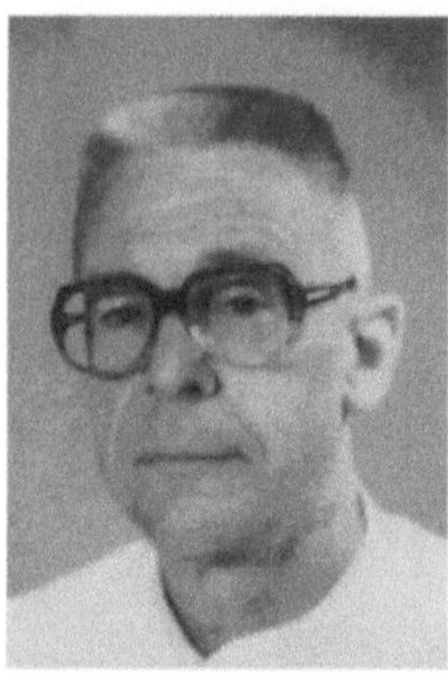

Business Address:
Department of Radiology
University Hospital of Groningen
Groningen
Holland
Brink 6 9482 VJ Tinaarlo meth. (home)
Oostersingel 59 Groningen meth. (work)

Specialty: Radiology

ISS Member 1980

Spouse: Johanna J.

Tohgo, Ohno M. D., D. M. Sc.

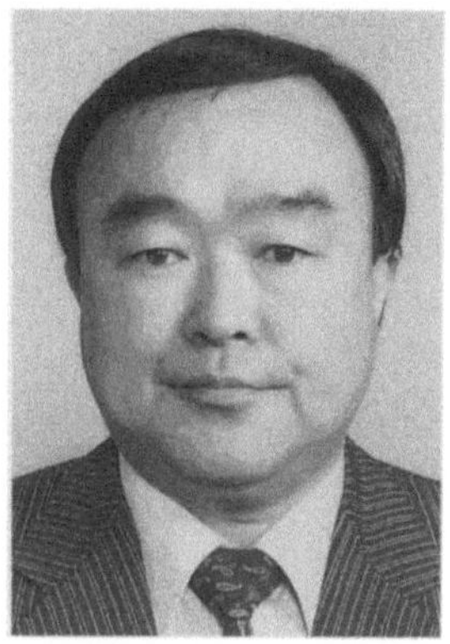

Academic Title: Professor

Position at Affiliation: Head of
Orthopedic Surgery

Business Address:
Dept. of Orthopedic Surgery
Teikyo University School of Medicine
Ichihara Hospital
3426-3, Anesaki, Ichihara City
Chiba Prefecture 299-01
Japan
0436-62-1211 ext. 2631 (work)
0436-62-1229 (fax)
nn9t-oon@asahi-net.or.jp (e-mail)

Home Address:
3-26-26, Natsumidai
Funabashi City
Chiba Prefecture
Japan 273
0474-30-1918 (home)
0474-90-8308 (fax)

Specialty: Orthopaedic Surgery

Education:
Tokyo University School of Medicine

ISS Member 1982

Spouse: Sachiko

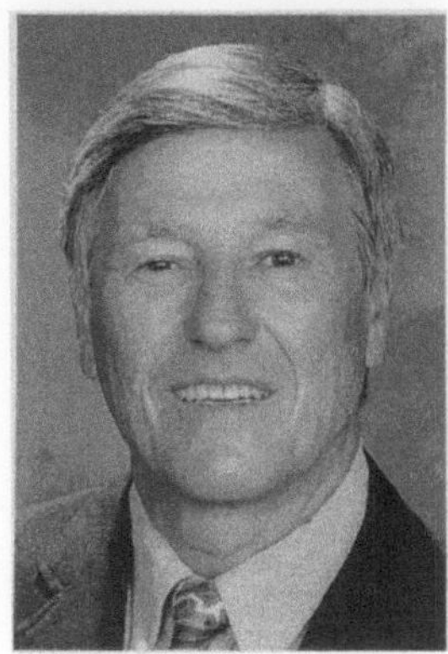

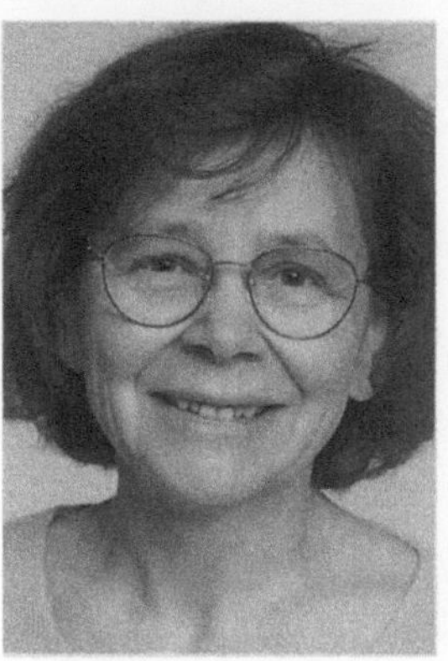

Birthdate: October 25, 1934

Academic Title: Professor Orthopedic Surgery

Position at Affiliation:

Business Address:
Joe Torg Center for Sports Medicine and Athletic Trauma
219 North Broad Street
Philadelphia, PA 19107
U.S.A.
215-762-5199 (work)
215-762-5150 (fax)
torgmd@aol.com (e-mail)

Home Address:
401 Conestoga Road
St. Davids, PA 19087
U.S.A.
610-688-2694 (home)

Specialty/Certification: Orthopedic Surgery, 1970

Education:
1957 – Haverford College
1961 – Temple Univ. School of Medicine (M.D.)

ISS Member 1990

Spouse: Barbara

Birthdate: February 6, 1941

Academic Title: Associate Professor

Position at Affiliation: Director of MR Center

Business Address:
University of Rochester Medical Center
Department of Radiology
Box 694, 601 Elmwood Avenue
Rochester, NY 14642
U.S.A.
716-275-2231 (work)
716-273-1033 (fax)
tot@rad.rochester.edu (e-mail)

Home Address:
195 Dunrovin Lane
Rochester, NY 14618
U.S.A.

Specialty/Certification: Radiology, 1974

Education:
1963 – University of Turku, Turku, Finland (B.Sc.)
1967 – University of Oulu, Oulu, Finland (M.D.)
1983 – University of Bergen School of Medicine, Bergen, Norway (Ph.D.)

ISS Member: 1996

Spouse: Arvid

Totty, William G. M.D.

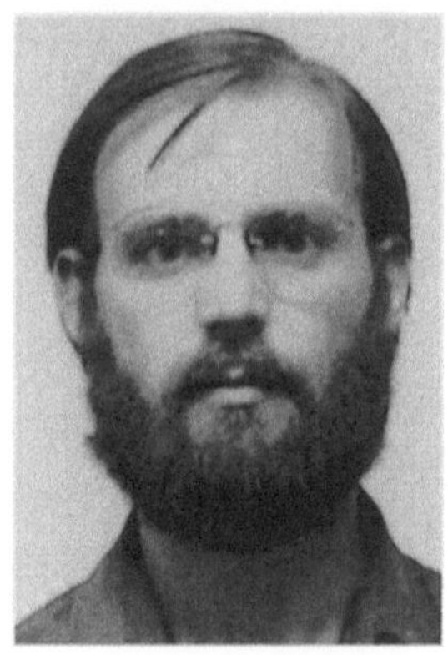

Birthdate: January 17, 1947

Academic Title: Professor

Position at Affiliation: Radiologist

Business Address:
Washington University, School of
Medicine
510 South Kingshighway Boulevard
St. Louis, MO 63110
U.S.A.
314-362-2910 (work)
314-362-4660 (fax)
totty@totty.wustl.edu (e-mail)

Home Address:
12810 Bourbon Red Drive
St. Louis, MO 63131
U.S.A.

Specialty: Radiology

Education:
1975 – University of Tennessee
1980 – Radiology

ISS Member 1984

Spouse: Helen

Tsuneyoshi, Masazumi M.D., Ph.D.

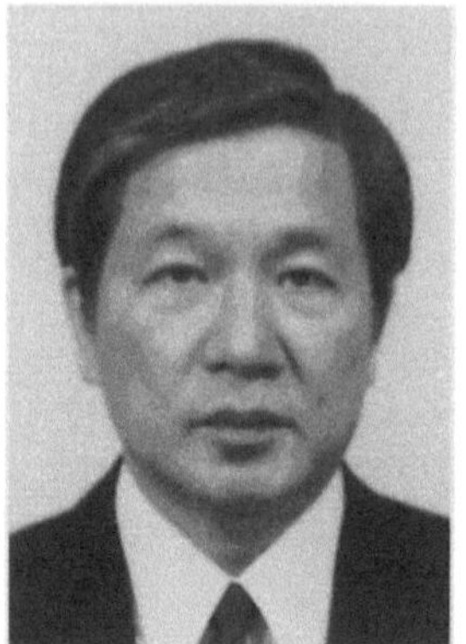

Birthdate: October 14, 1945

Academic Title: Professor

Position at Affiliation: Professor and
Chairman

Business Address:
Second Department of Pathology
Kyushu University, Faculty of Medicine
3-1-1 Maidashi, Higashi-ku
Fukuoka 812-82
Japan
92-642-6061 (work)
92-642-5968 (fax)
masazumi@surgpath.med.kyushu-u.ac.jp

Home Address:
3-14-5 Ropponmatsu, Chuo-ku
Fukuoka, 810
Japan
92-713-8164 (home)

Specialty/Certification: Pathology, 1981

Education:
Kyushu University, Faculty of Medicine

ISS Member 1992

Spouse: Kahoko

UEDA, YOSHIMICHI M.D., PH.D.

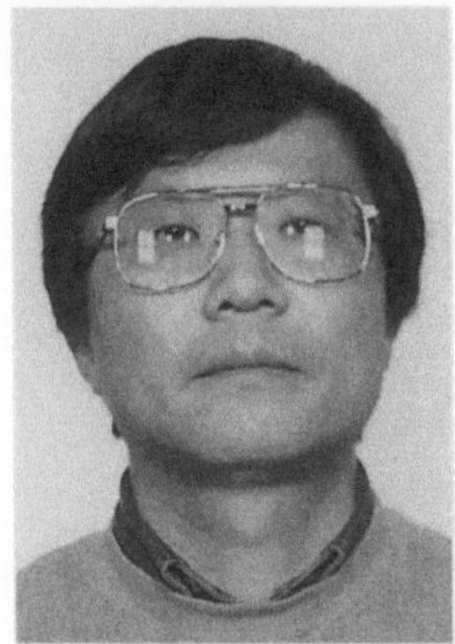

Birthdate: January 18, 1957

Academic Title: Associate Professor

Position at Affiliation: Associate Professor

Business Address:
Department of Pathology
Kanazawa Medical University
1-1 Daigaku, Uchinada-Machi
Ishikawa 920-02
Japan
81-762-86-2211 ext. 3622 (work)
81-762-86-2484 (fax)

Home Address:
No. 344
1-3 Daigaku
Uchinada-Machi
Ishikawa 920-02
Japan
81-762-86-4604 (home)

Specialty: Pathology

Education:
Kanazawa University
Tenri Hospital

ISS Member 1992

UNNI, KRISHNAN K. MB, BS

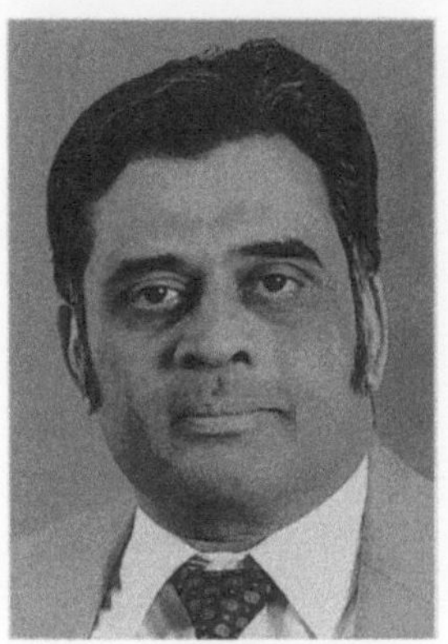

Birthdate: January 6, 1941

Academic Title: Professor

Position at Affiliation: Consultant
Pathology

Business Address:
Department of Surgical Pathology
Mayo Clinic
Rochester, MN 55905
U.S.A.
507-284-1193 (work)
507-284-1599 (fax)

Home Address:
855 Paxton Road S.W.
Rochester, MN 55902
U.S.A.
507-285-0226 (home)

Specialty: Pathology

Education:
A.I.I.M-S., New Delhi (M.D.)
Mayo Graduate School of Medicine
(Pathology residency)

ISS Member 1979

ISS Committees:
Nomenclature Committee, Chairman

Spouse: Chandrasheila

USHIGOME, SHINICHIRO M.D.

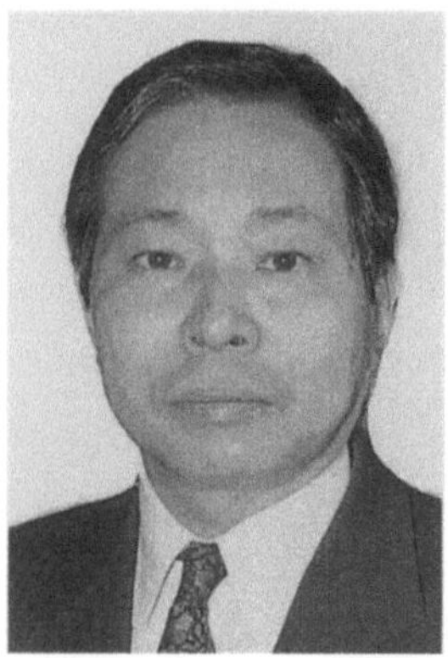

Birthdate: August 9, 1934

Academic Title: Professor

Position at Affiliation: Professor and Chairman

Business Address:
Department of Pathology (I)
Jikei University School of Medicine
3-25-8 Nishi-shinbashi
Tokyo 105, Minato-ku, Japan
81 3-3433-1111 x2230 (work)
81 3-3435-1922 (fax)

Home Address:
4-10-12 Takatanobaba
Shinjuku-ku
Tokyo 169, Japan
81 3-3362-0732 (home)

Specialty/Certification: Pathology, 1961

Education:
1956 – Tokyo Metropolitan University
1960 – Jikei University School of Medicine
1961 – The Tokyo First National Hospital (internship)
1968 – Baylor College of Medicine, Houston, TX (Pathology residency)

ISS Member 1982

ISS Committees:
Committee for the Promotion
of the Refresher Course Outside
of North America

Spouse: Yumiko

van HOLSBEECK, MARNIX T. M.D.

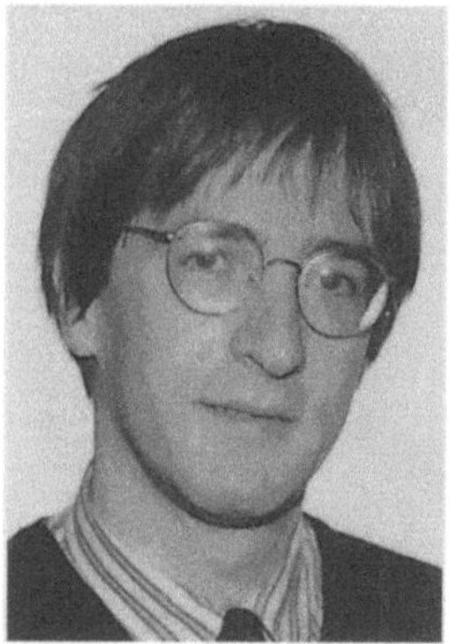

Birthdate: January 17, 1957

Academic Title: Associate Professor of Radiology

Position at Affiliation: Director, ER – Musculoskeletal Radiology

Business Address:
Musculoskeletal Radiology
Henry Ford Hospital
2799 W. Grand Blvd.
Detroit, MI 48202
U.S.A.
313-876-3325 (work)
313-556-9842 (fax)
MARNIX@rad.h/h.edu (e-mail)

Home Address:
41449 Woodridge Court
Northville, MI 48167
U.S.A.
810-348-6853 (home)

Specialty/Certification: Radiology, 1986

Education:
Catholic University Leuven, Belgium
Royal National Orthopaedic Hospital
London, United Kingdon
University of Michigan, Ann Arbor

ISS Member 1992

ISS Medals and Awards:
President's Medal, New Orleans, 1995

Spouse: Beatrice

Vanel, Daniel M.D.

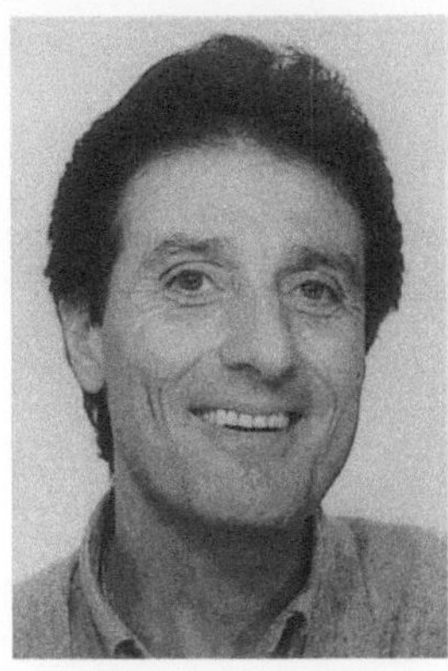

Birthdate: April 30, 1948

Position at Affiliation: Head of Department Responsible for Education and Training

Business Address:
Service de Radiodiagnostic
Institut Gustave-Roussy
39, rue Camille Desmoulins
94805 Villejuif
France
33 1 42 11 48 25 (work)
33 1 42 11 52 79 (fax)
vanel@igr.fr (e-mail)

Home Address:
18 avenue Foch
94340 Joinville Le Pont
France
33 1 48.83.84.38 (home)
33 1 48.83.84.38 (fax)

Specialty/Certification: Radiology, 1976

ISS Member 1984

ISS Medals and Awards:
President's Medal, Stockholm, 1992

ISS Committees:
Ad Hoc Committee Recruitment
of Skeletal Radiologists – 1988
Refresher Course Committee, New York –
1989
Liaison Planning Committee – 1992 – 93
Nomenclature Committee, 1992 – 97

Vigorita, Vincent J. M.D.

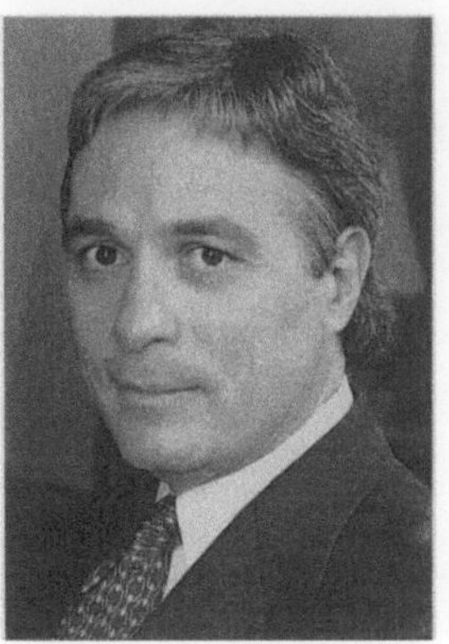

Birthdate: July 15, 1950

Academic Title: Professor of Pathology and Orthopaedic Surgery

Position at Affiliation: Medical Director

Business Address:
Lutheran Medical Center
150-55th Street
Brooklyn, New York 11201
U.S.A.
718-630-7380 (work)
718-630-6330 (fax)
vvigorita@lmcmc.com (e-mail)

Home Address:
101 Willow Street
Brooklyn, NY 11201
U.S.A.
718-875-7154 (home)

Specialty/Certification: Pathology, 1979

Education:
Williams College, Williamstown MA
New York Medical College, New York, NY
The Johns Hopkins Hospital, Baltimore,
MD (internship, residency)
Memorial Sloan-Kettering (fellowship)

ISS Member 1983

Spouse: Patricia

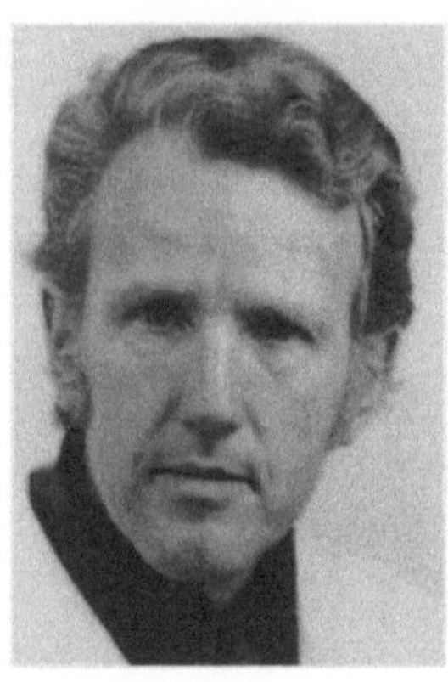

Business Address:
Radiology Department
Rontgeninstitut
Kantonsspital
600 Luzerne
Switzerland
041/47 14 10 (home)
041/25 46 51 (work)
041/25 44 11 (fax)

Specialty: Radiology

ISS Member 1974

Spouse: Rosmarie

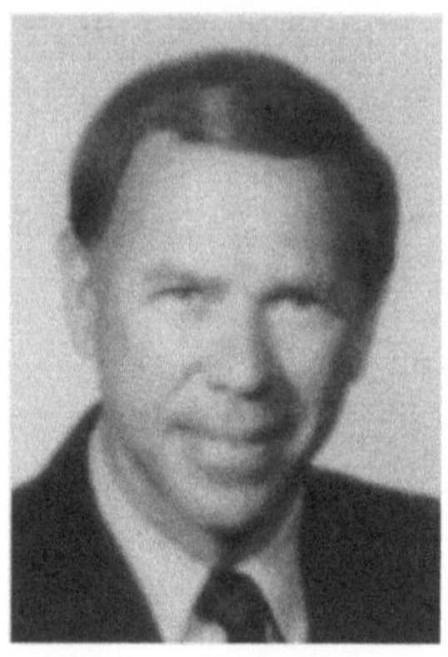

Business Address:
Division of Orthopaedic Surgery
The University of Arizona
Health Sciences Center
Tucson, AZ 85724
U.S.A.
602-626-7644 (work)
602-577-6900 (home)
602-626-2668 (fax)

Specialty: Orthopaedic Surgery

ISS Member 1987

Spouse: Ann

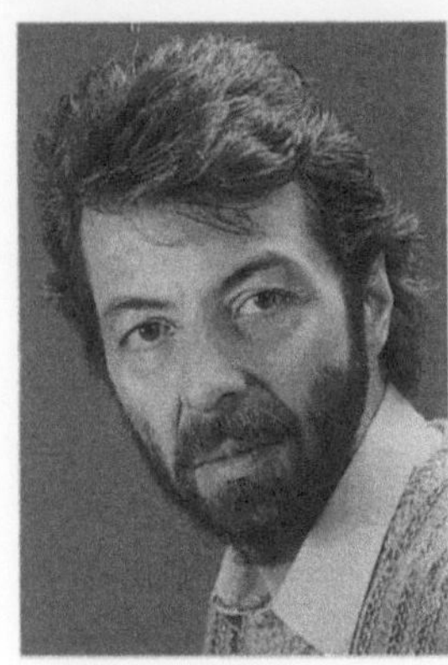

Birthdate: September 13, 1945

Position at Affiliation: Director

Business Address:
Pathologie Institut Enge
Tödistrasse 48
Postfach
8039 Zurich
Switzerland
1 287 3838 (work)
1 287 3839 (fax)

Home Address:
Clausiusstr. 48
CH-8006 Zurich
Switzerland
1-252-9963 (home)
1-252-9963 (fax)

Specialty/Certification: Pathology, 1980

Education:
Medical School – University of Western
Ontario, London Ontario Canada (M.R.)
University of Lausanne, Switzerland
(M.D.)
University of Hawaii (Surgery)
Dartmouth (Pathology)
University of Zurich, Switzerland,
University Hospital (Pathology)

ISS Member 1994

Spouse: Malihé

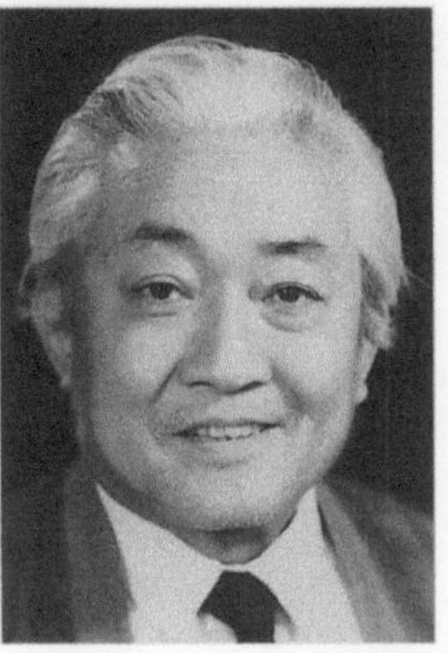

Academic Title: Professor

Position at Affiliation: Advisory Editor
of Chinese Journal of Radiology

Business Address:
Chinese Medical Association
42 Dongsi Xidajie
Beijing, 100710
People's Republic of China

Home Address:
31 East Street
Xin Jie Kou, Beijing 100035
People's Republic of China
86-010-6616-7631 ext. 365

Education:
1950 – Beijing Medical University
Medical College (M.D.)

ISS Member 1989

Spouse: Yingxiu

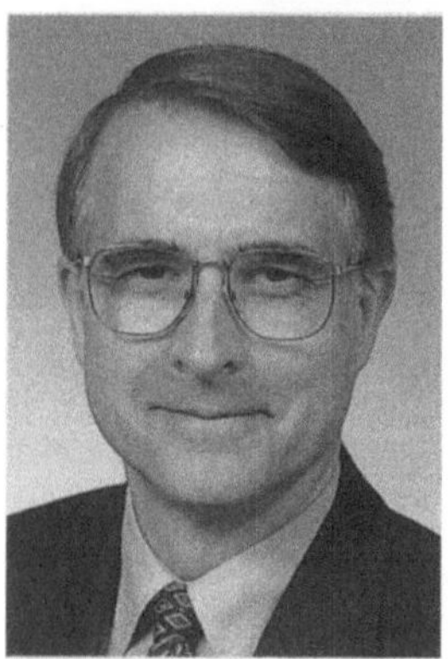

Academic Title: Dr.

Position at Affiliation: Consultant Radiologist

Business Address:
Department of Clinical Radiology
Bristol Royal Infirmary
Bristol, BS2 8HW
Great Britain
44 117 928 3854 (work)
44 117 928 3267(fax)
iain.watt@netgates.co.uk

Home Address:
Top Floor Flat, Regent House
Saville Place, Clifton
Bristol BS 8 4EJ
Great Britain
44 117 964 4212 (home)
44 117 964 4213 (fax)

Specialty: Radiology

Education:
1966 – University of London (M.B., BS)
1970–76 University of Bristol
(Radiology training)

ISS Member 1982

ISS Committees:
Ad Hoc Liaison Committee (Chairman)
Membership Committee
Editorial Board of Skeletal Radiology

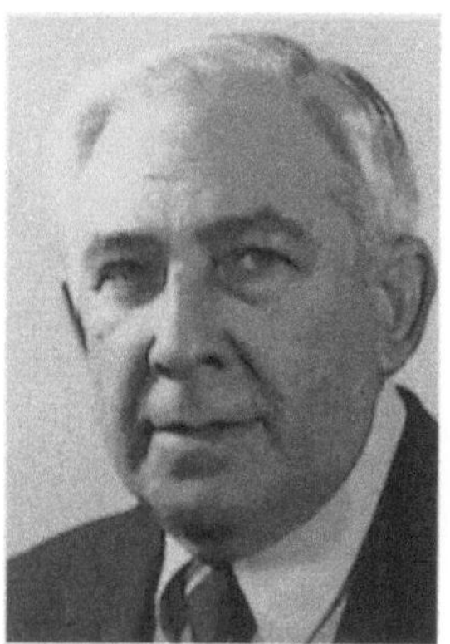

Business Address:
Veterans Administration Hospital
3200 Vine Street
Radiology Department
Cincinnati, OH 45220
U.S.A.
513-559-5077 (work)
513-731-9471 (home)

Specialty: Radiology

ISS Member Founding member

Spouse: Shirley

Weiss, Sharon M.D.	**Weissman, Barbara N. M.D.**

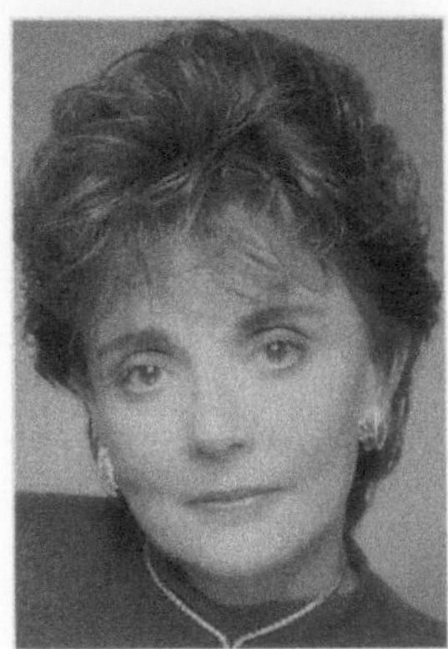 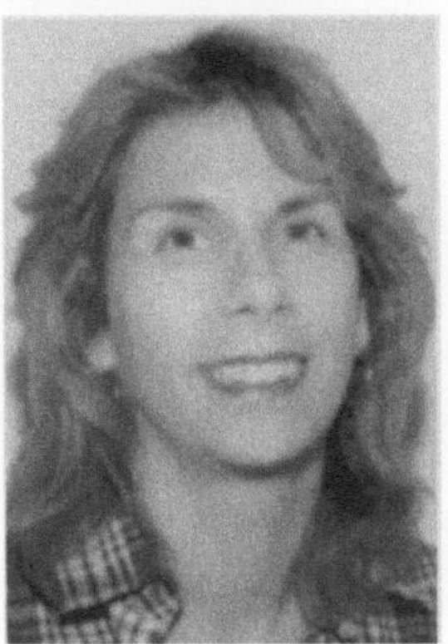

Weiss, Sharon M.D.

Birthdate: March 4, 1945

Academic Title: A. James French Professor of Pathology; Director of Anatomic Pathology

Position at Affiliation: Director, Anatomic Pathology; Chief, Surgical Pathology

Business Address:
Department of Pathology
University of Michigan Hospitals
1500 E. Medical Center Drive
Ann Arbor, MI 48105
U.S.A.
313-763-4035 (work)
313-936-6676 (fax)

Home Address:
245 High Orchard Drive
Ann Arbor, MI 48105
U.S.A.

Specialty/Certification: Anatomic Pathology, 1974

Education:
Wellesley College, Wellesley, MA (A.B.)
Johns Hopkins (M.D.)
Johns Hopkins Hospital (internship, residency)

ISS Member 1987

ISS Committees:
Closed Meeting Committee
Corinne Farrell Prize Committee

Spouse: Bernard Weiss

Weissman, Barbara N. M.D.

Academic Title: Professor of Radiology

Position at Affiliation: Chief, Musculoskeletal Section

Business Address:
Brigham and Women's Hospital
Bone Radiology Service
75 Francis Street
Boston, MA 02115
U.S.A.
617-732-6295 (work)
617-732-6336 (fax)
bnweissman@bics.bwh.harvard.edu (e-mail)

Home Address:
20 Gordon Road
Waban, MA 02168-1023
U.S.A.
617-9694-0720 (home)

Specialty/Certification: Radiology, 1974

Education:
Queens College, New York
Tufts University School of Medicine, Boston, MA (M.D.)

ISS Member 1980

ISS Committees:
American Member at Large, 1995
Liaison Committee of Future Planning

Spouse: Irving Weissman M.D.

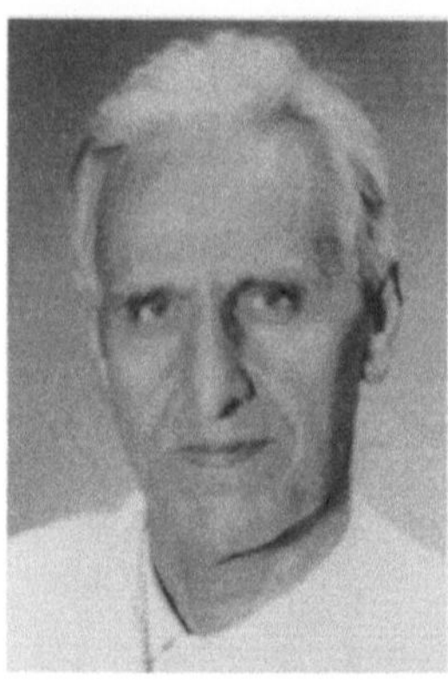

Business Address:
Accident Hospital Workman's
Compensation Company
"Berufsgenossenschaftliche Unfallklinik"
72076 Tübingen
Schnarrenbergstr. 95
Germany .
07071/606361 (work)
07071/606370 (fax)

ISS Member 1982

Spouse: Karin

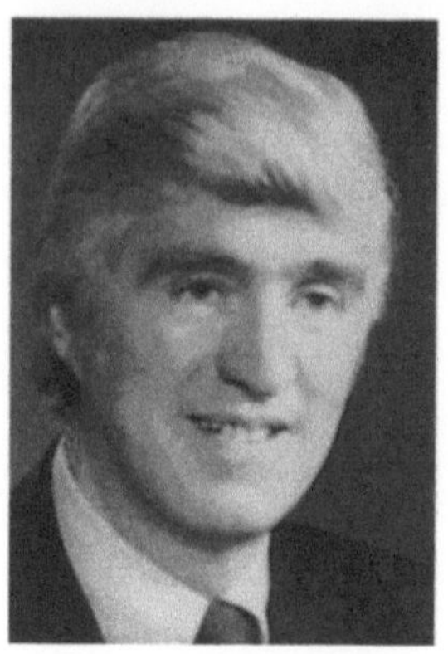

Business Address:
Department of Radiology
The New York Hospital
525 East 68th Street
New York, NY 10021
U.S.A.
212-746-2520,21 (work)
212-758-9107 (home)
212-746-8645 (fax)

Specialty: Radiology

ISS Member Founding member

Spouse: Liz

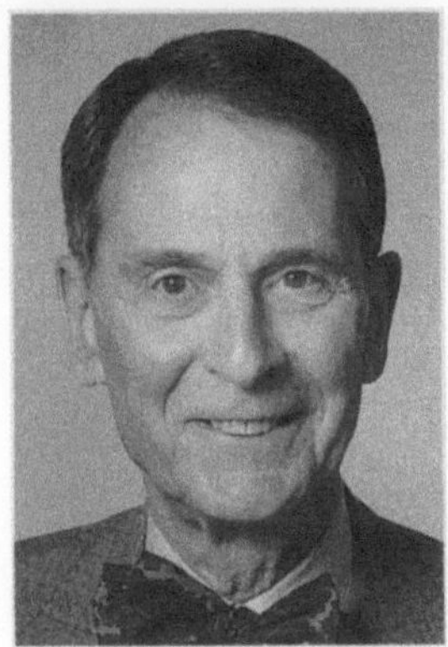

Birthdate: November 18, 1926

Academic Title: Professor of Radiology and Pediatrics

Position at Affiliation: Pediatric Radiologist

Business Address:
Radiology Department
Dartmouth-Hitchcock Medical Center
One Medical Center Drive
Lebanon, NH 03756, U.S.A.
603-650-5561(work)
603-650-5455 (fax)
robert.h.wilkinson @hitchcock. org
(e-mail)

Home Address:
8 Downing Road
Hanover, NH 03755, U.S.A.
603-643-2030 (home)

Specialty/Certification: Pediatrics, 1957; Radiology, 1967; recertified 1995

Education:
1947 Wesleyan University (B.A.)
1951 Cornell University Medical College (M.D.)
1952–56 Univ. of Michigan Med. Ctr. (Radiology residency)
1963–65
1965–67 Children's Hospital, Boston (Pediatric Radiology

ISS Member 1974

ISS Committees:
Membership Committee

Spouse: Linda

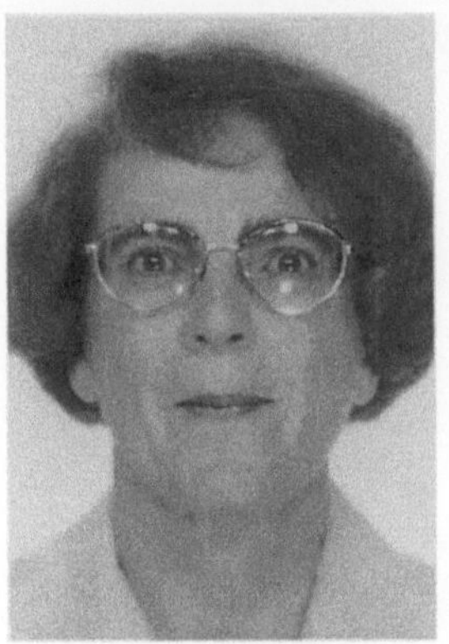

Academic Title: Associate Professor

Position at Affiliation: Senior Consultant, Assistant Professor

Business Address:
Department of Pathology and Cytology
University Hospital
S-221 85 Lund
Sweden
46-46-17-3409 (work)
46-46-14-3307 (fax)
helena.willen@pat.lu.se

Home Address:
Clemenstorget 4
222 21 Lund
Sweden
46-46-15-2722 (home)
46 46 15 27 22 (fax)

Specialty/Certification: Surgical Pathology,1972; Cytology, 1987

Education:
1966 – Charles University
Dissertation Lund University

ISS Member 1995

Spouse: Roger Willén M.D., Ph.D.

WILLERT, HANS GEORGE M.D.

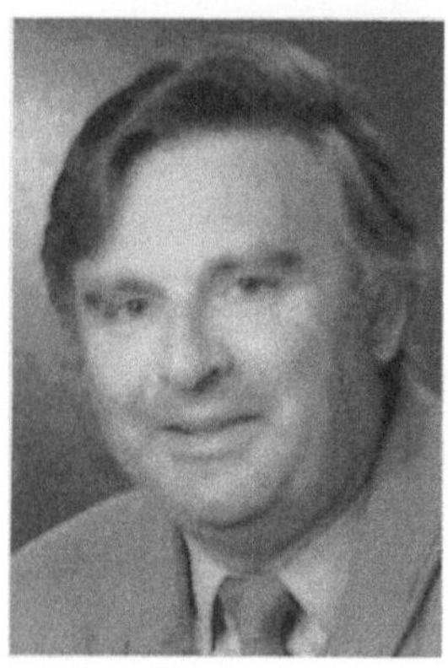

Business Address:
Direktor der Orthopadischen
Universitatsklinik Göttingen
Robert-Koch-Strasse 40
37075 Göttingen
Germany

ISS Member 1975

WILSON, ANTHONY J. MB, CHB.

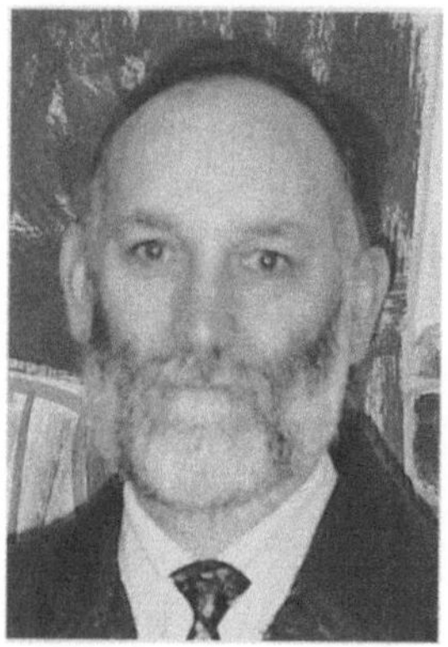

Birthdate: October 8, 1946

Academic Title: Professor

Position at Affiliation: Radiologist

Business Address:
University of Washington
Harborview Medical Center
325 39th Avenue
Seattle, WA 98104
U.S.A.
206-731-3561 (work)
206-731-8560 (fax)
wilsona@u.washington.edu (e-mail)

Home Address:
5644 39th Avenue West
Seattle, WA 98199
U.S.A.
206-270-8617 (home)

Specialty/Certification: Radiology, 1976

Education:
1972 – University of Otago, New Zealand
(MB ChB)
Auckland Hospital – (Radiology
residency)
1978 – 79 – University of Missouri
(fellowship, Skeletal Radiology)

ISS Member 1990

Spouse: Carolyn

WILSON DAVID J. FRCR, MRCP, MBBS, BSC

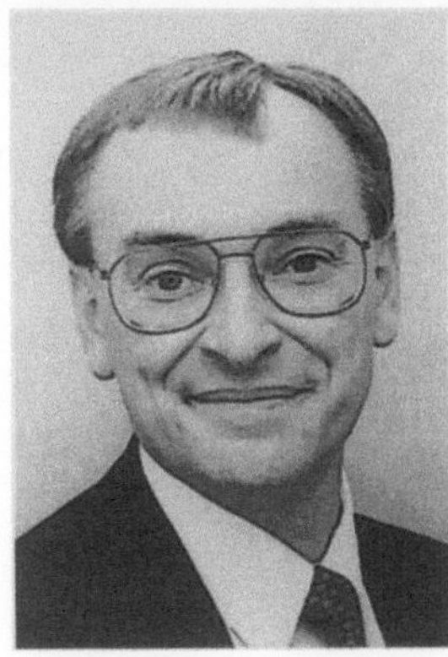

Birthdate: September 10, 1952

Academic Title: Senior Clinical Lecturer, University of Oxford

Position at Affiliation: Clinical Director

Business Address:
Nuffield Orthopaedic Centre
Consultant Radiologist
Headington, Oxford OX3 7LD
United Kingdom
44-1865-227257(work)
44-1865-227347(fax)
david.wilson@radiology.ox.ac.uk (e-mail)

Home Address:
3 Beckley Court
Beckley, Oxford OX39UB
United Kingdom
44-1865-351-276(home)
44-1865-351-005 (fax)

Specialty/Certification: Radiology,1984; Medicine, 1976

Education:
Kings College Hospital
University of London

ISS Member 1990

ISS Committees:
Editorial Board, Skeletal Radiology

Spouse: Barbara

WOLD, LESTER E. M.D.

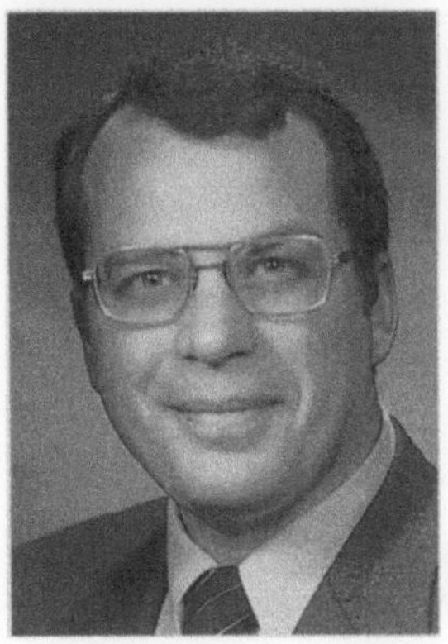

Birthdate: May 6, 1949

Academic Title: Professor

Position at Affiliation: Consultant/Chair, Department of Laboratory Medicine and Pathology

Business Address:
Mayo Medical Center
200 First Street SW HI 530
Rochester, MN 55905, U.S.A.
507-284-6095 (work)
507-284-1927 (fax)
lwold@mayo.edu (e-mail)

Home Address:
2505 Hillside Lane SW
Rochester, MN 55902, U.S.A.
507-289-0616 (home)

Specialty/Certification: Pathology, 1980

Education:
1967–71 St. Olaf College, Northfield, MN (B.A.)
1971–73 Cornell University, Ithaca, NY (M.S. Chemistry)
1973–77 University of Chicago, Chicago, IL (M.D.)
1977–80 Mayo Clinic Rochester, MN (residency)

ISS Member 1988

ISS Committees:
Membership Committee, 1994–96

Spouse: Patricia S. Simmons, M.D.

YANG, SEOUNG-OH M.D., PH.D.

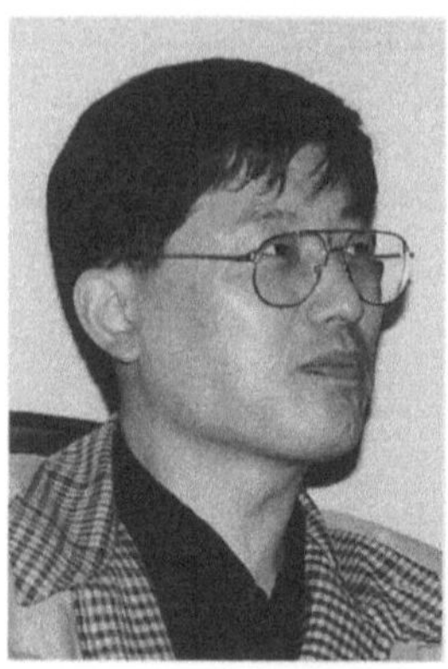

Birthdate: December 18, 1956

Academic Title: Associate Professor

Position at Affiliation: Associate Professor

Business Address:
Asan Medical Centre, Ulsan University
Dept. of Nuclear Medicine
Poonap-Dong, 388-1, Songpa-ku
Seoul, 138-736
Korea
82-2-224-4594 (work)
82-2-224-4588 (fax)
soyang@amc.ulsan.ac.kr (e-mail)

Home Address:
Songpa-ku
Songpa-Dong
Sam-Ik Apt. #212-501
Seoul
Korea
82-2-418-6858 (home)

Specialty/Certification: Radiology, 1985

Education:
Seoul National University, School of
Medicine (M.D.)
Seoul National University Hospital,
residency in Diagnostic Radiology;
fellowship in Nuclear Medicine)

ISS Member 1996

Spouse: Hwa-Sook Cha

YAO, LAWRENCE M.D.

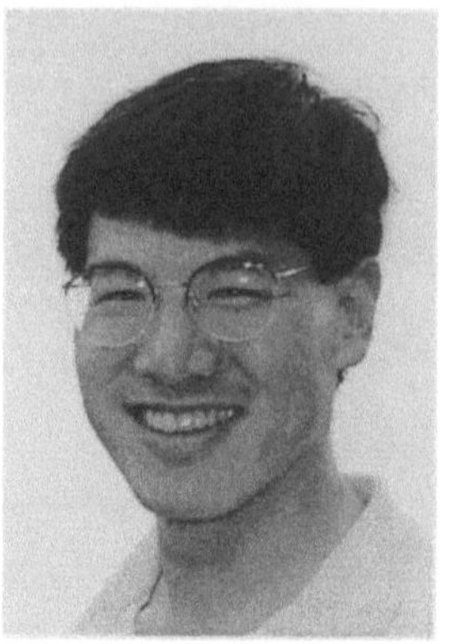

Birthdate: June 23, 1959

Academic Title: Assistant Professor

Position at Affiliation: Director,
Musculoskeletal MR Imaging

Business Address:
UCLA Department of Radiological
Sciences
200 UCLA Medical Plaza, #165-45
Los Angeles, Ca 90095-6952
U.S.A.
310-206-9378 (work)
310-794-1428 (fax)
lyao@mail.rad.ucla.edu (e-mail)

Home Address:
11044 Ophir Dr., #601
Los Angeles, CA 90024
U.S.A.
310-824-1872 (home)

Specialty/Certification: Radiology, 1990

Education:
1977–81 – Brown University, Providence,
RI (B.A.)
1981–85 – Brown University, Providence,
RI (M.D.)
1985–86 – Miriam Hospital, Providence,
RI (internship)
1986–90 – Albany Medical Center,
Albany, NY (Radiology residency)
1990–91 – UCLA, Los Angeles, CA
(fellowship)

ISS Member 1996

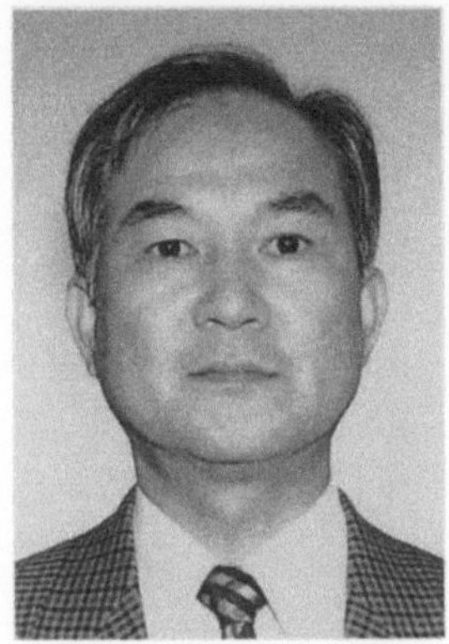

Birthdate: April 15, 1942

Academic Title: Professor

Position at Affiliation: Professor

Business Address:
College of Medial Care Technology
Pathology Section
Tottori University
133-2 Nishi-Machi
Yonago Tottori 683
Japan
0859-34-8325 (work)
0859-34-8073 (fax)
kinkai@grape.med.tottori-u.ac.jp

Home Address:
1131-19 Kamifukubara
Yonago, Tottori 683
Japan
0859-32-9003 (home)
0859-32-9003 (fax)

Specialty: Pathology

Education:
1961–67 Nagasaki University, Faculty of
Medicine (M.D.)
1967–72 Kyushu University, Graduate
School (Pathology)

ISS Member 1994

Spouse: Toshiko

Academic Title: Professor

Position at Affiliation: Chairman

Business Address:
Medical University of South Carolina
171 Ashley Avenue
Charleston, SC 29425
U.S.A.
803-792-7147 (work)
803-792-9503 (fax)

Home Address:
1965 Omni Blvd.
Mt. Pleasant, SC 29464
U.S.A.
803-856-0865 (home)

Specialty: Radiology

Education:
Oxford University, St. Thomas Hospital,
London
St. Bartholomews Hospital, London
(Radiology)
Royal National Orthopaedic Hospital,
London

ISS Member 1988

Spouse: Briony

Young, Lionel W. M.D.

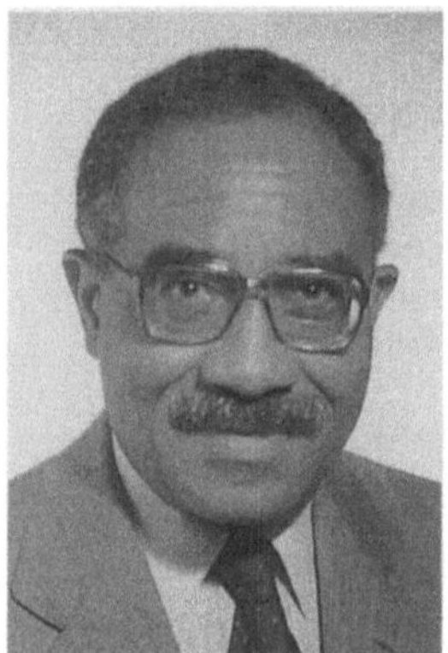

Birthdate: March 14, 1932

Academic Title: Professor of Radiology

Position at Affiliation: Director of Pediatric Radiology

Business Address:
Dept. of Radiology, Rm. 2605E
Loma Linda University Medical Center
11234 Anderson Street
Loma Linda, CA 92354
U.S.A.
909 824-4281 (work)
909 478-4266 (fax)
lionel_young@ccmail.llu.edu (e-mail)

Home Address:
909 335-8735 (home)
909 35-2397 (fax)

Specialty/Certification: Radiology,1964; Pediatric Radiology, 1994

Education:
1953 – Benedictine College (B.S.)
1957 – Howard University College of Medicine (M.D.)
1961 – University of Rochester (Radiology residency)
1965 – Cincinnati Children's Hospital (Pediatric Radiology)

ISS Member 1984

Spouse: Florence

Zafiroski, George J. M.D., Ph.D.

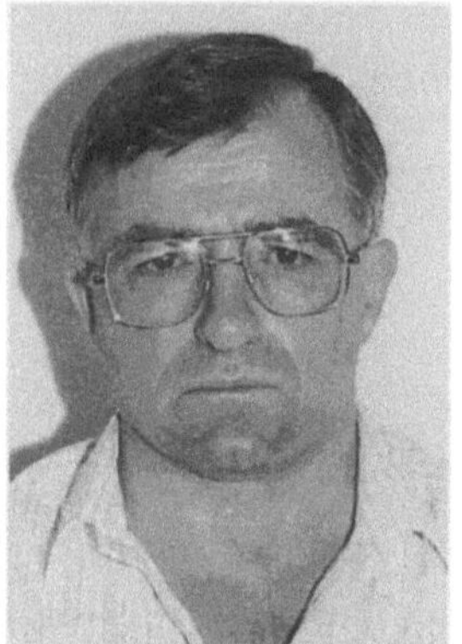

Birthdate: November 28, 1945

Academic Title: Professor

Position at Affiliation: Professor, President of MOTA

Business Address:
Department of Orthopaedic Surgery
University of Skopje
Medical University Centre
91 000 Skopje
Republic of Macedonia
Yugoslavia
389 91 235 137 or 427 068 (work)
389 91 427 068 (fax)

Home Address:
"Nikola Parapunov" br.1/19
91 000 Skopje
Republic of Macedonia
Yugoslavia
389 91 362 280 (home)

Specialty: Orthopaedic Surgery

Education:
Medical Faculty
Orthopaedic Surgeon
Orthopaedic Oncology

ISS Member 1988

Spouse: Angja

ZÍDKOVÁ, HELENA M.D., PH.D.

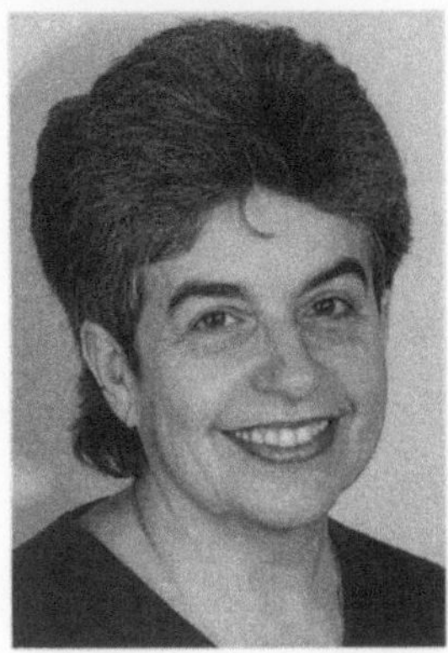

Birthdate: January 7, 1943

Academic Title: Professor

Position at Affiliation: Professor of Radiology

Business Address:
Postgraduate Medical School
University Hospital Bulovka
18081 Praha 8-Liben
Czech Republic
02/822431 (work)
02/822431 (fax)

Specialty: Radiology

Home Address:
26705
Nizbor 213
Czech Republic
02/361120 (home)

Specialty/Certification: Radiology, 1972, 1976

Education:
Charles University, Medical Faculty, Praha
Postgraduate Medical School, Praha

ISS Member 1991

Spouse: Milos Zídek

ZLATKIN, MICHAEL B. M.D.

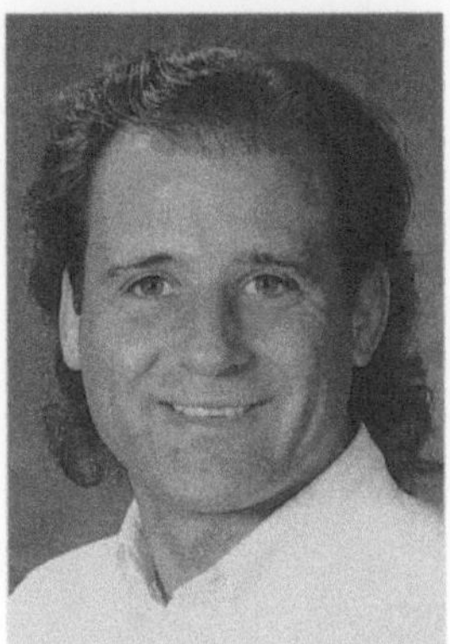

Birthdate: March 20, 1957

Academic Title: Clinical Associate Professor

Position at Affiliation: Director of MRI and Musculoskeletal Imaging

Business Address:
Department of Radiology
Memorial Regional Hospital
3501 Johnson Street
Hollywood, FL 33332
U.S.A.
954-985-5886 (work)
954-967-2945 (fax)
mbzlat@aol.com

Home Address:
2689 Meadewood Court
Ft. Lauderdale, FL 33332
U.S.A.
954-389-3998 (home)
954-384-8676 (fax)

Specialty/Certification: Radiology, 1987

Education:
McGill University (B.S.)
Queens University, Kingston, Ontario (M.D.)
McGill University (Diagnostic Radiology)
University California San Diego, (Musculoskeletal Radiology fellowship)

ISS Member 1992

Spouse: Marilyn

ISS Honorary Members

AEGERTER, ERNST M.D.,

RD #1
CHALFONT, PA 18914
U.S.A.

ALEXANDER, COLIN J. M.D., EHB, FRCR, FRACR

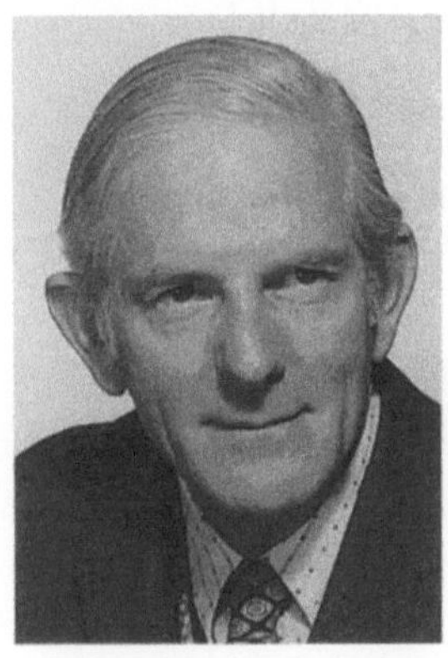

Birthdate: April 10, 1920

Academic Title: Professor Emeritus

Position at Affiliation:
Emeritus Professor

Business Address:
Department of Anatomy with Radiology
School of Medicine
University of Auckland
Private Bag
Auckland
New Zealand

Home Address:
49 Richard Farrell Avenue
Remuera
Auckland
New Zealand
09 5201 682 (home)
c.alex@xtra.co.nz (e-mail)

Specialty/Certification:
Radiology, 1948

Education:
Auckland Grammar School
University of Otago, New Zealand
St. Mary's Hospital, London

ISS Member 1973

ISS Committees:
Membership Committee

Spouse: Susan

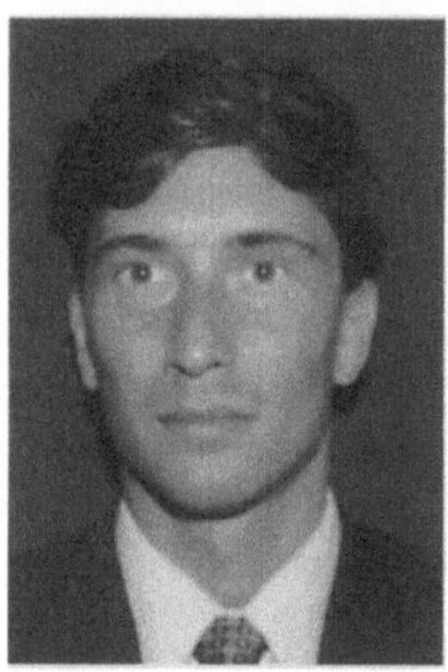

Birthdate: June 9, 1963

Position at Affiliation: Chief of Service

Business Address:
Sanatorio Pargue
Orono 860
2000 Rosario
Argentina
5441-200245/5441-259800 (business)
5441-491820 (fax)

Home Address:
Ituzaingo 849
2000 Rosario
Argentina
5441-492488 (home)
5441-491820 (fax)

Specialty/Certification: Radiology, 1989

Education:
Universidad Nacional de la Plata
School of Radiology of Fundacion
"Dr. J. Roberto Villavicencio"

ISS Member 1993

Spouse: Laura Gabriela Ochoa

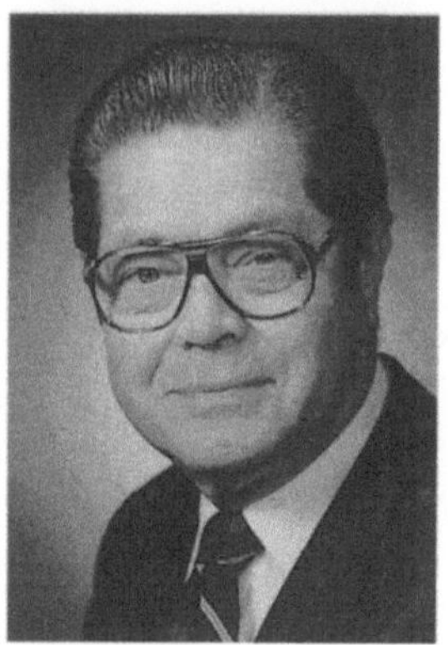

Birthdate: September 3, 1917

Academic Title: Emeritus Professor
of Surgical Pathology

Position at Affiliation: Emeritus
Professor of Surgical Pathology

Business Address:
Mayo Clinic
Surgical Pathology
200 First Street S.W.
Rochester, MN 55902
U.S.A.
507-284-2691 (business)
507-284-5036 (fax)

Home Address:
618-14th Avenue S.W.
Rochester, MN 55905
U.S.A.
507-289-5014 (home)

Specialty/Certification:
Pathology, 1948

Education:
1940 – Rush Medical School (M.D.)
1942–45 – U.S. Army Medical Corps
1945–48 – Mayo Clinic (resident in
Pathology)

ISS Member: Founding Member

ISS Medals and Awards:
Founders' Gold Medal, New York, 1989

Dijian, Albert M.D.

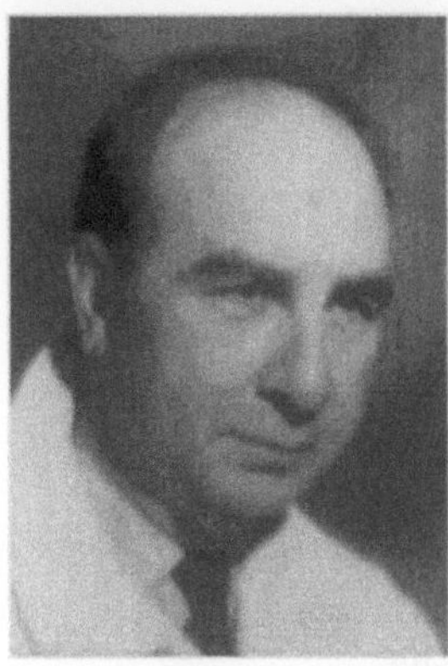

4 Rue Albert Samain
75017 Paris
France

Davidson, John K. OBE, MD, FRCP
(Edin & Glasg), FRCR, Hon.FACR,
Hon.FRACR

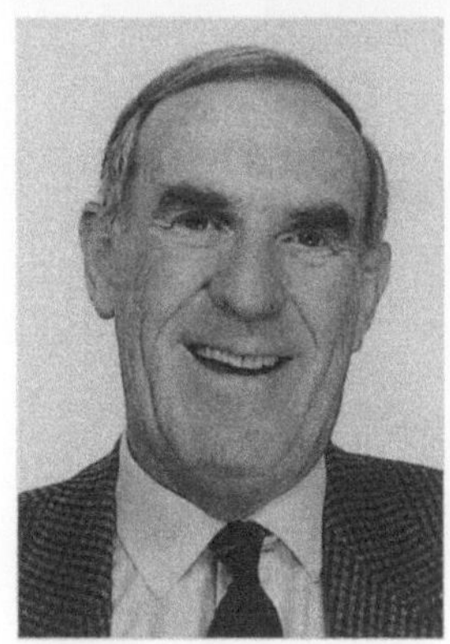

Academic Title: Dr.

Position at Affiliation: Consultant Radiologist

Business Address:
15 Beechlands Avenue
Netherlee
Glasgow G44 3YT, Scotland
0141-637-0290 (business & fax)

Home Address:
15 Beechlands Avenue
Netherlee
Glasgow G44 3YT, Scotland
0141-637-0290 (home & fax)

Specialty/Certification: Radiology, 1958

Education:
University of Edinburgh (Medical School)
Edinburgh Royal Infirmary
St. Bartholomews Hospital, London
(Radiology Training)

ISS Member: Founding member

ISS Medals & Awards:
Medal of the ISS (Silver), Stockholm, 1992

ISS Committees:
Executive Committee, 1990-92 Member at Large
Chairman, Refresher Course, Edinburgh 1985
Co-Chairman, Refresher Course, Cannes 1987

Spouse: Edith

ENNEKING, WILLIAM F. M. D.

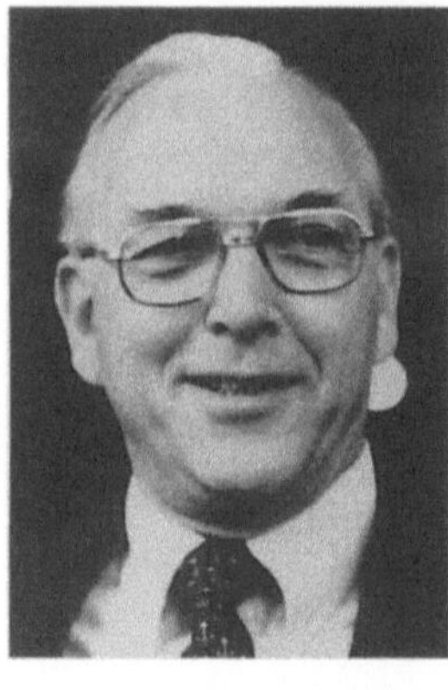

Academic Title: Distinguished Service Professor Emeritus

Position at Affiliation: Professor meritus Orthopedic Surgery

Business Address:
Department of Orthopaedics
Box 100246 JHM Health Center
University of Florida
Gainesville, FL 32610-0246
U.S.A.
352-392-4251 (business)
352-392-7868 (fax)
catie.orthoped@mail.health.ufl.edu
(e-mail)

Home Address:
Box 444
Melrose, FL 32666
U.S.A.
352-475-2712 (home)

Specialty: Orthopaedic Surgery

Education:
1946 – University Wisconsin (BS)
1949 – University Wisconsin (MD)
1955 – University of Chicago
(Orthopedic Surgery)

ISS Member 1974

Spouse: Margaret

FAIRBANK, T. J. M. D.

10 Cranmer Road
Cambridge CB3, 91BL
England

GORLIN, ROBERT M. D.

Oral Pathology
University of Minnesota
School of Medicine
136 Owre Hall
Minneapolis, MN 55455
U.S.A.

GÖTZE, HEINZ
DR. PHIL. DR. MED. H.C. MULT.

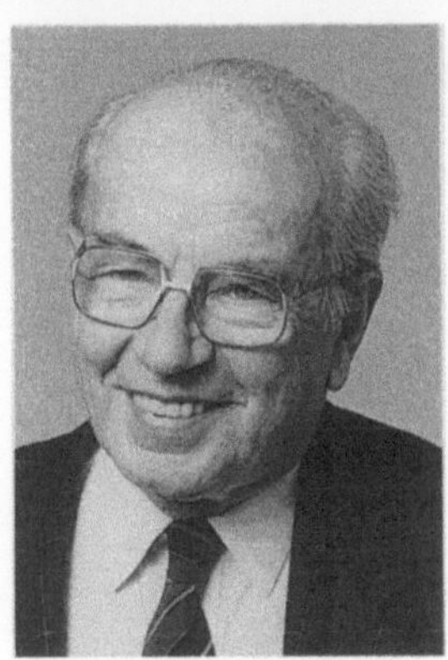

Position at Affiliation: Co-Owner of
Springer-Verlag

Business Address:
Springer-Verlag
Tiergartenstrasse 17
69121 Heidelberg
Germany
06221-486225 (business)
06221-487546 (fax)

Home Address:
Ludolf-Krehl-Strasse 41
69120 Heidelberg
Germany
06221-470717 (home)

Education:
1938 – Doctorate of Philosophy, Leipzig
(Ph.D.)

ISS Member 1983

ISS Medals and Awards:
Medal of the ISS (Silver), Salzburg, 1990

Spouse: Linde

HEUCK, FRIEDRICH H. W. M.D.

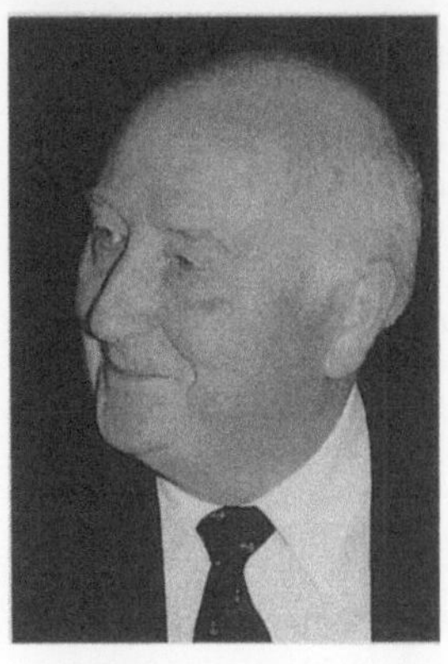

Birthdate: January 20, 1921

Academic Title: Professor of Radiology,
(University of Tubingen; Hon. Prof.
Biom. Img. (University of Stuttgart)

Position at Affiliation: Retired 1986,
Medical Director (Chairman)

Home Address:
Hermann-Kurz-Str. 5
D-70192 Stuttgart
Germany
49-711-257-3250 (home)

Specialty: Radiology, Nuclear Medicine

Education:
1944 – University of Berlin (approbation)
1944 – Medical Academy of Danzig
(Dr. med.)
1951 – University of Kiel (Radiology and
Nuclear Medicine)
1957 – Christian-Albrecht-University,
Kiel (habilitation)

ISS Member: 1974

Offices Held in ISS and Dates of Service:
President elect, 1982 – 84
President, 1984 – 86

ISS Medals and Awards:
Founders' Lecture, Salzburg, 1990
Founders' Gold Medal, New Orleans,
1995

ISS Committees:
Executive Committee, 1979, 1982 – 90
Board of Trustees of the Endowment
Fund 1988 – 95
Program Committee 1978 – 81;1988 – 90
Refresher Course Committee 1978 – 80;
1982 – 84; 1988 – 90
Membership Committee 1978, 1986 – 88
Editorial Committee 1986 – 92
Awards Committee (Chairman) 1986 – 92
Advisory Committee on Convention
Planning 1986 – 92
Continuation Course Committee 1978–82
Committee for Future Planning 1986 – 90
Committee for Promotion of Refresher
Course outside of North America
1986 – 92
Nomenclature Committee 1988 – 90
Chairman, Munchen Meeting, 1979
Chairman, Salzburg Meeting, 1990

Spouse: Ingeburg

JOHNSON, LENT C. M.D.

Armed Forces Institute of Pathology
Washington, DC   20105
U.S.A.

JACOBS, PHILIP M.D.

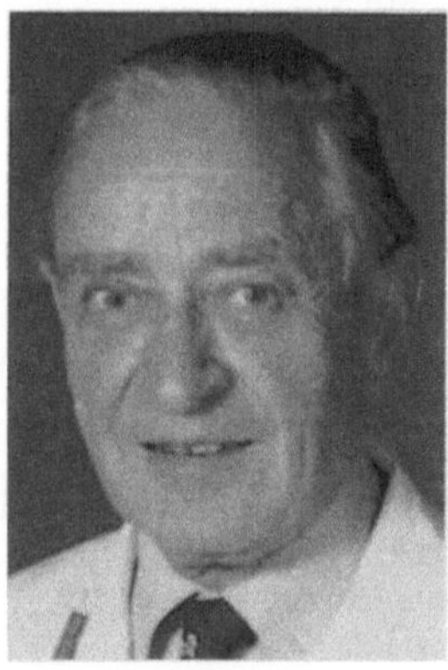

30 Longdon Croft
Copt Heath
Knowle, Solihull
West Midlands B93 9LJ
England

KNICKERBOCKER, W. JAMES M.D.

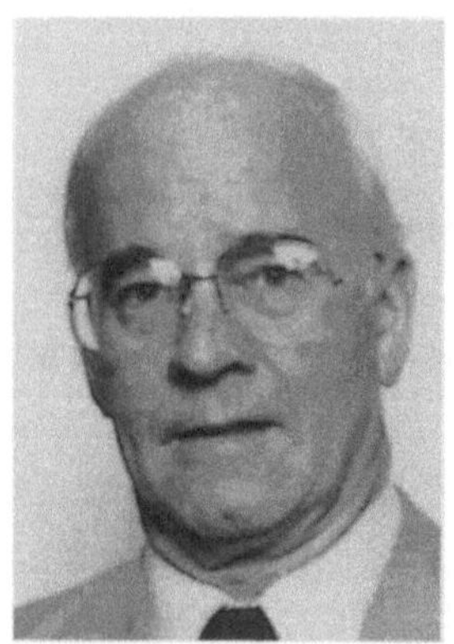

Business Address:
7888 Angus Drive
Vancouver, B.C.
V6P5K5
Canada
504-228-7080 (business)
604-263-6807 (home)

ISS Member 1979

Spouse: Betty Ann

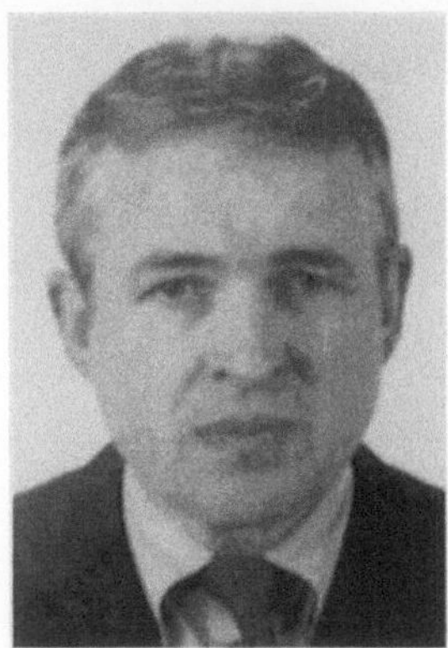

President, AGFA Photo Division
Sr. Vice President, Agfa Corp.
100 Challenger Road
Ridgefield Park, NJ 07660
U.S.A.

ISS Medals and Awards:
Medal of the ISS (Silver),
New York, 1989

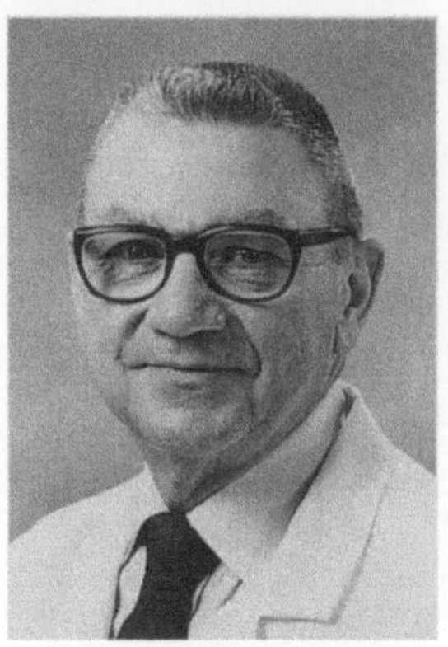

Academic Title: Professor

Position at Affiliation: Chief,
Orthopaedic Oncology

Business Address:
M.D. Anderson Cancer Center
1515 Holcombe Blvd.
Houston, TX 77030
U.S.A.
713-792-8828 (business)
713-794-1940 (fax)

Home Address:
2335 Bellefontaine
Houston, TX 77030-3203
U.S.A.
713-668-6156 (home)

Specialty/Certification: Orthopaedic
Surgery 1967,1983,1993

Education:
1954 – Western Reserve University (B.S.)
1958 – University of Pittsburgh School of
Medicine (M.D.)
1958 – 63 – Baylor College of Medicine
(residency Orthopaedic Surgery)

ISS Member 1991

Spouse: Kathryn

SILVERMAN, FREDERIC M.D.

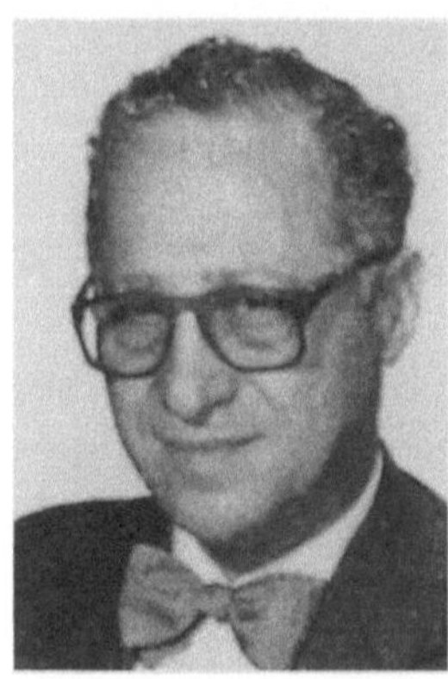

Radiology Department
Stanford University School of Medicine
Stanford, CA 94305
U.S.A.

SISSONS, HUBERT A. M.D.

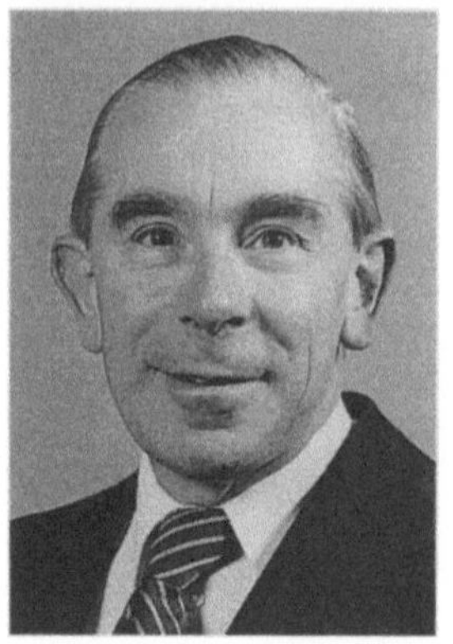

Academic Title: Professor

Position at Affiliation: Consultant

Business Address:
Histopathology Unit
Imperial Cancer Research Foundation
Laboratories
35-43 Lincoln's Inn Fields
London WC2A 3PN
England
171-269-3087 (business)
171-269-3091 (fax)

Home Address:
8 The Glebe
Chislehurst
Kent BR7 5PX
England
181-467-2122 (home)

Specialty: Histopathology

Education:
University of Melbourne
(M.B., B.S., M.D.)
Alfred Hospital, Melbourne, Australia
(resident)
Royal College of Surgeons, London, U.K.
(research fellow)

ISS Member Founding Member

ISS Medals and Awards:
Founders' Lecture, Sydney, 1988

Spouse: Patricia

van Rijssel, Theodorus G. M. D.

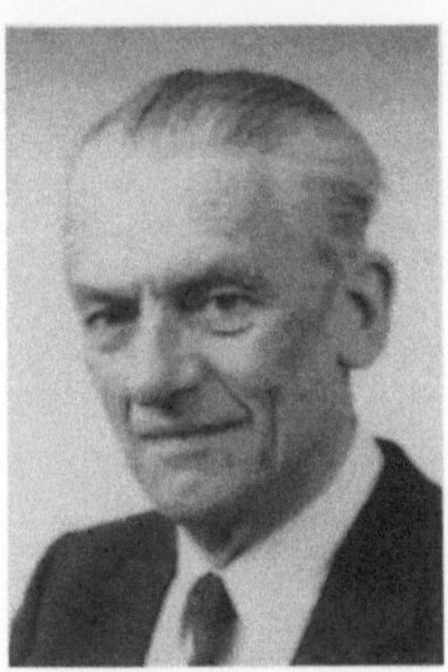

Pathologisch Laboratorium
der Rijksuniversiteit
Wssenaarseweg 62
Leiden
The Netherlands

Wood, Philip M. D.

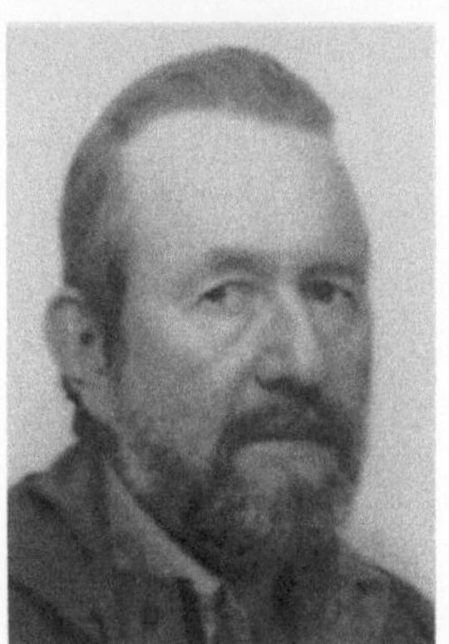

157 Buxton Old Road
Higher Disley
Stockport SK12 2BX
England

New Members 1997

Karl Gunnar Astrom
Sweden

Helen Carty
United Kingdom

Jean-Luc Drape
France

Mercedes Roca Espiau
Spain

Bernard Hindman
USA

Hiroshi Iwasaki
Japan

Josef Kramer
Austria

Bi Ling Liang
China

Clement Charles McCormick
Australia

Michael E. Mulligan
USA

Antonio G. Nascimento
USA

Christian H. Neumann
USA

Simon Ostlere
United Kingdom

Reinhard V. Putz
Germany

Douglas K. Smith
USA

Luke Michael Vaughan
USA

In Memoriam

Michael Bonfiglio M.D.
Crawford J. Campbell M.D.
William P. Cockshott M.D.
Corrinne Farrell M.D.
John Gwinn M.D.
Philip Hodes M.D.
John F. Holt M.D.
John Ivins M.D.
John Kirkpatrick Jr. M.D.*
Mamed Mesgarzadeh M.D.
William Meszaros M.D.
Sir J. Howard Middlemiss M.D.
Jacob Mulder M.D.

Ronald O. Murray M.D.*
Olof Norman M.D.
William M. Park M.D.
Hanno Poppe M.D.
Charles H. F. Price M.D.
Walter G. Putschar M.D.
Fritz Schjowicz M.D.
Howard Steinbach M.D.
Elias Theros M.D.
J. R. Von Ronnen M.D.
Charles Warrick M.D.
John Windsor Weston M.D.
Issa Yahmai M.D.

* Former Presidents of the ISS

MIX
Papier aus verantwortungsvollen Quellen
Paper from responsible sources
FSC® C105338

If you have any concerns about our products,
you can contact us on
ProductSafety@springernature.com

In case Publisher is established outside the EU,
the EU authorized representative is:
Springer Nature Customer Service Center GmbH
Europaplatz 3, 69115 Heidelberg, Germany

Printed by Libri Plureos GmbH
in Hamburg, Germany